Hazardous Waist

TACKLING MALE WEIGHT PROBLEMS

Edited by
ALAN WHITE
and
MAGGIE PETTIFER

Forewords by
PETER BAKER
and
MICHAEL KIMMEL

Radcliffe Publishing
Oxford • New York

Radcliffe Publishing Ltd
18 Marcham Road
Abingdon
Oxon OX14 1AA
United Kingdom

www.radcliffe-oxford.com
Electronic catalogue and worldwide online ordering facility.

British Library Cataloguing in Publication Data

A catalogue record for this book is available from the British Library.

ISBN-13 978 184619 103 9

Typeset by Ann Buchan (Typesetters), Middlesex
Printed and bound by TJI Digital, Padstow, Cornwall

Contents

Forewords   v
Peter Baker
Michael Kimmel

Preface   ix
Alan White and Maggie Pettifer, Editors

About the editors   xi

About the contributors   xii

PART 1: THE CHALLENGE OF MALE WEIGHT PROBLEMS   1

1   The research base for male obesity: what do we know?   3
    David Wilkins

2   The causes of male obesity and associated health problems   12
    David Haslam

3   Male obesity: policy and context   22
    Alan White

4   Using body image to help men manage weight problems   36
    Ewan Gillon and Kerri McPherson

5   Men, obesity and the media   48
    Claire Mac Evilly

6   Men, masculinities and health   55
    Brendan Gough

PART 2: TACKLING MALE WEIGHT PROBLEMS   65

7   Managing male obesity in primary care   67
    Caroline Gunnell

8   Working with men in groups – experience from a weight   75
    management programme in Scotland
    Jim Leishman

9   Weight management in men – community pharmacy   87
    approaches
    Kurt Ramsden and Julie Hunter

10   Commercial slimming groups in the management of weight
     problems in men   92
     Amanda Avery

11   Tackling weight problems in men in the workplace   103
     Steve Deacon

12   Weight problems in boys and young men   112
     Paul Gately and Duncan Radley

13   Tackling weight problems in older men   125
     Kate Davidson

14   Fit for inclusion: working with overweight and obese   135
     men with disabilities
     Sue Catton

15   Promoting exercise to men   150
     Jim McKenna

16   Counselling the man beyond the weight problem   159
     Richard Bryant-Jefferies

17   Communicating the risks of obesity to South Asian men   166
     Jenne Dixit

18   Weight management in men with mental health problems   173
     Alison Sullivan

19   Working with men via the internet   186
     Jim Pollard

20   Innovation in obesity services for men   198
     Jane DeVille-Almond

21   The Australian experience   205
     Garry Egger

Afterword: The way forward   213
David Wilkins

The Men's Health Forum   220

Index   221

Foreword

Male weight problems were first highlighted as a major health issue by the Men's Health Forum (MHF) in 2004. Our analysis of the available research showed that, contrary to widespread belief, men are more likely than women to be overweight but are much less likely to perceive themselves as overweight or to wish to take any action to lose weight. Men are also much less likely to take part in weight management programmes in primary care or provided by the commercial organisations, such as Slimming World or Weight Watchers. Even though obesity had become a major public concern by 2004, it seemed to us that male weight problems were being largely overlooked, by men themselves as well as by health policymakers and practitioners.

We believed it was important for the public health community to understand more about male weight problems, especially the issues that are specific to men, and how to work with men effectively. We also wanted to make 'the man in the street' more aware of his weight, how to maintain a healthy weight and, if necessary, how to lose weight.

The MHF therefore decided to take four major steps. The first was to focus National Men's Health Week in June 2005 on men and weight. The Week, which has been run by the Forum every year since 2002, provides a good opportunity to draw men's health issues to the attention of the policymakers, practitioners, politicians, the press and, last but not least, the general public (and especially men).

Second, as part of the Week, we worked with Haynes and a large number of other partner organisations to publish *HGV Man*, a definitive guide to weight for men. This book was designed to look like a car maintenance manual in order to increase its appeal. The book was edited by Dr Ian Banks, the MHF President, and a huge debt is owed to him not just for his work on this definitive book but also for his commitment over many years to supporting the Forum and improving men's health.

The MHF's third step was to approach BT, the telecommunications company, with a proposal to run a lifestyle change programme for its staff with a focus on diet, physical activity and weight loss. This led to the Work Fit initiative, launched in September 2005, an ambitious and innovative intervention delivered almost entirely online. Over 16,000 out of 90,000 BT staff registered for the 16-week programme and, in line with the company demographic, the majority (72%) were male. Of the 5,700 Work Fit participants who could be tracked, three-quarters lost an average of 2.3 kg in weight.

Fourth, the MHF organised the first-ever national conference on men and weight. Supported by the Department of Health and held in London on 13 June 2005, the first day of National Men's Health Week, this conference was aimed at a wide-ranging group of health professionals including GPs (general practitioners), practice nurses, occupational health practitioners and health promotion specialists. It aimed to increase understanding of the scale of male weight problems and its consequences for health, to raise awareness of the need to develop policy and practice that includes men and boys, and to develop and disseminate good practice in tackling weight problems in men and boys. This book stems from this event and is essential reading not only for anyone wishing to improve policy and practice on tackling obesity but also for those who need to comply with the new legal duties.

Our approach to male weight has clearly shown that, like so many other major health issues, it is a 'gendered' issue that requires a 'gendered' response. This message will, we hope, resonate even more strongly with policymakers and practitioners as the new gender equality duty is implemented from April 2007. Health services can no longer be delivered – for weight problems and virtually any other area – on a 'one size fits all' basis. The MHF will continue to work with government, the National Health Service (NHS) and others to develop appropriate policy and practice for men.

Finally, on behalf of the MHF, I would like to thank Alan White and Maggie Pettifer for their foresight, energy and commitment in editing and producing this book. I know it has not been easy, especially given the number of contributors (all busy people with huge commitments) and the many other demands Alan and Maggie have had on their time. However, they have succeeded in producing a definitive and seminal book that will change the way male weight problems are tackled in the UK and beyond.

About the Men's Health Forum

The MHF was established in 1994 and became a registered charity in 2001. Its mission is to provide an independent and authoritative voice for male health and to tackle the issues affecting the health and well-being of boys and men in England and Wales. It envisions a future in which all boys and men have an equal opportunity to attain the highest possible level of health and well-being.

The MHF aims to achieve this through:
- policy development
- research
- providing information services
- stimulating professional and public debate
- working with MPs (members of parliament) and government
- developing innovative and imaginative projects
- professional training
- collaborating with the widest possible range of interested organisations and individuals
- organising the annual National Men's Health Week.

For more information about the MHF, visit www.menshealthforum.org.uk.

Peter Baker
Chief Executive, Men's Health Forum, London
July 2007

Foreword

Twenty years ago I read an article in the *New York Times* about our relationship with our bodies. The headline read: 'Women Unhappy with Body Image'. The article went on to 'discover' what feminists and therapists had been discussing for years – the frightening rise of anorexia and bulimia among teenaged girls and young women. Since that time, such articles have become commonplace, and women's problematic relationship with their bodies a staple of self-help mania.

But that's not why I bring this up. I remember this article because the subheading read 'Men Tend to see Themselves as Just About Perfect'.

If you were to ask me what's changed in the past 20 years, *that* is what I would point to. Men no longer tend to see themselves as 'just about perfect'. Men have been encouraged to view their bodies in similar ways as women have – as too fat, too skinny, not buff enough. We've seen our bodies displayed in countless adverts since Calvin Klein made every man feel inadequate compared with one man splayed across a Santorini streetscape in his underwear. And men have dutifully trooped off to the gym to pump up, work out, and otherwise transform their bodies into ectomorphic hypermuscular specimens.

Men no longer see themselves as 'just about perfect'. Men have also become enslaved to what psychologists call 'The Adonis Complex' – the constant measurement of our bodies against some Greek God-like measure. Men are fully capable of objectifying themselves.

Just as some men have become compulsive toners and shapers, other men have become slothful couch potatoes, whose only exercise is reaching for another beer or the remote. Yet even among those men, there's a touch of resentment in their sloth, a hint of resentment at the sorts of cultural expectations about their bodies. Not taking care of yourself can become an expression of men's resistance to their objectification.

They're two sides of the same coin. Compulsive exercisers and chronic couch potatoes are both screwing around with their health. In this breakthrough volume, Alan White and Maggie Pettifer have assembled a group of experts who can advise men on exactly what the dangers of male weight problems might be.

The consequences, we learn, are not just medical, although the list of ailments for which men are susceptible at elevated risk is long and frightening. It's not just longevity, but quality of life: obese men are less happy, less productive, and live less satisfying lives.

Men need to develop a healthy relationship with their bodies – recognising what they can do and what they cannot do – and both accept their limitations and resist lethargic surrender. This is not going to be easy: we've been taught from an early age to never admit weakness, to pretend our energy is limitless, and that our bodies are either out of control aliens or simple instruments of our will (or, occasionally, both). Confronting men's weight problems means confronting our cultural definitions of masculinity – definitions that set up standards that would be impossible for anyone to meet and simultaneously let us off the hook within nanoseconds, so we don't have to actually put up much of a struggle.

This book provides the beginning of a conversation in that elusive middle ground – the ground of healthy and engaged conversations about our bodies. Conversations with each other, and conversations with ourselves about what we expect of ourselves. We owe this to ourselves. Our lives could depend on it.

Michael Kimmel
Department of Sociology
SUNY at Stony Brook, New York
Editor, *Men and Masculinity*
July 2007

Preface

Men's weight is becoming a serious public health issue. With men laying down their fat around their abdomen, in a form that increases the chance of developing hypertension, hyperlipidaemia, diabetes and the fat-related cancers, and with the prospect of three-quarters of British men being overweight by the year 2010, the need for urgent action is now recognised as paramount. Coupled to this, the middle-aged spread (now seen as a very 'hazardous waist') that most men expect to develop as they enter into their thirties and forties is now occurring much earlier with even boys and young men developing life-limiting weight problems.

A main part of the 2005 National Men's Health Week, organised by the Men's Health Forum, was the first ever conference on men and their weight. With a multidisciplinary focus the day saw the bringing together of 300 academics, practitioners and politicians in an attempt to make sense of why men were so at risk and what could be done to tackle the problem. This book drew upon the presentations at that conference. The scant attention that was being given to this very gendered problem and the lack of any academic text that has focused on men and their weight made this book an essential component of the Forum's commitment to tackling this serious health issue.

Of the 21 chapters, 16 are based upon original conference presentations, updated and rewritten for the book's audience in 2007 and beyond and five have been written *de novo* to give the book an even broader perspective than the conference. It is noticeable as you move through the book that different styles of presentation have been adopted, some very practice based, some with a heavier academic feel and some with more of a personal perspective. To a large extent this is unavoidable in a text that has attempted to focus on issues that for some are breaking into new territory.

The first part of the book focuses on the causes of weight problems in men and their consequences. Within the opening chapters we explore what is currently known on men's weight and its effects on health. We then move into an appraisal of the state of health policy that is meant to be addressing the challenges posed by obesity. How men view their weight and their bodies is both a product of their psychology and also their socialisation, leading to chapters addressing the impact of men's psychological make-up and the influence of masculinity on their weight and the influence of the media.

The second part comprises chapters written by specialists in their respective fields who tackle the broad spectrum of issues that surround the management of men's weight. The breadth of the chapters highlights the complexity that surrounds men and their health with such factors as the impact of disability, mental health problems, ethnicity and age being discussed along with the role that primary healthcare, counselling and exercise can play in managing men with weight problems.

Targeting men where they are rather than waiting for them to come to the health professionals in their health centres has been recognised for some time as a key component of successful work with men in relation to their health. That this maxim has been adopted by those working with men and their weight is evident within a number of the chapters: the use of the internet; initiatives based within pharmacies and the workplace; organised commercial slimming services and through the direct work with men as developed by practitioners who have specialised in men's health.

In this ground-breaking text many authors have provided practical guidance for readers based on their experience of what appears to work well in their setting. Equally, though, it is clear to all the contributors, and will also be clear to our readers, just how little gender-specific research there is in the field of men and weight problems. Thus the book is as much a guide to what we do *not* know, and will provide a signpost to all those in the broader academic community towards the need for focused research into men and their weight. For sure, we urgently need research programmes that address how men's relationship with food, diet and exercise influences the risk of becoming overweight and obese and what can be done to help those who are afflicted.

In April 2007, the Equality Act 2006 became law and it is now a legal requirement that health policies and practices should be seen to be meeting the differing needs of men and women. This new Duty requires all to deliver gender-sensitive care in a way that has been sadly lacking up to now. Rarely has such an important health issue been so badly neglected. If the predictions are true, and the implications of the obesity epidemic are potentially so catastrophic, then this book must be seen as a wake-up call to recognising that a gender-sensitive approach is essential and that men need to be targeted specifically and in a male-focused manner.

Professor Alan White
Maggie Pettifer
July 2007

Neither editor has received a royalty from the publication of this text and they have elected to donate these towards the Men's Health Forum, a Registered Charity.

About the editors

Professor Alan White, Leeds Metropolitan University
Professor Alan White was the world's first Professor of Men's Health and is the Director of the Centre for Men's Health at Leeds Metropolitan University, which is a focus for research and education on the health of men. Alan is the Chair of the Board of Trustees for Men's Health Forum (England) and is on the Executive Committee of the European Men's Health Forum (EMHF).

His research includes the *Scoping Study on Men's Health* for the Department of Health in 2001, the *Report on the State of Men's Health Across 17 European Countries* (for the EMHF), which was launched at the European Parliament in 2003, and he has recently completed a study into *Patterns of Mortality for Young Men and Women (Aged 15–44 years) Across 44 Countries*. Alan's work includes studies into men's experiences of illness, including coronary heart disease, diabetes and prostate cancer. Other ongoing research includes the evaluation of *Self Care for People* and *Self Care for Primary Health Care Professionals* as part of the NHS Working in Partnership Programme of work and a study on the Bradford Health of Men initiative (www.healthofmen.com). The latter is the subject of a book published by Radcliffe Publishing in 2007: *Men's Health – how to do it*, edited by David Conrad and Alan White.

Maggie Pettifer
Maggie Pettifer has a background in healthcare publishing and conference development. In 1993 she organised the first national conference on men's health in London, bringing together academics, politicians and men's health workers. Her interest in men's health continued during the later 1990s in her role as Head of Publishing at the British Association for Counselling and Psychotherapy (BACP).

Upon leaving BACP, Maggie was invited by Men's Health Forum to organise a national conference on male weight problems in 2005. This event ('Hazardous Waist?'), which was the highlight of the 2005 National Men's Health Week, took part at Savoy Place Conference Centre in London and all 300 tickets were sold before the day. It seemed to uncover a huge gap not only in practitioner education and understanding but also in the research literature and in healthcare policy and provision. There was much to build on after the conference.

Thus, later in 2005, Maggie began working with Alan White to invite selected speakers to contribute chapters to this book, commissioning new chapters in the light of issues raised at the conference. The aim was to publish the first book on male weight problems in 2007.

About the contributors

Amanda Avery
For the past 18 years Amanda has worked as a community dietician in Southern Derbyshire. During a secondment within the public health department, Amanda was given the remit to produce a local obesity strategy, undertaking a comprehensive mapping exercise to look at local examples of good practice. During this secondment the opportunity arose to look at the feasibility of the NHS working in partnership with the commercial slimming sector, Slimming World headquarters being situated in Derbyshire. Amanda co-ordinated the feasibility study for partnership working and has subsequently worked part time for Slimming World as a partnerships co-ordinator, overseeing an increase in the number of 'slimming on referral' schemes across the country.

Richard Bryant-Jefferies
Richard Bryant-Jefferies trained as a person-centred counsellor/psychotherapist in the early 1990s and then spent eight years working in the NHS as a counsellor in primary healthcare settings. He has had 20 books published on counselling themes, including *Counselling for Eating Disorders in Men*, *Counselling for Eating Disorders in Women* and *Counselling for Obesity*, and offers workshops and talks on counselling themes. He believes strongly that often eating disorders are rooted in dysfunctional relational experiences and that offering a constructive therapeutic relationship in line with the principles of the person-centred approach is key to enabling the person to re-define themselves and break free of their disordered eating pattern. Details of his books and other writings can be found at www.bryant-jefferies.freeserve.co.uk. He is currently working as an Equalities and Diversity Manager at an NHS mental health trust in London.

Sue Catton
Since graduating from Loughborough University in Physical Education (PE) and Sports Science, Sue Catton has been heavily involved in the sport and leisure industry, including teaching, event and project management and consultancy services. Sue is the National Director of the Inclusive Fitness Initiative (IFI), one of the largest nationally networked projects supported by the Sport England Lottery Fund. Receiving over £8 million of investment, the IFI scheme is an innovative and ground-breaking project that ensures that disabled people can access safe and appropriate fitness services in their local community. It is leading the global fitness industry

with solutions to meet the inclusion agenda. Sue is also a Director of Montgomery Leisure Services, the IFI Project Management Agents.

Kate Davidson

Kate Davidson is a Senior Lecturer in Social Policy and Sociology in the Department of Sociology, and is Co-Director of the Centre for Research on Ageing and Gender (CRAG) at the University of Surrey. She is President of the British Society of Gerontology, a Governor of the Centre for Policy on Ageing, Vice Chair of Age Concern Surrey and Chair of the Gerontological Society of America's Special Interest Group for 'Men's Issues'. In collaboration with Age Concern Surrey and Surrey Social and Market Research (SSMR), Kate recently completed a Big Lottery Fund research project examining the needs of lone older men in the community. Prior to this she was involved with a European Union (EU) project examining food choices for older people (Senior-Foods: Quality of Life) in eight countries, and a research project on *Older Men: their social worlds and healthy lifestyles* as part of the Economic and Social Research Council (ESRC) Growing Older Programme.

Steve Deacon

Steve Deacon is Group Medical Director at Scottish Power. At the time of writing this chapter he was Head of Health at Royal Mail. Steve is a senior occupational health physician with many years' experience in a wide range of UK and international manufacturing and service industries. He is active in postgraduate medical education and has been published widely in medical and scientific journals.

Jane DeVille-Almond

Jane DeVille-Almond is an independent nurse consultant in primary care and a freelance journalist. She develops new ways of working with men and obesity, highlighting both areas through medical journals, books, the media and working with primary care teams around the UK. She also runs one of the first accredited courses for obesity training in primary care. Jane runs surgeries for men in a range of 'male-dominated environments'. Her weight management clinic that she ran at the back of a barber shop for two years, and the Harley-Davidson showroom surgery, have both been featured in a BBC2 documentary about weight. She has also appeared on several obesity programmes both for ITV and the BBC. She has won several awards for her innovation to nursing, is Vice President/Vice Chair of Men's Health Forum and a director of the National Obesity Forum.

Jenne Dixit

Jenne Dixit has a background with Media Reach Advertising – an ethnic specialist agency reaching out to people from black and minority ethnic communities. She headed the public relations (PR) team for the agency, working with the ethnic media to devise campaigns for mainstream companies to get their messages out to hard-to-reach communities. Clients included British Telecom and the Department of Health. For the past four years Jenne has been working for Diabetes UK as an Equality and Diversity Advisor, to improve cultural awareness within Diabetes UK, influence the provision of more culturally appropriate diabetes care, production and dissemination of information, and to increase diabetes and Diabetes UK awareness among diverse communities. This includes people from black and minority ethnic backgrounds, people with diabetes and mental health or learning disabilities, and people with diabetes in institutional care.

Garry Egger

Garry Egger is an Australian health scientist and consultant to governments and the World Health Organization (WHO) on obesity and health promotion. He is the author of 25 books and almost 100 scientific publications. In 1991 he developed the GutBusters 'Waist Loss' programme for men in Australia, the biggest of its kind in the world, and has now developed Professor Trim's Weight Loss for Men programme.

Paul Gately

Paul Gately is Carnegie Professor of Exercise and Obesity at Leeds Metropolitan University. His primary research interest is childhood obesity treatment strategies. His PhD at Leeds Metropolitan University evaluated a residential weight loss camp as an intervention for the treatment of overweight and obese children. In addition he is the Director of Carnegie Weight Management, which runs the successful Carnegie International Camp and community-based weight loss afterschool and primary care trust (PCT) clubs throughout Britain. Paul was a contributor to the International Obesity Task Force/WHO report on childhood obesity and is a frequent consultant to government agencies, health organisations and corporations throughout the UK and internationally.

Ewan Gillon

Ewan Gillon is a Chartered Counselling Psychologist. He is Director of the Edinburgh Psychology Centre and is developing mens-talk.co.uk, a portal website designed to support men address a range of psychological concerns. He is also a part-time Lecturer in Psychology at Glasgow Caledonian University.

Brendan Gough

Brendan Gough is a Senior Lecturer at the Institute of Psychological Sciences and is currently Deputy Director for the Centre for Interdisciplinary Gender Studies, both at the University of Leeds. His research and publications to date have mainly centred on issues around men and masculinities, including recent research on men's health. His research is informed by critical psychological theory and qualitative research methods, and he is co-founder and co-editor of the journal *Qualitative Research in Psychology*. Current research projects include analyses of men's health promotion materials and media representations of gender and health.

Caroline Gunnell

Caroline Gunnell has a background in nursing. She is currently Clinical Lead (Nursing and Allied Health Professionals) East of England Primary Care Research Network, Research Governance Coordinator for West Essex PCT and Chair of the Management Group for the EPCRDO (Essex Primary Care Research and Development Office). She is a member of the NHS R&D Forum Primary Care Group, of the UK Federation of Primary Care Research Networks Steering Group, and the Royal College of Nursing (RCN) Research Society, among others. Her research interests include patient experience of service delivery and care, and men's health and professional development. Caroline sits on the All Parties Men's Health Policy Steering Group and has been a member of the Men's Health Forum for many years.

David Haslam

David is a full-time practising GP as well as being Clinical Director of the National Obesity Forum, and is involved with many other organisations in the field of obesity including the charity foundations, PCOS UK (for polycystic ovary syndrome), and groups such as Counterweight and MEND (Mind, Exercise, Nutrition … Do It!). He took charge of formulating the guidelines for obesity management in primary care and was part of a four-man working party convened by the Royal College of Paediatrics and Child Health (RCPCH) which developed the first guidelines for management of childhood obesity in primary care. David has written widely in books, journals and papers and speaks internationally on obesity and related subjects. He is co-author with Dr Ian Campbell of a book in the Your Questions Answered series, and has several other volumes on the shelves or in press.

Julie Hunter

Julie Hunter is a Pharmacy Assistant and 'TROCN 3' trained weight management adviser. Julie provides one-to-one weight reduction services for both men and women.

Jim Leishman

Jim Leishman works as a charge nurse within the town of Falkirk, Central Scotland. In February 2001 he co-developed a service aimed at improving the health of men. Since then the service has gone from strength to strength. Known nationally as the Forth Valley model, the Camelon Centre is viewed by many, including the Scottish Executive, as the way ahead for improving the health of Scotland's men. Jim's work has featured in numerous publications. He regularly presents at national and international conferences and in partnership with the Men's Health Forum Scotland provides training on men's health issues.

Claire Mac Evilly

Claire Mac Evilly completed her undergraduate nutrition degree in University College Cork and followed this with a Master's in Nutrition Communications from Tufts University, Boston. She is currently working as the Communications Manager for the Medical Research Council Human Nutrition Research in Cambridge. Her main activities include handling media calls, developing communications strategies and outreach programmes for health professionals, academics and industry on nutrition issues.

Jim McKenna

Jim McKenna is Professor of Sport at the Carnegie Faculty of Sports and Education at Leeds Metropolitan University. He is an ex-PE teacher. His research interests range from exercise in elderly people, to counselling for behaviour change in exercise, nutrition and injury rehabilitation. Recently he has developed a strong interest in qualitative methods of enquiry and particularly focuses on using interviewing and focus group techniques. He is widely published in healthcare and sports sciences journals.

Kerri McPherson

Kerri McPherson is a Chartered Health Psychologist and Lecturer in Psychology at Queen Margaret University, Edinburgh. Her work in the area of weight-related psychology in men began with her PhD, which was entitled 'Psychological correlates of overweight in a group of Scottish men'. She is particularly interested in the development of body image (dis)satisfaction in men and the relationship this shares with other weight-related psychological phenomena, including cognitive/dietary restraint. Much of her work has used the theories of evolutionary psychology to explore and explain men's body image.

Jim Pollard

Jim Pollard is the editor of malehealth.co.uk as well as other websites for the Men's Health Forum and European Men's Health Forum. A health editor of *Maxim* in its pre-top-shelf days and the only-ever health columnist on the *Daily Star*, he also writes for newspapers and magazines. He is the author of seven books, six of them about health and the other a novel about punk rock.

Duncan Radley

Duncan Radley is Research Fellow for the Carnegie Research Institute at Leeds Metropolitan University. His primary research interest is body composition measurement in overweight and obese children. His work within Carnegie Weight Management focuses on the evaluation of the effectiveness of weight loss interventions for these children.

Kurt Ramsden

Kurt Ramsden is a community pharmacist in Redcar with an interest in public health, particularly with regard to increasing the access of public health services through community pharmacy. He is also a spokesperson for the Royal Pharmaceutical Society, and a qualified hypnotherapist.

Alison Sullivan

Alison Sullivan is Chief Dietician and Head of Service for the Nutrition and Specialist Dietetics Service of the West London Mental Health Trust, which includes the high-secure hospital Broadmoor, as well as low- and medium-secure sites, provision for adults, older people, children and adolescents with mental health needs, in the community and in hospitals. Alison has worked in community dietetics and in private practice, lectured at the University of North London (now London Metropolitan) and been a frequent contributor to journals and popular magazines such as *Men's Health*, *Essentials*, *Sugar*, *B* and *Company*. She is currently studying for a part-time PhD at King's College London, researching factors around weight gain in men with mental health needs.

David Wilkins

David Wilkins has held the post of policy officer at the Men's Health Forum since 2002. He previously worked for 11 years in the NHS, for the last three years of which he was lecturer/practitioner in health promotion on a joint appointment with Bournemouth University. David's previous work experience included local authority social services and youth work, and several years as a community worker in Southampton. He has been interested in men's health for many years and has published a number of articles on the subject. David is an experienced trainer and has a long track record of involvement in community organisations.

PART 1

The challenge of male weight problems

The research base for male obesity: what do we know?

David Wilkins

Men are getting fatter – there's no doubt about that. The most recent statistics, published in 2004, show that two-thirds (65.4%) of English men have a BMI (body mass index) of more than 25 compared to just over half of women (55.5%) (Department of Health, 2004), and that 23% of men are obese. A recent World Health Organization study of 40 countries found that the UK had the eighth highest rate of obesity in men (compared with the eleventh highest for women) (Swinburn *et al.*, 2003). Some 31% of English men now have a waist circumference of over 102 cm (Department of Health, 2003). If present trends continue, more than three men in every four will be overweight by 2010 and almost one man in three will be obese.

Only three or four decades ago, any suggestion that matters could reach this stage this quickly would have been dismissed as absurd. Indeed the 1990 *Health of the Nation* targets included a plan – to reduce the level of obesity in men from the then baseline of 8% to 6% by 2005 – that now looks laughably naive. The only reason that we are not amazed by the shape of the typical British bloke in 2007 is that – rather like an expanding waistline itself – the present situation has crept upon us gradually, inch by inch.

If this is hard to conceptualise, imagine that the first ever episode of *Doctor Who* in 1963 had seen the Tardis land on a crowded, real-life, British beach in summer 2007. The immediate reaction of the Doctor's young companions would have been to gape in disbelief at the sheer size and number of bellies overhanging waistbands. The normal-weight world of 40 years before could never have prepared them for such a startling sight. They would have assumed perhaps that the nation, and especially its men, had been struck by some dreadful belly-expanding epidemic – which, in a way, it has …

What do we know about male attitudes?

The little that is known about men's attitudes to weight tends to be concentrated on identifying obstacles rather than developing solutions. Nevertheless, knowing where the obstacles are is a helpful prerequisite to dismantling them.

The first problem is men's difficulty in coming to grips with the idea that their weight is something about which they should concern themselves. A recent National Opinion Polls (NOP) survey conducted on behalf of one of the leading pharmaceutical companies found no significant differences between men and women in terms of the perceived disadvantages of being overweight in relation to health (around one-fifth of both sexes believing that poor health is the most worrying consequence of being overweight) but found that 42% of men (compared to only 27% of women) took the view that being overweight 'wouldn't bother me at all' (NOP, 2005).

A charitable interpretation of such a view is that it represents nothing more damaging than complacency, and should be relatively easy to challenge. Unfortunately, there is good evidence to suggest that the problem is rather more deep-rooted. Many overweight men refuse to acknowledge that they are so. The now sadly defunct Australian GutBusters programme (certainly the world's most successful weight loss programme for men to date – *see* Chapter 21) found that 'denial' was commonplace among potential users of its service (Egger, 2000). More worrying still, it seems probable that many men simply have no idea that they have become overweight in the first place. A Canadian study found, for example, that around half of men who are overweight may consider themselves to be of normal weight (the reverse of this proposition is true for women) (McCreary and Sadava, 2001).

This latter point highlights the second of the obstacles to be overcome – that of 'gender stereotyping', which tends to associate 'bigness' in men with good health and physical attractiveness. The same Canadian study found that overweight men are much more likely than overweight women to consider themselves physically attractive (McCreary and Sadava, 2001). Similarly, a detailed psychological study of overweight Swedish men, all aged 51, suggested that, despite measurably poorer physical health being experienced by all men in the study group, simply being overweight (by BMI) was positively correlated with relatively high levels of self-esteem (Rosmond and Bjorntorp, 2000). This suggests a connection between increased body size and feeling positive about oneself.

The final attitudinal problem is the 'feminisation' of weight as an issue of personal concern. A few years ago I was involved in a study in which men aged over 40 were invited to discuss their attitudes to weight. In addition to consistently echoing the themes outlined above, that study suggested that, by and large, men believe that pre-occupation with weight loss is a 'women's thing' (Wilkins, 2001) – and, frankly, no academic research is really needed to conclude that most men and women subscribe to this same popular notion, at least to some degree.

The difficulty here is that the pervasiveness of this way of looking at the matter is very damaging to the health of men. Virtually all industrialised countries have a highly developed and widely understood network of support systems for women who want to lose weight. This network encompasses elements as diverse as the routine expectation of empathy and encouragement from friends and relatives, ready access to 'female-friendly' advice from the mass media, multinational companies running nationwide chains of weight loss classes, and 'calorie-counted' foodstuffs in every supermarket. This firmly established socio-cultural context results in a vicious cycle. That is to say, men do not regard attempting to lose weight as a 'male activity', and the consequent lack of demand discourages the development of a 'male-friendly' infrastructure of support, whether that is from social networks, commercial providers or the NHS.

In these discouraging circumstances it is therefore perhaps not surprising that the GutBusters' experience further suggests that Australian men's most serious limitation in attempting to lose weight is lack of basic knowledge on how to go about it (Egger, 2000). Things are unlikely to be different in the UK. A study focused specifically on the nutritional knowledge of Scottish men, for example, found 'glaring gaps' between what men knew and what they needed to know to make even the most basic decisions about healthy eating in accordance with official recommendations (McPherson and Turnbull, 2004).

What do we know about the attitudes of health providers?

It is natural to assume that the commonly held preconception about weight being largely an issue of concern for women does not affect the NHS. The NHS has principles of equity at its heart after all. Disappointingly, a glance at some of the evidence suggests otherwise.

The *Counterweight* programme (www.counterweight.org) is a multicentre, nurse-led obesity management project being conducted in seven regions of the UK. Since 2000 it has been offering structured programmes to patients in 80 general practices. A computerised audit of almost 120,000 medical records in 26 of the participating *Counterweight* GP practices revealed that male patients were less likely than female patients ever to have been routinely weighed in the surgery (57.0% against 69.2%) or to have had their BMI recorded (57.7% against 70.6%) (Counterweight Project Team, 2004b). This suggests unconscious collusion between health professionals and male patients in seeing being overweight as less of a concern for men than women.

Since men are less likely to be identified as overweight, it might not be unexpected for them to be under-represented as participants in NHS weight loss programmes. Even so, the scale of the discrepancy between the sexes is surprising. An analysis of 1,256 patients taking part in *Counterweight* programmes across 58 of the participating practices in 2004 found that only 26% of those attending the programmes were men (Counterweight Project Team, 2004a). (Incidentally, men who did take part lost weight as effectively as women.) Similarly, while recommendation 357 from the Health Select Committee's 2004 report on obesity (House of Commons Health Committee, 2004) (that NHS organisations should consider partnerships with commercial slimming organisations) has been enthusiastically embraced by a number of primary care trusts (PCTs) (Carlisle, 2005), the most structured pilot programme so far to use this approach achieved only 12% participation by men (Slimming World, 2004).

It should perhaps be remembered at this point that significantly more men are overweight than women. In other words, a service that aspired to equitable take-up would expect to involve *more* men than women. The figures in the paragraph above need to be viewed in this context and not simply measured against a rough sense that 50/50 would be about right.

All this is against a background in which broad popular prejudices against both men and women who are overweight are already believed to affect detrimentally the way such people are perceived and treated by health professionals (Association for the Study of Obesity). Even those specialising in obesity are not exempt; a comprehensive study of delegates (admittedly, not UK-based) attending a clinical obesity conference in Quebec in 2001, for example, found a significant association of the stereotypes 'lazy', 'stupid' and 'worthless' with obese people (Schwartz *et al.*, 2003).

There is good evidence in relation to women that obesity is a factor in predisposing patients to avoid deliberately some interactions with health services. Large-scale studies have shown that obese female patients are less likely to attend routinely for cervical or breast screening (Wee *et al.*, 2001). This suggests that a combination of embarrassment about their bodies and a sense of potential prejudice against them may be putting them off. There is no equivalent research to draw on for male patients, but how much worse, potentially, might this situation be for overweight men, when men are well known to be less likely to seek help and support from health professionals in the first place?

What do we know about the social context for male weight problems?

Weight problems in both men and women are essentially a phenomenon of very recent times, and of the developed world. Levels of obesity in men in England have trebled since 1986, for example (British Heart Foundation, 2003), and the average waist circumference of English men grew by 3.8 cm between 1994 and 2003 (from 93.8 to 97.6 cm – an increase of 4%) (Johnson, 2005). The problem affects men of all racial backgrounds (with the exception of men of Chinese origin) and is particularly marked in the white population and the Afro-Caribbean population (Hansard, 2006). Weight problems among boys are also increasing. The Health Survey for England 2002, which had a particular concentration on the health of children, found that 30% of boys aged under 15 are now overweight or obese by the customary BMI measures applied to adults (although if the alternative, international classification system designed specifically for children is applied, this figure falls to 21.8%) (Department of Health, 2003).

Such changes in weight at the population level are unprecedented in recorded history and, of course, cannot be explained by changes in the gene pool or by the increased incidence of underlying physiological causes ('slow metabolism', for example). It is often asserted that the western world has created an 'obesogenic' environment. Is this the case?

The western world has an abundance of food. Modern manufacturing processes and the twin commercial imperatives of keeping production costs low while making food taste as appealing as possible mean that much of this food is supplied in an energy-dense form (high in fat and high in sugar). Mass advertising campaigns exhort people to eat foods of this kind and some biological research has even suggested an inborn preference for high-fat and high-sugar foods (Levine *et al.*, 2003) – a characteristic that may be more marked in men (Rolls *et al.*, 1991).

High-fat, high-sugar foods are particularly popular with children, and the ethical issues associated with directly marketing such foods to children have been the subject of a great deal of public debate in recent years. A review of the research literature commissioned by the Office of Communications (OFCOM) noted that several studies have found that the food choices of adolescent boys are more likely to be affected by advertising than those of girls (Livingstone and Helsper, 2004).

Along with these changes to food supply and consumption, the developed world has experienced massive technological changes over the past century. These changes have resulted in unprecedented shifts in the pattern of work, transportation and communication. American studies suggest that the population-level increase in men's BMI began in the late nineteenth century when the amount of physical effort involved in work began to decline. Physical work gradually became less demanding and fewer men were required to be engaged in it. This continuing shift towards sedentary occupations for men was paralleled by a five-fold increase in obesity between the beginning and end of the last century (Helmchen, 2001).

This effect may be particularly marked for men in the UK where working hours are the longest in Europe. Some 27 per cent of men with full-time jobs in the UK work more than 48 hours a week (compared with 11% of women) and 11% of men work more than 60 hours a week (Hogarth *et al.*, 2003). Long working hours are not only, in most cases, hours spent in sedentary activity, they also severely limit the time and energy available for physical activity in leisure time.

What do we know about physical activity and diet in men?

Weight gain at an individual level has only one simple cause – an excess of energy intake over energy expenditure. Energy is measured in calories and is taken into the body in the form of food and drink. Energy is expended in all forms of human activity (even sleeping burns calories) but expenditure increases in proportion to the level of vigorousness.

Men tend to be more physically active than women but even so, even in the youngest age group, less than 50% of men undertake enough physical activity each week to derive a positive health benefit. Overall, one man in five is effectively inactive. (*See* Table 1.1.)

TABLE 1.1 Numbers of days per week (p.w.) of men's participation in at least 30 minutes of activity of at least moderate intensity (Great Britain).

Age	19–24 (%)	25–34 (%)	35–49 (%)	50–64 (%)	All ages (%)
1 or 2 days p.w.	21	12	20	30	21
2 or 3 days p.w.	14	21	27	28	24
3 or 4 days p.w.	17	21	19	18	19
5 days p.w. or more*	49	46	34	24	36

* = Recommended level
Source: Office for National Statistics, 2004.

TABLE 1.2 Estimated Average Requirements (EARs) for men.

Men, by age	EAR (kcal per day)
19–59	2,550
60–64	2,380
65–74	2,330
74+	2,100

Source: Department of Health, 1991.

The energy intake required to meet the average requirements of particular population groups was estimated by the Committee on Medical Aspects of Food Policy (COMA) in 1991. These average requirements are expressed as EARs ('Estimated Average Requirements'). The EARs for men are shown in Table 1.2 (Department of Health, 1991).

Surprisingly, given the prevalence of weight problems across all age groups, men average an energy intake of only 92% of the EARs (Office for National Statistics, 2004). There is, however, significant variation in energy intake between individual men – for example, for men aged 50 to 64, the range is from 1,110 kcal per day to 3,409 kcal per day (Office for National Statistics, 2004). It is also very important to note that surveys which rely on self-reporting of energy intake – that is to say, practically all such surveys – are accepted to be subject to an under-estimation rate of up to 25%, with overweight subjects more likely to under-report their energy intake than people of normal weight (Rennie *et al.*, 2004).

It must also be observed that 27% of British men drink more than 21 units of alcohol each week, and around 8% drink more than 50 units (General Household Survey, 2003). A pint of beer is usually around two units of alcohol and contains roughly 180 calories. A man drinking (say) two pints of beer each day (28 units per week) is therefore consuming the equivalent of one day's energy requirements each week in beer alone.

What do we know about the health risks of being overweight?

The risks to men's physical health are dealt with elsewhere in this book – but it is perhaps worth summarising them here. We can thus remind ourselves that a proper (and very pressing) concern with public health remains the primary reason for tackling the problem of overweight men. Whether or not we can develop successful policy and practice is – quite literally – a matter of life or death for many men.

For physiological reasons, overweight men tend to accumulate fat around the abdomen. Abdominal fat is strongly associated with the most damaging consequence of obesity, *metabolic syndrome*, one of whose components, type 2 diabetes, is 10 times as common in people with a BMI of 30 or higher (Diabetes UK, 2005). Metabolic syndrome greatly increases the risk of developing heart and circulatory problems, approximately tripling the risk of death from coronary heart disease and doubling the risk of death from cardiovascular disease (Lakka *et al.*, 2002). Men are also more likely to die earlier in life from heart disease or stroke, conditions which are more prevalent in those who are overweight whether they suffer from metabolic syndrome or not.

Obesity is strongly linked with significantly greater risk of several cancers (obesity is second only to smoking as the most important preventable risk factor for cancer). Obesity is most strongly correlated with increased risk of colorectal cancer, oesophageal cancer and kidney cancer (Key et al., 2002). All three of these latter cancers are much more common in men than women (Men's Health Forum, 2004). Prostate cancer, although it is not linked specifically to weight gain, is known to be strongly associated with a diet that is high in fat, high in sugar and low in fruit and vegetables (Key et al., 2002) (i.e. it is associated with a diet that also predisposes the individual to being overweight).

Weight problems are also associated with other long-term health risks, some of which are less obvious than those mentioned above. An important longitudinal study found a strong link between weight problems in mid-life and an increased risk of dementia in old age, for example (Whitmer et al., 2005), and a large-scale US study recently found that obesity significantly increases the risk of death in road traffic accidents – an effect specific to men (Zhu et al., 2006). Excess weight is additionally a very common – but effectively unquantifiable – cause of chronic, misery-inducing conditions such as low back pain, breathing difficulties (e.g. sleep apnoea) and permanent damage to weight-bearing joints like the knees and hips.

Conclusion

In short, this is a problem whose importance it would be difficult to exaggerate – and we have reached a crucial point in dealing with it. Obesity not only causes disease, it is in many ways a disease in itself. It is not therefore an intrusion into individual liberty to seek to change the attitudes and conditions that underpin its advance, anymore than it is to seek to save lives by imposing speed limits on the roads. Unless we act rapidly to tackle the epidemic of overweight males, families will continue to lose fathers and grandfathers unnecessarily, and large numbers of men will never experience optimum health and well-being.

Asking 'What do we know?' is important. It is the first step towards deciding how best to frame the action that we need to take – although the most immediate and honest answer to the question is undoubtedly, 'not enough'. Nevertheless, we can say with reasonable confidence that the predisposing factors for becoming and remaining overweight vary between the sexes and that the overall risk is significantly greater in men. Men know less about diet than women and are more likely to drink alcohol to excess. Men are more likely to be physically active than women – but most are nevertheless nowhere near physically active enough to gain a health benefit. Men are more likely to be prevented from taking exercise by long working hours spent in sedentary occupations. Men are less likely to be concerned about becoming overweight, more likely to fail to notice that they have gained weight, and more likely to deny that they have a problem once they are overweight. Men are less likely to be offered participation in weight management programmes and less likely to take up the offer when it is made.

We need to change the way services are delivered and to tackle the structural issues that underpin the obesogenic environment. We also need to try to change men's attitudes and – perhaps more importantly – to change public perceptions so that men feel encouraged and supported when they do decide to lose weight. In taking these steps we need consciously to develop approaches that are in tune with male sensibilities and that reflect a male world-view. Strategies predicated on the assumption that what works with women will work with men will never be as successful as we need them to be – and we are in desperate need of some success.

References

Association for the Study of Obesity. *The Social and Psychological Consequences of Obesity.* Online factsheet at www.aso.org.uk (accessed 7 March 2007).

British Heart Foundation. Written evidence to the Health Select Committee, London. April 2003.

Carlisle D. Profit in loss. *Health Development Today.* 2005; **26**: 18–19.

Counterweight programme website: www.counterweight.org (accessed 15 March 2007).

Counterweight Project Team. A new evidence-based model for weight management in primary care: the Counterweight programme. *Journal of Human Nutrition and Dietetics.* 2004a; **17**(3): 181–2.

Counterweight Project Team. Current approaches to obesity management in UK primary care: the Counterweight programme. *Journal of Human Nutrition and Dietetics.* 2004b; **17**(3): 183–90.

Department of Health. *Dietary Reference Values for Food Energy and Nutrients for the United Kingdom.* London: HMSO; 1991.

Department of Health. *Health Survey for England 2002.* London: The Stationery Office; 2003.

Department of Health. *Health Survey for England 2003.* London: The Stationery Office; 2004.

Diabetes UK. *A Heavy Burden: type II diabetes and obesity.* London: Diabetes UK; 2005.

Egger G. Intervening in men's nutrition: lessons from the GutBuster men's 'waist loss' program. *Australian Journal of Nutrition and Dietetics.* 2000; **57**(1): 46–9.

General Household Survey. Cited in: Wanless D. *Securing Good Health for the Whole Population: population health trends.* London: HM Treasury; 2003.

Hansard. Answer to a parliamentary question from Keith Vaz MP. *Hansard.* 2006; 1 March, Column 767W.

Helmchen L. *Can Structural Change Explain the Rise in Obesity? A Look at the Past 100 Years.* Discussion paper for the Population Research Center at NORC and the University of Chicago. Chicago, IL: University of Chicago; 2001.

Hogarth T, Daniel WW, Dickerson AP *et al. The Business Context to Long Hours Working (Employment Relations Research Series No. 23).* London: Department of Trade and Industry; 2003.

House of Commons Health Committee. *Third Report of the Session 2003–2004: obesity.* London: The Stationery Office; 2004.

Johnson M, MP, Parliamentary Under Secretary for Public Health in answer to a parliamentary question, 7 February 2005.

Key T, Allen N, Spencer E, Travis R. The effect of diet on the risk of cancer. *The Lancet.* 2002; **360**(9336): 861–8.

Lakka HM, Laaksonen DE, Lakka TA *et al.* The metabolic syndrome and total and cardiovascular disease mortality in middle-aged men. *Journal of the American Medical Association.* 2002; **288**: 2709–16.

Levine AS, Kotz CM, Gosnell BA. Sugars and fats: the neurobiology of preference. *Journal of Nutrition.* 2003; **133**: 831–834.

Livingstone S, Helsper E. *Advertising Foods to Children: understanding promotion in the context of children's daily lives.* London: Media@LSE; 2004.

McCreary D, Sadava S. Gender differences in relationships among perceived attractiveness, life satisfaction, and health in adults as a function of body mass index and perceived weight. *Psychology of Men and Masculinity*. 2001; **2**: 108–16.

McPherson KE, Turnbull JD. Scottish men's nutritional knowledge and the Scottish Executive's current dietary targets: they don't match up. *British Nutrition Foundation Nutrition Bulletin*. 2004; **29**(3): 183–7.

Men's Health Forum. *National Men's Health Week 2004 Briefing Paper: men and cancer*. London: Men's Health Forum; 2004.

National Opinion Polls. Conducted by National Opinion Polls in January 2005. Unpublished (quoted with permission).

Office for National Statistics. *National Diet and Nutrition Survey Volume 5*. London: The Stationery Office; 2004.

Rennie R, Coward A, Wright A, Jebb S. *Estimating Under-Reporting of Energy Intake in a British National Dietary Survey*. Poster presentation; 2004.

Rolls BJ, Federoff IC, Guthrie JF. Gender differences in eating behavior and body weight regulation. *Health Psychology*. 1991; **10**(2): 133–42.

Rosmond R, Bjorntorp P. Quality of life, overweight, and body fat distribution in middle-aged men. *Behavioural Medicine*. 2000; **26**(2): 90–4.

Schwartz MB, O'Neal Chambliss H, Brownell KD *et al*. Weight bias among health professionals specializing in obesity. *Obesity Research*. 2003; **11**: 1033–9.

Slimming World with Greater and Central Derby Primary Care Trusts. *Tackling Obesity in Primary Care. A feasibility study to assess the practicalities of working in partnership with the commercial slimming sector*. Alfreton: Slimming World; 2004.

Swinburn B *et al*. Draft report for the World Health Organization cited in the British Heart Foundation's written evidence to the Health Select Committee. April 2003.

Wee C, McCarthy E, Davis R, Phillips R. Screening for cervical and breast cancer: is obesity an unrecognized barrier to preventive care. *Annals of Internal Medicine*. 2001; **132**(9): 697–704.

Whitmer RA, Gunderson EP, Barrett-Connor E *et al*. Obesity in middle age and future risk of dementia: a 27 year longitudinal population based study. *BMJ*. 2005; **330**: 1360.

Wilkins D. Keeping it up. In: Davidson N, Lloyd T, editors. *Promoting Men's Health*. London: Baillière Tindall; 2001.

Zhu S, Layde PM, Guse CE *et al*. Obesity and risk for death due to motor vehicle crashes. *American Journal of Public Health*. 2006; **96**(4): 734–9.

CHAPTER 2

The causes of male obesity and associated health problems

David Haslam

Obesity has been documented for the last 25,000 years (Bray *et al.*, 1997). Prehistoric fertility symbols accurately portray obese women – ironic as we now know that obesity reduces fertility in women. Hippocrates recognised that corpulence led to premature death. But obesity has been a rare phenomenon up until the last 30 years, and so it was not a topic for discussion, study or treatment among early physicians. Gradually, as numbers of cases increased, it became worthy of study, and patterns began to emerge, and it became apparent that obesity affected different people in different ways, men in a different way to women.

The wealthy Venetian, Luigi Cornaro (Cornaro, 1558), was born in 1464, and is one of the most famous fat men in history. In a story not unfamiliar to many men, he spent 40 years as a glutton, overindulging in 'sensual pleasures, adulation, ceremony, heresy and intemperance', until in middle age he faced the prospect of premature death:

> ... *a heavy train of infirmities, which had not only invaded, but even made great inroads in my constitution ... different kinds of disorders, such as pains in my stomach, and often stitches, and spices of the gout; attended by, what was still worse, an almost continuous low fever, a stomach generally out of order, and a perpetual thirst.*

In his autobiography he denounced gluttony, which: 'kills every year as great a number as would perish during the time of a most dreadful pestilence, or by the sword or fire of many bloody wars', eventually exclaiming, 'Put a stop to this abuse for God's sake, for there is not, I am certain of it, a vice more abominable than this in the eyes of the divine Majesty'. Remarkably, his autobiography was finished nine years before his eventual death at the age of 102.

Cornaro's story is both a message of warning, and of hope, to fat men everywhere. It is a perfect illustration of the sinister influence of obesity upon health, in his case leading to joint and stomach disorders, and quite possibly diabetes. Obesity leads to an average nine-year reduction in life expectancy, a fact which did not escape Cornaro, who wrote with regret that:

Friends and associates, men endowed with splendid gifts of intellect and noble qualities of heart ... fall in the prime of life, victims of this dread tyrant; men who were they yet living, would be ornaments to the world, while their friendship and company would add to my enjoyment in the same proportion as I was caused sorrow by their loss.

But his is also a very clear message that obesity need not be a death sentence, and can be managed successfully over a sustained period. Sadly for the literary world, Cornaro's change in lifestyle seemed also to convert him into a crashing bore, as his writings demonstrate. Although we should be grateful to him for enlightening us to the cause of his remarkable longevity, the religious fervour with which he preached is tedious. Nonetheless, we should heed his advice; Luigi Cornaro's life was changed by the decision to take a trip to see his doctor – one act which gives two vital messages which 21st-century man should take to heart. The first message is that obesity, especially abdominal obesity, is a serious chronic medical condition, and the second is that the doctor's surgery is an appropriate port of call.

Understanding the physiology of obesity

Regulation of weight and appetite is very precisely controlled by the body, and obesity is the result of this highly accurate mechanism being catastrophically disrupted (Haslam *et al.*, 2006; Ronti *et al.*, 2006). The science of appetite regulation, especially with regard to obesity, is complicated and far from being comprehensively understood.

The brain has a continuous dialogue with the gut, so that the brain can govern the amount of food eaten, compared to the amount required by the body. The brain receives messages from all five senses via the cerebellum: the sight of a sumptuous feast, the sound of bacon sizzling, the smell of garlic from the kitchen, the feel of food being prepared, and of course the taste of a favourite dish. Just like Pavlov's dogs, which salivated at the sound of the dinner bell, these sensations induce the desire to eat, as the brain sends messages through the autonomic nervous system, telling the stomach to prepare itself.

The gut also has ways of communicating to the brain that it needs food, so it is time to go hunting for some. Messages to and from the gut travel via the autonomic nervous system, which leads to increased activity of the gut muscles, increasing peristalsis, rumbling, and hunger pangs, and by way of hormones released from the gut, such as ghrelin, which stimulate hunger and increase food intake.

In response to all these heightened sensations, we eat. The gut then contacts the brain in different ways; the nerve endings in the stomach wall transmit impulses directly via the vagal nerve to inform it that food has arrived. In addition, with increasing amounts of food entering the bowel, the cells of the gut produce a number of hormones (PYY 3-36, obestatin, cholecystokinin), which are released into the blood stream and circulate around the body. These hormones are monitored by the brain stem, and the hypothalamus, which responds by producing messenger chemicals called neuropeptides (NPY, AgRP), which give us the sensation of being satisfied, and full, so we should stop eating.

The desire to eat and the sensation of hunger, however, are distinct and different phenomena, and it is possible to override the effects of these chemicals, so we can eat when we are not actually hungry because of the external cues which make eating enjoyable. These sensations are governed by chemicals in the brain called neurotransmitters, which control eating behaviour, the most important being serotonin, which is the target for one of the anti-obesity drugs available in the UK. However, a system called the endocannabinoid system has recently been discovered, the partial blockade of which alters eating behaviour, inducing weight loss as well as specific improvements in cholesterol and control of blood sugar.

Once a person has become overweight or obese, the dialogue between the gut and the brain is joined by a third party: fat. Far from being merely an inert mass, adipose tissue is one of the most active glands in the body, but unlike other glands, fatty tissue is highly toxic. It produces chemicals called cytokines, such as tumour necrosis factor-α, and interleukin-6, which cause inflammation, particularly in the lining of the blood vessels, which leads to heart disease, but also in other organs such as the liver. Adipose tissue also secretes a hormone called leptin, whose function is to tell the brain how much energy is stored in the body. Obese people have high levels of leptin, but may be resistant to its action.

Fatty tissue also absorbs, alters and releases sex hormones leading to infertility, prostate and testicular disease, and, in women, polycystic ovaries.

There are three main elements to the way we use up energy: physical activity, thermogenesis (the energy produced by burning off food) and basal metabolic rate. We all know of people who seem to be able to eat what they like without gaining an ounce, while others merely look at food and put on weight, so it seems there must be a genetic element controlling our metabolism. However, it is a myth that overweight people have a slower metabolism. In fact the metabolic rate is higher in obese people, and slows down with weight loss. It is thought that certain foods such as coffee and chilli peppers increase the metabolic rate.

A medical condition responsive to treatment

Many people, doctors and nurses included, view obesity as a social issue, and prefer to de-medicalise the condition. They say that its cause is sedentary behaviour and overeating, modern lifestyle, and the so-called 'toxic' obesogenic environment. They say that until the environment changes, obesity levels will not change, and change in the environment is the government's job. The point, though, is not how the obese condition came about, but what the consequences are; not what leads to obesity, but what obesity leads to. Even the most cynical doctor must recognise that the expanded waistline is a physical sign of serious underlying pathology. Put simply, fat, especially within the abdomen, causes a whole catalogue of diseases, and must therefore be assessed and managed in that context. The cause of obesity certainly needs addressing, and preventative measures put in place, not only by the government, but by food, advertising and retail industries, schools and so on.

The fact of the matter is that if preventative measures were 100% successful with immediate effect, and not one more person became obese, and those already obese individuals did not gain a single extra ounce, we would still witness an epidemic of diabetes within a decade, followed by epidemics of heart disease and early death, as people progressed through the 'latent' phase of the illness towards overt disease (Haslam *et al.*, 2006). Therefore treatment of obesity must be prioritised alongside prevention, otherwise we will condemn an entire 'lost generation'.

The WHO (www.who.int/dietphysicalactivity/publications/facts/obesity/en/) describes obesity as 'one of today's most blatantly visible – yet most neglected – public health problems', which 'threatens to overwhelm both developing and developed countries'. In the UK we currently have an epidemic of obesity, but not the worst one in the world; certain Pacific Islanders and American Indians hold that position. We are not even the worst in Europe, but here in the UK we are climbing the obesity league table faster than anyone. Different sections of the population are not affected in the same way by obesity; the problem is far worse in deprived areas, and much more significant among some ethnic minority populations, e.g. South East Asians, who may succumb to type 2 diabetes at a much lower BMI than their non-Asian counterparts.

Men are especially at risk

The other subsection of the population to have their own unique risks and predisposing factors to obesity-related co-morbidities are men. The risk of carrying excess weight for men is so great that they even have a form of obesity named after them: 'android' obesity. Overweight and obese individuals are known as either 'apples' or 'pears'. Pear-shaped people are generally women, who carry their excess weight around their thighs and buttocks, hence the term 'gynoid' obesity. Apples are usually men, who carry their fat abdominally: android obesity (Vague, 1947).

Unfortunately for men, the android form is the dangerous sort. Abdominal obesity refers not to subcutaneous fat beneath the skin of the abdomen, but to visceral fat, which surrounds the omentum of the bowel. The amount of visceral fat inside the abdomen is directly proportional to the waist circumference, implying that waist circumference is a more accurate measure of the dangers of obesity than BMI, as BMI can be elevated to obese levels in superfit athletes.

Young and middle-aged men are notoriously poor at looking after themselves, and fail to present themselves to the local provider of medical care until it is too late. They do not have occasional pregnancies, and regular pill checks, to have their BMI and blood pressures measured. Affluent men will have private health checks, and can afford to go to the gym if they need to, but the at-risk group will not. In 1811, Thomas Jameson described ages 28 to 58 as the height of male perfection. However, at the height of their perfection men must also pay some thought to staying perfect from age 59 onwards.

Long-term problems in men if obesity is not treated

The problem with the obese abdomen, and expanded waistline, has nothing to do with its cosmetic appearance, but its function. Far from being an inert mass of blubber, used to store excess energy, adipose tissue represents a dangerous metabolically active organ. Most glands in a man's body are beneficial, and produce hormones and other chemicals that are helpful in some way: the thyroid, pancreas and testicles, for instance. Fat – specifically that inside the abdomen, wrapped around our bowels and core blood vessels – acts as a 'bad gland', secreting harmful hormones and chemicals. The bigger it gets, the more damage it does. The fundamental flaw in obese men, which leads to illness, is insulin resistance. When sugar is absorbed from the stomach into the blood stream, insulin is the hormone produced by the islet cells of the pancreas, which enables skeletal muscle to take up sugar to be used as energy. If a man is resistant to insulin, the level of sugar in the blood tends to rise, and the body's initial response is for the pancreas to produce extra insulin to compensate: a condition known as hyperinsulinaemia. Eventually the β-cells of the pancreas fail to maintain insulin production, and impaired glucose control and frank diabetes develop.

Insulin resistance only occurs in muscle, liver and adipose tissue. Other organs of the body have been described as 'innocent bystanders' (www.cacr.ca/news/2000/0009reaven.htm) of the hyperinsulinaemic state, and react in different ways. The liver, for example, develops fatty deposits, leading eventually to fibrosis, cirrhosis, and sometimes even cancer, but the most important casualty of the abnormal metabolism in obese men is the heart and circulation: cardiovascular disease (CVD). The initial damage in CVD is inflammation of the walls of the arteries due to the combination of high insulin and inflammatory toxins produced by fatty tissue. This is aggravated by the cholesterol abnormalities caused by the release of fatty substances by adipose tissue which in turn leads to plaque formation in the arterial wall. The plaques subsequently rupture, causing blood to clot, a thrombus to form, and heart attack or stroke ensues. Even the blood is sticky in obese individuals – hypercoagulability – making thrombosis more likely to occur. Well over a third of all deaths in the UK are caused by cardiovascular disease, 35% in men (British Heart Foundation, 2004), and obesity, along with the abnormal metabolism it causes, is the leading factor, along with smoking.

High cholesterol is almost universal in obese individuals, and the lipid picture is a particularly dangerous one. The protective HDL (high-density lipoprotein) cholesterol is reduced, the dangerous triglycerides are increased, and the 'bad' LDL (low-density lipoprotein) cholesterol is present in small dense particles, conferring higher risk. There is a very close link between obesity, particularly abdominal obesity, and high blood pressure; up to two-thirds of cases of hypertension are linked with obesity (Cassano *et al.*, 1990). Obese people have over five times the risk of developing hypertension, and people who are 20% overweight are eight times more likely to develop it. The finding of high cholesterol levels and hypertension in obese children as young as nine has led to the concept of childhood obesity 'casting a shadow' on future health and increasing morbidity and mortality in adulthood, even if the obesity itself is remedied.

The connection between obesity and type 2 diabetes is so strong that attempting to treat diabetes properly without managing any co-existing obesity is almost futile. The association between the conditions is so close that many experts consider obesity and type 2 diabetes to be different ends of the same spectrum, and that obesity should be treated as a 'pre-diabetes'. The term 'diabesity' is increasingly being used by some experts (Sims *et al.*, 1973). Statistics emphasise the point: 85–90% of diabetics have type 2 diabetes, and approximately 80–85% of type 2 diabetics are obese. A staggering 12% of people with a BMI of over 27 have type 2 diabetes. A waist circumference of over 100 cm in men increases the risk of diabetes 3.5 times (Chan *et al.*, 1994).

On a Monday morning GP surgery, if a patient with a BMI of 35 or more walks through the door they are up to 93 times more likely to develop type 2 diabetes than the lean person next on the list (Colditz *et al.*, 1995). There are estimated to be over one million undiagnosed diabetics in the UK, giving a high probability that any particular obese patient is either one of the missing million, or soon will be, and an absolute certainty that sooner rather than later one of the obese patients on a doctor's books will become diabetic.

The fact that certain illnesses clustered together in the same individual was recognised long before the exact science was discovered, and the clustering of diabetes, blood pressure and high cholesterol was rather melodramatically called 'syndrome X' or the metabolic syndrome. Metabolic syndrome is not something that the average bloke talks about in the pub, which is odd, because at least a quarter of men suffer from the condition, and among the male, pub-going population, the percentage is considerably higher, so it is something they could have in common to discuss. It is actually incredibly easy to attain the qualifications to be diagnosed as having metabolic syndrome: waist 102 cm, blood pressure (BP) 135/85, and slightly raised cholesterol are enough, and if recent criteria by the International Diabetes Federation (www.idf.org/home/index.cfm?node=1429) are adopted, almost 70% of the population will be labelled as having the condition. But its ramifications are staggering. The 15-fold increased risk of type 2 diabetes is well known, as is the quadruple risk of heart disease, and the danger of high blood pressure, high cholesterol and stroke. But less well known is the risk of up to 20 different sorts of cancer, including colon, prostate and testicular; the increased likelihood of arthritis, not just in the weight-bearing joints, but even in the wrists and elbows; the danger of sleep apnoea which leads to daytime somnolence and vastly increased number of fatal RTA (road traffic accidents); and the risk of liver failure; obesity has the same effect on the liver as excess alcohol. And worst of all the premature death. A young obese black male from a deprived inner city area will lose up to 20 years of life because of obesity.

The problem is for men to recognise the problem!

According to Jameson (1811), 'Corpulency steals imperceptibly on most men, between the ages of 30 and 57. In many cases the belly becomes prominent …'. Speaking in the context of the age in which he wrote – when a degree of fat indicated the lack of any serious disease – he continued, 'A moderate degree of obesity is certainly a desirable state of body at all times, as it indicates a healthy condition of the assimilating powers … diminishes the irritability of the system, since fat people are remarked for good humour'.

Many obese men are characterised by good humour, and many have the wrong attitude towards their bellies; they treat them like a constant faithful companion, and, like a dog, give them the occasional pat. Rotund, plethoric men are the very embodiment of conviviality, standing at the bar, holding court to the assembly of drinkers. They joke about their waistline as a sign of affluence – 'It's all paid for' – and to lose it would be nothing less than a bereavement. It is as though their humour and *joie de vivre* are seated in their belly, and to lose it they would be like Samson without his hair. The belly may be equated to a suit of armour, a protection against a hostile environment.

This demeanour seems to be mainly associated with men. Obese women tend to suffer more from depression and mental health problems, and have worse educational, employment, financial and marriage prospects. This concept was nicely explained in *Crow Magazine* (quoted in Gilman, 2004): 'Excess weight is just as damaging to men's health as to women's, but for men to attract women, they don't need to be fit, or healthy, or even have hair. They just need to be men. Rich, successful men choose from the cream of the crop, discarding and replacing, as each mate ages and fattens.' Dr Albert Stunkard (1976), one of the foremost medical authorities on obesity, on the other hand quoted a female patient as feeling like '… a great mass of gray-green amorphous material. Then at times I feel like a sloth. And just now, when I got up on the examining table, I felt like an elephant'.

A major study in 2000 tested the relationship between body weight and depression, suicide ideation and suicide attempts in over 40,000 people, with remarkable results. In women obesity increased the risk of being diagnosed with severe depression by 37%, but in men obesity *decreased* the risk by 37%. A 10-unit increase in body mass index increased the risk of suicide ideation and suicide attempts in women in the past year by 22%, but in men by 26 and 55% respectively (Carpenter *et al.*, 2000). In men, being underweight is associated with higher risk of depression and suicide. Although obese men should count themselves extremely fortunate not to have to suffer similar experiences to the same degree as women, their lack of concern does prevent them from seeking help for their weight. More awareness about their own weight would make a considerable difference to their consultation rates, and allow clinicians to gain access to their target population.

But men could help themselves more

Rather than sit back and let the environment slowly change for the better, as the cycle of government policy invention grinds on, along with the food industry's gradual grudging changes, each man, in order to be successful in his fight against excess weight, must create his own micro-environment. Physical activity has been removed from men's work and leisure lives. We can send an email to the person in the next room, switch the TV on and off by remote. We do not have to get up to answer the phone, we do not even have to push doors, as they open automatically; escalators and elevators take the strain, and there are more cars, TVs and computers per household than ever before.

The current generation of men is the first in history not to experience shortage of food. Since post-war rationing, food has become plentiful, ubiquitous, cheap, available all day and night, unhealthier in quality, and served in ever-bigger portions. Unfortunately the environment has evolved millions of times more rapidly than our metabolisms, and in the 30 years it has taken for the obesity epidemic to take hold, we have not had the chance to evolve to protect ourselves, and have no instinct to avoid food and increase beneficial activity. If we get up in the morning and jump onto the conveyor belt, which is our modern environment, eat what is in front of us, and use technology as it is intended, most of us will become obese, which is why the majority of the men suffer from excess weight.

In order to avoid excessive weight gain, we have to behave un-naturally, by creating a bubble around ourselves, protecting us from the world around us. Natural selection has played a dirty trick on us. Those individuals who had the capacity to lay down excess food as energy stores in fatty tissue were able to cope with times of fast and famine in ages gone by, and therefore had superior genetic predisposition and were programmed to survive. Now, however, it is the identical phenotype which, faced with an abundance of food, and no innate ability to modify intake, is being selected to die prematurely. As it will take at least a generation for policymakers and industry to induce a significant environmental shift, it falls to the individual to sculpt his own personal protective environmental bubble around himself. He should create his own rules and regulations, and be aware that whenever food is presented, or technology raises its ugly head, that he himself is the only person who cares about his health, fitness, or longevity, so it is up to him to control intake and output. Presented with a bag of crisps or an apple, his radar should identify the fruit. Presented with a lift, or staircase, the steps provide an ideal opportunity to increase the activity in the daily routine. Shoe-horning physical activity into the day-to-day schedule need not be time-consuming; it is quicker to walk up an escalator than to ride; time on the mobile phone is wasted without getting up and walking while the conversation continues.

Micro-activity is defined as the small individual movements which make up an action. The journey from home to work is made up of a series of steps, turns of the steering wheel, etc. Micro-activity is vital activity. Some studies have shown that even fidgeting of the arms and legs is protective against weight gain. So park the car as far from the platform as possible; walk to the far end of every tube station platform while the train comes. Eating a meal at a table burns up more energy than eating in front of the TV because of gestures and gesticulations. Every little bit counts.

Weird and wonderful or the sensible middle ground?

To keep a balanced view on life it is essential to keep an eye out for the unbalanced minority view, whether in politics, religion or any other of life's sidewaters. In other words, beware of the weirdo with bizarre yet compelling opinions. Health-promoting lifestyle is no different to politics or religion; there is a sensible, middle path we can take, which may well prove to be beneficial in the long term, or a weird and wonderful digression which will end up doing more harm than good.

A balanced diet, combined with a sensible physical activity regime, is the gold standard. However, these rules are frequently flaunted for a quick buck by the inventor of a new, supposedly better regimen. Each new diet launched is based upon a new selling point or idiosyncrasy, which is the exact reason why we should treat the new concept with profound cynicism. For example, in the 16th century, the physician

Cardan (Dick Humelbergius Secundus, 1829) absolutely condemned physical activity as prejudicial to health. His proof was that, by comparing the longevity of trees to the ordinary duration of animal life, he attributed the longevity of the former to their immobility. Esop invented a specialist diet for himself, eating only birds' tongues, and limiting intake further by avoiding birds that couldn't speak. Compared to the Esop, diets such as Atkins and the Last Chance Diet seem reasonable, but still contain unacceptable elements. Low carbohydrate diets, and low glycaemic load diets, are perfectly acceptable in the appropriate circumstances. William Banting, the coffin-maker to the royal family in the mid-19th century, is credited with first publicising low-carb (Banting, 1864), or in his case reduced intake of 'farinaceous food'. He was cured of deafness by weight loss, which had been caused by pressure of fat around his neck and face on his airways. Reduction in refined carbohydrate makes perfect sense in individuals with insulin resistance, but it is senseless to allow the introduction of increased saturated fat, as some low-carb diets do. Meal replacements and low, and very-low, calorie diets are excellent in their place, but the Last Chance Diet went a step too far; the total lack of nutritional intake, apart from a protein supplement, led to a dramatic fatality count.

Men and obesity: a new model of care

Weight problems and obesity can be treated. It is not always easy and not always successful, but a combination of nutrition and lifestyle advice, with today's excellent anti-obesity pharmacotherapy, and in extreme cases surgery, can very often produce a successful outcome and prevent co-morbidity and early death. But thereby hangs the other massive problem that men must overcome. The standard medical model for provision of medical care, in particular relating to obesity and its co-morbidities, simply does not work for this high-risk group. The answer therefore is to look outside the standard medical model, and let the mountain come to Mohammed. If blokes won't come to see their doctor, then occupational health must provide superior levels of medical care within the workplace to select and treat those at highest risk. Companies themselves must take responsibility for providing the chance for employees to become fitter: healthy canteen food options, stairs that are not hidden behind the lifts, cycle parks and showers, tax redemption schemes for gym members.

These may seem outlandish, but such models can be successful. Men and weight have a peculiar and dangerous relationship. 'Fat as a feminist issue' (Orbach, 1986) has set men's health back three decades, but men must, at last, assume control of their apple-shaped bodies to avoid the effects of obesity and the otherwise inevitable consequences.

The news is not all bad. Weight loss of 10% of total body weight equates to a loss of 30% of the dangerous visceral fat within the abdomen, and therefore a vast improvement in risk. If a person has an increased waist circumference, borderline blood pressure, borderline cholesterol, and borderline blood sugar, their traditional treatment would have been monitoring over the course of several years, until one of these factors became frankly abnormal and needed treating. Nowadays it is being increasingly recognised that a series of borderline risk factors adds up and accumulates to equate to a high actual risk, requiring treatment, ideally of the underlying obesity. A trip to the GP is changing from a simple prescription for a complaint to a consultation to have one's risk managed. This concept will take some getting used to by doctors and patients alike.

Luigi Cornaro managed it, and so have countless others in the intervening centuries, but we now have a far more sinister obesity problem, which needs urgent action by healthcare professionals, government, schools and industry. While they get their collective acts together, however, it is every man for himself.

References

Banting W. *Letter on Corpulence Addressed to the Public.* 1864. New York: Cosimo; 2005.

Bray GA and Claude Bouchard. *Handbook of Obesity: etiology and pathophysiology* (2e). New York: Marcel Dekker Inc.; 1997.

British Heart Foundation. *Coronary Heart Disease Statistics, 2004 Edition.* British Heart Foundation Statistics Database; 2004. www.heartstats.org (accessed 7 March 2007).

Carpenter KM, Hasin DS, Allison DB, Faith MS. Relationships between obesity and DSM-IV major depressive disorder, suicide ideation and suicide attempts. *Am J Pub Health.* 2000; **90**: 251–7.

Cassano PA, Segal MR, Vokonas PS *et al.* Body fat distribution, blood pressure and hypertension. *Annals of Epidemiology.* 1990; **1**: 33–48.

Chan JM, Rimm EB, Colditz GA *et al.* Obesity, fat distribution and weight gain as risk factors for clinical diabetes in man. *Diabetes Care.* 1994; **17**: 961–9.

Colditz GA, Willett WC, Rotnitzkya A, Manson JE. Weight gain as a risk factor for clinical diabetes. *Annals of Internal Medicine.* 1995; **122**(7): 481–6.

Cornaro L. *The Art of Living Long.* Padua, Italy. 1558.

Dick Humelbergius Secundus. *Apician Morsels: Tales of the table, kitchen and larder.* London: Whittaker, Treacher & Co.; 1829.

Gilman S. *Fat Boys.* Lincoln NE: University of Nebraska Press; 2004. p. 6.

Haslam D, Sattar N, Lean M. Obesity – time to wake up. *BMJ.* 2006; **333**, 23 September: 640–2.

Jameson T. *Essays on the Changes of the Human Body at its Different Ages.* London: Longman; 1811.

Orbach S. *Fat is a Feminist Issue.* New York: Berkley Publishing Group; 1986.

Ronti T, Lupattelli G and Mannarion E. The endocrine function of adipose tissue: an update. *Clin Endocrinol.* 2006; **644**: 355–65.

Sims EAH, Danforth E, Horton ES *et al.* Endocrine and metabolic effects of experimental obesity in man. *Recent Prog Hormone Res.* 1973; **29**: 457–96.

Stunkard AJ. *The Pain of Obesity.* Boulder, CO: Bull Publishing Company; 1976.

Vague J. Sexual differentiation, a factor affecting the forms of obesity. *Presse Méd.* 1947; **30**: 339–40.

CHAPTER 3

Male obesity: policy and context

Alan White

> *It is now accepted that obesity is caused by a combination of gluttony (driven by cheap, palatable, heavily promoted energy-dense foods) and sloth (driven by energy-saving devices, motorised transport, sedentary work, TV viewing and computing). These provide us with plenty of targets for action.*
> (PRENTICE, 2004)

When a health issue emerges that can be seen to have widespread and significant impact on the public's health, then policy, backed up with legislation, quickly follows. This has been seen with the recent threat of bird flu, but perhaps has been most visible in relation to diseases such as smallpox, malaria, HIV/AIDS (human immunodeficiency virus/acquired immune deficiency syndrome) and the problems of smoking, alcohol, drugs, etc. The problem of being overweight and obese, however, is more complex and is creating more of a challenge.

There is a need to recognise the dilemmas in addressing what has been identified as a 'global epidemic' by the World Health Organization (WHO) and of such significance that it is now seen as a greater threat to health than that posed by smoking. This chapter will explore the role of policy in directing health strategy and, through an analysis of activity within the WHO, the European Commission and our own government, provide the context for the activity which is now being seen at a local level. This analysis will incorporate a broader discussion on how gender is (or, in many cases, is not) incorporated into policy.

What the chapter will argue is that there is a high level of awareness and concern about the problems of being overweight and obese, but there is not a clear way forward on how to tackle what was previously seen as an issue of individual choice within a rapidly changing society. The chapter will highlight a tension between the recognition that men have a specific problem with being overweight and obese – and hence the need for gender-sensitive policy – and the traditional population-based approach. The lack of appreciation of men's relationships between diet, nutrition and body image, as a result of the male socialisation process, by those engaged in policy creation will also be considered.

Gender mainstreaming

The Beijing 'Platform for Action' at the 1995 United Nations (UN) International Conference for Women saw the first global commitment to recognising the importance of gender within the framing of policy. This event was followed by a series of meetings that saw the idea of 'gender mainstreaming' develop beyond ensuring that women's concerns and experiences became incorporated into all aspects of an organisation – from employment issues, through to organisational governance, delivery and outcomes (Derbyshire, 2002) into the broader health arena.

During these early days certain key concepts emerged that have helped guide thinking about the importance of gender within policy development.

> *Mainstreaming gender:*
> *'Integration of gender concerns into the analyses, formulation and monitoring of policies, programmes and projects, with the objective of ensuring that these reduce inequalities between women and men.'*
>
> *Gender equality:*
> *'Absence of discrimination on the basis of a person's sex in opportunities and the allocation of resources or benefits or in access to services.'*
>
> *Gender equity:*
> *'Fairness and justice in the distribution of benefits and responsibilities between women and men. The concept recognises that women and men have different needs and power and that these differences should be identified and addressed in a manner that rectifies the imbalance between the sexes.'*
> (WHO, 1998)

In reality the debate was focused mainly on the discrimination that women experienced and was not seen as being directed towards men's issues. In more recent times it has been recognised that this drive for equality must incorporate the health concerns that seem to have a more detrimental effect on men, such that all health policy should really be viewed through a lens that recognises both men and women (O'Brien and White, 2003). But what will become apparent as the discussion develops below is that there is still a tendency to create population-based policy with little regard for the differences between men and women (White and Lockyer, 2001), and this includes policy on weight problems and obesity.

This is a particular problem in the UK as this lack of strategic guidance causes significant problems at the practice level with the passing of the Equality Act in 2006, which came into force in April 2007. This Act creates a Gender Duty that applies to all public and private bodies providing a public service and '... require[s] public authorities – as employers or service providers – to actively consider whether they are treating women and men fairly and meeting their different needs' (DTI 2006, p.14). The Equal Opportunities Commission (www.eoc.org.uk) has developed a Statutory Code of Practice to accompany the Act, which includes the requirement for all authorities affected by the Act to conduct and publish a Gender Impact Assessment of each 'major' development in policy and services.

This new Act is in response to the frustration many found with the Sex Discrimination Act 1975. Although individuals could bring action, these did not resolve the problems of discrimination and gendered inequalities that existed as a result of poor policies and practices. The new Act is also admissible in evidence in any legal action under the Sex Discrimination Act 1975, or Equality Act 2006 in criminal or civil proceedings before any court or tribunal.

The position of obesity as a topic for policy

Governments have always been interested in the nation's diet, with the supply of good quality food being an absolute necessity (European Commission, 2002) to avoid malnutrition (though it is possible to argue that the current weight problems of many are also a result of 'malnutrition') and ensure that the masses were supplied with sufficient food through a safe supply chain.

In the past, health challenges caused by poor nutrition led to policies to ensure that individuals had a sufficiently balanced diet to prevent the occurrence of diseases such as scurvy and rickets, for instance by ensuring calcium levels for children were appropriate through the provision of school milk. These, however, were problems of deficiency and not excess.

The problems of excessive food intake, inactivity and weight problems were those of the wealthy, and indeed were signs of prosperity and affluence, and to a large extent, even if health problems were identified, they were not seen as being within the domain of health policy.

The corpulent individual was known to have joint and muscle difficulties and other health problems, such as gout and poor fitness, but as their condition was seen as a consequence of personal lifestyle choice it was not seen as a political concern. Indeed many of the policymakers over the centuries were themselves male and overweight and it could be argued that they would be unlikely to impose health policy against their own way of life.

Over the last 10 years there has been an awakening of concern relating to the problem of being overweight and obese such that it has now captured the attention of politicians. Action should ensue (Reeves, 2003), but this is not as straightforward as it may seem.

The causes of the problem

Current government drivers for health policy are focused on personal choice, with a reluctance to be seen to be directing how individuals live their lives. This approach supports the notion that obesity and being overweight is a matter of individual free will and not a subject for state intervention, i.e. each individual putting on weight has made a personal decision to eat those foods or to adopt a sedentary lifestyle. Thus it should be sufficient to offer healthcare based on that individual seeking appropriate support. The American 'fat lobby' would go further and say that they are defending their right to be fat.

The food manufacturers put pressure on governments to prevent state intervention on the basis of loss of revenue, while at the same time exerting their own influence on eating patterns. For every £1 the now-replaced Health Education Authority spent on trying to promote healthy diets, the food industry spent £800 encouraging us to eat their products (Reeves, 2003). Furthermore, much of the energy-dense food on the market is quicker to prepare and more tasty to eat than much of what would be classed as 'healthy food' to the untrained palate.

The counter-argument is that the significant changes in weight in the last decade indicate a structural rather than individual problem. The Obesity in Europe report from the International Obesity Task Force (IOTF, 2002) states very clearly that the problem of weight problems and obesity is a societal one and not the fault of the individual, listing the principal causes as:

> 1 *An increased abundance of 'energy dense' foods and drinks which promote excessive 'calorie' consumption and support a ubiquitous 'snacking' culture. New evidence highlights the ready evasion of appetite control by these foods, drinks and their frequency of consumption. This leads to a pervasive 'passive over-consumption' of energy.*
> 2 *The systematic public and commercial developments which restrict opportunities for physical activities – leading to an almost sedentary life-style.* (IOTF, 2002, p. 9)

It is ironic that the need to protect the food chain and individual nations' food production capacity in part has added to this problem. The creation of the Common Agricultural Policy (CAP) – with the original objectives of ensuring food security – had as a central goal a public health agenda, but the massive subsidies aimed at helping maintain the food chain and the living standards of the farming community actually prevented the public health agenda from coming to the fore.

Examples include the subsidies aimed at maintaining prices by the withdrawal and destruction of good quality fruit and vegetables (€117 million per year), consumption aid for butter (€460 million per year), consumption aid for high-fat milk products in schools (about €50 million per year), subsidies for distillation of surplus wine (€650 million per year), and subsidies to promote sales of high-fat milk products and wine (€10 million every two years).

Changes in CAP that could promote public health include a phasing out of subsidies which currently support consumption of high-fat dairy products, focusing support to schools on low-fat content milk products (a switch from high- to low-fat milk in schools would reduce fat consumption by 1.5 kg per child per year), introducing similar school support for fruit and vegetable consumption, and redistributing agricultural support in favour of fruit and vegetables (WHO, 2003, p. 11).

This is compounded by the fact that in many countries energy-dense foods – oils, margarine and sugars – are very cheap per calorie as opposed to fresh fruits and vegetables, which can increase the food budget by 5,000% per calorie (Ulrich, 2005). Changes in work patterns are also resulting in more reliance on calorie-dense convenient foods (Ulrich, 2005).

We have seen a reduction in physical education in schools, in part through a change in the national curriculum, but also through the selling off of school and other municipal playing fields. There has been an increase in cash-strapped schools accepting contracts from vending machine companies. There are radical changes in the way children get to school with a marked decrease in the numbers walking. Children are losing their traditional after-school activities in favour of sedentary pastimes, such as watching the television and playing computer games, with boys spending substantially more money (ONS, 2002) and time on both.

There are additional factors, such as the legislation to stop smoking. This is leading to an increase in obesity as one craving replaces another. Indeed, we are now seeing the emergence of new conditions as a result of changes in society, including the Binge Eating Disorder (BED).

Can policy impact on an individual's lifestyle?

There is a problem in adopting current government thinking on managing weight loss through promoting personal choice. The public have been inured by the media that there are simple solutions to reducing excess weight (Cottam, 2004), involving either weight-reducing medicines or surgery to circumvent the more stringent public health action that is needed. The IOTF (2002), noting this trend, has warned that health ministers have not been nurturing the public, the media or indeed the political sector to gain backing for the type of change that is needed.

The notion of relying on an individual choosing a healthier lifestyle has also been criticised by the UK Public Health Association (UKPHA): 'There should be a recognition that choice is a spurious, and largely irrelevant, concept in public health and that health education will make a negligible, and possibly harmful, difference to health status and inequalities' (UKPHA, 2005). They go on to argue, 'Public health is principally about organising society for the good of the population's health; at this level of concern, it is no more a matter of individual choice than the weather'. Though this brings complaints of a 'nanny state', there are a number of successful examples where a reluctant public has accepted change, for instance the introduction of seat-belt legislation, the compulsory wearing of crash helmets on motorbikes, and the move to ban smoking in public places.

Cottam (2005, p. 1594) argues that it is the responsibility of the government to move to 'protect us from that version of us prayed on by the worst excesses of the market' and that this needs to be tackled at a policy, public health level rather than relying on persuading individuals to change.

The rising awareness of policymakers to the issues of weight problems and obesity

The implications of weight problems and obesity to the health of a large proportion of the world population have only recently become apparent to policymakers. The changes that have occurred within the last decade have come as a shock to many and the rising tide of concern can be mapped in the key policy documents of the last 10 years. This next section will map these changes at the level of the WHO, the European Commission, our own government and at the local level of politics and health strategy development. What will become apparent through this analysis is the absence of gender as an issue.

World Health Organization (WHO)

The joint WHO–UNICEF (UN Children's Fund) conference in 1978 led to the Alma Alta Declaration for 'Health for all the people of the world by the year 2000'. This gave the steer that to tackle the world's major health problems there was a need to adopt public health measures aimed at programmatic areas rather than diseases, to encourage community and self-reliance and participation, to have an emphasis on prevention, and to have a multisectoral approach. The WHO has continued this approach by bringing to the attention of the world key health issues and through mainly consensus measures has driven national policies on most of the major health challenges.

The problem of being overweight and obese has now been recognised by the WHO as a 'global epidemic' (i.e. more than 15% of the population affected) for, with 115 million people now identified as overweight or obese, the numbers are rising faster than those of the 170 million under-nourished (WHO, 2003).

> *At the other end of the malnutrition scale, obesity is one of today's most blatantly visible – yet most neglected – public health problems. Paradoxically coexisting with undernutrition, an escalating global epidemic of weight problems and obesity ('globesity') is taking over many parts of the world. If immediate action is not taken, millions will suffer from an array of serious health disorders.* (WHO, 2003)

The problems are now being seen increasingly in developing as well as developed countries with this New World Syndrome (WHO, 2000), following the increased tendency to urbanisation, reduction in manual labour and the move to more westernised diets creating the ideal conditions for a sedentary and overweight population.

Over the last six years there have been three key publications from the WHO on this issue. In 2000 *Obesity: Preventing and Managing the Global Epidemic* (WHO, 2000) gave a comprehensive overview of the causes and implications of the problem. The WHO 2002 Annual Report (WHO, 2002), which focused on risk and risky lifestyles, gave a clear steer to the problems of how modern-day society was becoming increasingly problematic in relation to the world's health. The 2004 *Global Strategy on Diet, Physical Activity and Health* (WHO, 2004) has become the definitive document guiding nations on their own domestic policy. If the WHO had highlighted the differential impact of weight problems and obesity on men then their policy steer might have seen more gender-appropriate services developed in the nation states. However, in their defence much of the guidance is directed at more structural problems as outlined below.

The main recommendations from these reports are that the WHO member states, UN agencies, civil society and the private sector should address the role of non-communicable disease prevention in health services, food and agriculture policies, fiscal policies, surveillance systems, regulatory policies, consumer education and communication including marketing, health claims and nutrition labelling, and school policies as they affect food and physical activity choices. The recommendations also suggest limiting the intake of sugars, fats and salt in foods, and increasing the consumption of fruits, vegetables, legumes, whole grains and nuts.

A downside to the policy, apart from the absence of gender as an issue, is that though this strategy constitutes a significant pressure on the nation states and all 'stakeholders' to adopt their recommendations and gives the 'green light' to take co-ordinated action (WHO, 2004), the WHO has not issued it as a convention and therefore there is no compulsion to act. By not making the member states accountable the WHO has lost a significant opportunity to force change through.

This is noticeable by the majority of the major food producers apparently ignoring the advice, with only 10 of the companies examined in a study on the effect of this global strategy having made any reduction in the salt content of their products, only five reducing sugar content, and only four reducing their fat content (Lang *et al.*, 2006). Those few countries that have adopted fiscal policies on this issue have seen marked improvements in their countries' health, with the North Karelia project in Finland being a prime example of what can be achieved where annual coronary heart disease mortality fell by 73% over 25 years through community-based activity encouraging a healthier diet (WHO, 2003, p. 8).

The European Commission (EC)

The European Commission is similarly blind to the issue of gender within its policy initiatives, but it is well aware of the implications to the population:

> *Obesity results in higher risk factors for diabetes, cardiovascular disease, hypertension and some types of cancer: this leads to the Member States bearing heavy economic, public and social costs. The distribution of healthy diets and the education of the consumer to choose an appropriate diet and increase physical activity remain a challenge requiring Community action.*
> (EUROPEAN COMMISSION, 2002, p. 8)

Within the European Commission there has been a lot of activity in developing policy on the issues of weight problems and obesity (European Commission, 2000, 2002, 2005). The European Commission issued a Green Paper in 2005 on *Promoting Healthy Diets and Physical Activity: a European dimension for the prevention of overweight, obesity and chronic diseases*. This document will pave the way for a much more interventionist approach to tackling what it acknowledges to be the leading cause of avoidable illness and premature death.

The European Commission is mandated to protect human health and with that authority will be able to set in place instruments to direct member states to act on the problem of being overweight and inactive. The line these mandates may take will be determined by the responses to the consultation process and hopefully give further support to public health measures.

The European Platform for Action on Diet, Physical Activity and Health was created in 2005 through the International Obesity Task Force with the intention of producing a non-legislative action plan to secure binding and verifiable commitments aimed at halting and reversing current trends in being overweight and obese within the member states.

Action by the British government

The 1991 *Health of the Nation* White Paper had as one of its main objectives the goal of having fewer than 7% of the adult population obese (DoH, 1991, p. 39). However, it was soon realised that this target would not be met with the 1996 National Audit Office (NAO, 1996) appraisal of progress on the Health of the Nation targets showing that the trend was increasing rather than decreasing. With Labour coming to power in 1997, their White Paper, *Our Healthier Nation* (DoH, 1998) gave an opportunity to tackle this growing problem, but it was not highlighted as being a specific concern, with only a passing mention made of the importance of diet. This was the same year that Dr Susan Jebb, head of obesity research at the Medical Research Council's Dunn Clinical Nutrition Centre, was reporting that 'Obesity is the greatest public health problem in the UK today and the rate of increase in the prevalence among all age groups is alarming'. With about 15% of men and 16% of women classified as obese, the cost to the NHS of treating the health-related problems was in excess of £1 million a week (BBC, 1998).

In 1999 Tessa Jowell, the then Public Health Minister, set in motion a 'wide ranging plan of action' (DoH, 1999), which included:

- Healthy Schools Programme
- Safe and Sound Challenge – to increase activity levels in children
- healthy living centres to be established
- exercise on prescription
- increased information for the public, so they can make 'informed choices'.

The National Audit Office report (2001) brought home the message that these approaches were not working as they recognised the more deep-seated structural changes in society, which they saw as:

- changes in eating patterns
- increasingly sedentary lifestyle
- decline in manual labour
- reduction in walking
- reduced opportunity for exercise
- alcohol consumption
- long working hours.

The Chief Medical Officer in his Annual Report of 2002 (DoH, 2002) certainly recognised the problem we were facing:

> *The growth of weight problems and obesity in the population of our country – particularly amongst children – is a major concern. It is a health time bomb with the potential to explode over the next three decades into thousands of extra cases of heart disease, certain cancers, arthritis, diabetes and many other problems. Unless this time bomb is defused the consequences for the population's health, the costs to the NHS and losses to the economy will be disastrous.* (DoH, 2002, p. 44)

The *Choosing Health* White Paper (DoH, 2004a) demonstrated this shift in awareness with two of the over-arching principles of the policy being 'Reducing obesity and improving diet and nutrition' and 'Increasing exercise'. 'Sensible drinking' was another principle in the White Paper and is closely related to the problems of an overweight population. But the focus was on getting the individual to change their behaviour rather than on tackling the deeper causes. Where more direct action could have been contemplated, for instance with the Food and Drink Federation setting out a manifesto to reduce salt, sugar and fat in food, this was left as voluntary.

The White Paper did recognise that direct intervention was needed with regard to the health of children and the plans to ban food advertising to schools. It pushed further the 'Healthy Schools' campaign with its emphasis on adequate diet, the importance of sports fields, playgrounds and increased activity, and tackling the problem of vending machines and 'tuck shops' in schools.

The 2005 *Choosing a Better Diet* report (DoH, 2005), which sets out the best practice guidance, was based on the consultation exercise following the publication of the 2004 *Choosing Health? Choosing a better diet* report (DoH, 2004b). This guidance did call for action on the banning of broadcasting to the young, but again fell short of committing to nutrient standards, unlike Scotland, which has instigated a £63.5 million programme (Anderson, 2005).

As a consequence of the increasing interest, the UK government has set up four cross-government Public Sector Agreements (PSAs) in relation to obesity and childhood obesity (*see* Table 3.1). These are being used to create Local Delivery Plans that will monitor progress against the obesity target.

As part of the first target the Department of Health instigated a National Childhood Obesity Database, which reported on its first year findings in December 2006. Though there were flaws in the data, with improvements planned for the coming year in the way the data is collected, there were still worrying findings, with 12.3% of girls and 13.4% of boys in Reception Year found to be overweight, and 9.2% of boys and 10.7% of girls in the same year group obese. In Year 6, 13.8% of boys and girls were overweight, and 15.4% of girls and 18.9% of boys were obese (Crowther *et al.*, 2006).

Other activity in the fight against obesity includes that of the new Food Commission (www.foodcom.org.uk), an independent organisation that has tasked itself with monitoring and challenging both government and food manufacturers over the state of the nation's diet and nutritional status. The Food Standards Agency (www.food.gov.uk) is an independent government department established in 2000 with the responsibility for ensuring food safety and healthy diets. However, when the strategic plan for 2005–10 is explored, it has retained the notion that adopting a healthy diet is a matter for personal choice:

■ to continue to reduce food-borne illness
■ to reduce further the risks to consumers from chemical contamination including radiological contamination of food
■ to make it easier for all consumers to choose a healthy diet, and thereby improve quality of life by reducing diet-related disease
■ to enable consumers to make informed choices.

This, as has already been stated, is problematic as it puts the overall responsibility

TABLE 3.1 The four Public Sector Agreements on obesity and childhood obesity.

PSA	Responsibility
Halt the year-on-year rise in obesity among children under 11 by 2010 (from the 2002–4 baseline) in the context of a broader strategy to tackle obesity in the population as a whole.	Department of Health Department for Education and Skills Department for Culture, Media and Sport
By 2008, increase the take-up of cultural and sporting opportunities by adults and young people aged 16 and above from priority groups by: • increasing the number who participate in active sports at least 12 times a year, by 3% • increasing the number who engage in at least 30 minutes of moderate intensity level sport at least three times a week, by 3%.	Department for Culture, Media and Sport
Further enhance access to culture and sport for children and give them the opportunity to develop their talents to the full and enjoy the full benefits of participation by: • enhancing the take-up of sporting opportunities by 5 to 16 year olds by increasing the percentage of school-children who spend a minimum of two hours each week on high-quality PE and school sport within and beyond the curriculum, from 25% in 2002 to 75% by 2006 and 85% by 2008 in England, and at least 75% in each School Sport Partnership, by 2008.	Department for Education and Skills Department for Culture, Media and Sport
Ensure people have decent places to live by improving the quality and sustainability of local environments and neighbourhoods, reviving brown-field land, and improving the quality of housing: • leading the delivery of cleaner, safer and greener public spaces and improvement of the quality of the built environment in deprived areas and across the country with measurable improvement by 2008.	Office of the Deputy Prime Minister

of being overweight back onto the individual, rather than acknowledging the broader societal pressures that need tackling.

The new National Institute for Health and Clinical Excellence Guidelines on Obesity (NICE, 2006) have been long awaited, as there has been a need for a national strategy setting the agenda for managing the problem. It is welcome to see that they have made both clinical and public health recommendations recognising the broad base of action that is required. Nevertheless they have failed to recognise the gendered nature of being overweight and they still seem to be focused onto localised action and promoting individual choice rather than tackling the broader structural issues that are causing the crisis in the first place.

The individual practitioner and the problems of obesity

It is interesting to dwell on the impact of all this policy on the individual practitioner's management of the overweight and obese patient. There is evidence from around the country of innovative and very effective work with men who have a weight problem. The question is how much of this work has been driven by personal interest and how much has been a strategic, and therefore centrally funded, initiative.

Though there are the Public Sector Agreements, up to the launch of the NICE guidelines there has been little compulsion for the healthcare practitioner to act on obesity. The General Medical Services (GMS) Contract that governs the workload of doctors, along with the Quality and Outcomes Framework (QOF) guidelines, when they were first introduced in 2005, did not really give sufficient importance to an individual's weight, with obesity not seen as a clinical domain in its own right and the measurement of weight only important for those with diabetes (NOF, 2005). This has now changed and work in the field of obesity can achieve eight points, but this is limited to the setting up of an 'obesity register'. Though this is a very useful move as it is needed to support the formulation of public health policy, it primarily involves the recording of the BMI and waist circumference of at-risk patients and is not directed towards setting up specific weight management strategies.

This is despite the Royal College of Physicians (RCP), Royal College of Paediatrics and Child Health, and Faculty of Public Health Working Party on Obesity's (2004) own report on obesity, *Storing Up Problems: the medical case for a slimmer nation*, calling for national action. Interestingly, again, this report does not mention treatment options or therapeutic services for the obese as there appears to be a fear that this should not be seen as a problem that can be cured by the GP who would be 'swamped' by having to manage all those with difficulties (Prentice, 2004). Indeed, in Suffolk there has been a decision to stop joint replacement surgery on obese patients, and a survey has found that 40% of doctors felt rationing was appropriate for obese patients (*The Lancet*, 2006).

There is, however, another aspect to this debate and that is the ability of practitioners to recognise the health of men as problematic, not just from the biological perspective, but also in relation to their health beliefs and behaviour. Until the curriculum of health professionals includes the serious examination of gender as a key variable in the health of the population then practitioners cannot be expected to understand why care may need to be framed in a different way for men.

Conclusion

It appears that there is a major challenge in tackling weight problems and obesity in men as currently there are two principal problems that affect the way that policy is being formulated.

The first is that there is still a strong lobby that argues that weight gain is an issue of individual choice and that attention should be focused on changing individuals' dietary and exercise habits. This chapter has argued that the difficulties we are now seeing with regard to men and their weight are as much a consequence of massive social change and as such cannot be seen as an individual's sole responsibility. For three-quarters of men to be at risk of being overweight by 2010 cannot be because three-quarters of men have become feckless with regard to their diet and activity levels. Structural change in society has created the environment that has led to such high levels of being overweight and obese and therefore policies addressing these changes are needed.

The second is that though it was hoped that gender mainstreaming would start to permeate down from the WHO and the EC into its own policy formation and that of the member states, it is noticeable in its absence through all the obesity documents.

Though reports have identified that the problem of obesity is an issue for men, for instance a distinction being drawn between the problem of 'android obesity' and the 'less problematic gynoid fat distribution' (WHO, 2000, p. 6) and the recognition that men have on average twice the amount of abdominal fat that is generally found in pre-menopausal women, the WHO Global Strategy limits its recognition of gender to noting it as a factor to be taken into consideration.

The disappointment with the new NICE guidelines on obesity (2006) is that they show a similar lack of awareness of men being at specific risk of the effects of being overweight and obese. Or that men's problems go beyond the biological to recognise the very different relationship men have to diet, nutrition and weight than that of women.

As such, current national and international policy gives no steer to health professionals to develop gendered approaches to tackling the problem. For it must be remembered that just as the current policy will fail to address men's needs it also has missed the opportunity to address women's specific issues with regard to their weight. In light of the requirements of the Equality Act this has to be seen as a great loss.

The way forward

The Vienna Declaration on Men's Health (EMHF, 2005) provides an important statement on the need for men and their health to be taken seriously within policy decision making at all levels, with its call for EU, national governments, providers of health services and other relevant bodies to:

■ recognise men's health as a distinct and important issue
■ develop a better understanding of men's attitudes to health
■ invest in 'male-sensitive' approaches to providing healthcare
■ initiate work on health for boys and young men in school and community settings
■ develop co-ordinated health and social policies that promote men's health.

The Men's Health Forum in 2005 (MHF, 2005) gave a significant steer on how policy relating to men and their weight should be developed, offering five points of action that are needed to see change occur.

1   Politicians, policymakers, practitioners, the media and the public need to recognise that weight is a male issue too.
2   It is important to understand male attitudes and behaviour in relation to weight and weight loss.

3   There must be investment in new 'male-sensitive' approaches, particularly in primary care and health promotion.
4   It is essential to develop work on weight issues with boys in pre-school, schools and community settings.
5   Ultimately, a wide-ranging national strategy on weight problems and obesity must be developed.

Adopting this framework would be a useful first step in addressing the cost, both personal and economic, of an ailing male population, for unless we start to address men's plight with regard to their weight the consequences are unimaginable.

References

Anderson AS. Obesity prevention and management – evidence and policy. *Journal of Human Nutrition and Dietetics*. 2005; **18**: 1–2.

BBC. *The Health of the Nation*. 1998. http://news.bbc.co.uk/1/hi/events/nhs_at_50/special_report/123233.stm (accessed 8 March 2007).

Cottam R. Obesity and culture. *The Lancet*. 2004; **364**: 1202–3.

Cottam R. Is public health coercive health? *The Lancet*. 2005; **366**: 1592–4.

Crowther R, Dinsdale H, Rutter H, Kyffin R. *Analysis of the National Childhood Obesity Database 2005–06. A report for the Department of Health by the South East Public Health Observatory on behalf of the Association of Public Health Observatories*. London: Department of Health; 2006.

Derbyshire H. *Gender Manual: A practical guide for development policy makers and practitioners*. London: DFID; 2002.

Department of Health. *The Health of the Nation*. White Paper. London: HMSO; 1991.

Department of Health. *Our Healthier Nation*. White Paper. London: HMSO; 1998.

Department of Health. *Government Action to Tackle Rising Levels of Obesity*. Press release. 1999. www.dh.gov.uk/PublicationsAndStatistics/PressReleases/PressReleasesNotices/fs/en?CONTENT_ID=4025462&chk=Kg8zDs (accessed 8 March 2007).

Department of Health. *Chief Medical Officer Annual Report*. London: Department of Health; 2002.

Department of Health. *Choosing Health: making healthy choices easier*. White Paper. London: HMSO; 2004a.

Department of Health. *Choosing Health? Choosing a better diet*. London: Department of Health; 2004b.

Department of Health. *Choosing a Better Diet: a food and health action plan*. London: Department of Health; 2005.

Department of Trade and Industry (DTI). *Advancing Equality for Men and Women: government proposals to introduce a public sector duty to promote gender equality*. London: Women & Equality Unit, Department of Trade and Industry; 2006.

European Commission. *EURODIET Nutrition & Diet for Healthy Lifestyles in Europe Science & Policy Implications*. 2000. http://ec.europa.eu/comm/health/ph_determinants/life_style/nutrition/report01_en.pdf (accessed 8 March 2007).

European Commission. *Status Report on the European Commission's Work in the Field of Nutrition in Europe October 2002*. Luxembourg: European Commission; 2002.

European Commission. *Promoting Healthy Diets and Physical Activity: a European dimension for the prevention of overweight, obesity and chronic diseases*. Green Paper. 2005. http://europa.eu.int/comm/health/ph_determinants/life_style/nutrition/documents/nutrition_gp_en.pdf (accessed 8 March 2007).

European Men's Health Forum (EMHF). *The Vienna Declaration on the Health of Men and Boys in Europe*. Brussels: European Men's Health Forum; 2005. www.emhf.org (accessed 8 March 2007).

International Obesity Task Force (IOTF). *Obesity in Europe: the case for action*. London: European Association for the Study of Obesity; 2002.

The Lancet. The weighty matter of care for all. Editorial. *The Lancet.* 2006; **367**: 876.

Lang T, Rayner G, Kaelin E. *The Food Industry, Diet, Physical Activity and Health: a review of reported commitments and practice of 25 of the world's largest food companies.* London: Centre for Food Policy, City University; 2006. www.city.ac.uk/press/The%20Food%20Industry%20Diet%20Physical%20Activity%20and%20Health.pdf (accessed 8 March 2007).

MHF. *Hazardous Waist: Tackling the epidemic of excess weight in men.* (Policy Report.) Men's Health Forum, London; 2005. www.menshealthforum.org.uk/uploaded_files/Hazardouswaist.pdf

National Audit Office (NAO). *Health of the Nation: a progress report.* London: National Audit Office; 1996.

National Audit Office (NAO). *Tackling Obesity in England.* London: National Audit Office; 2001. www.nao.org.uk/publications/nao_reports/000–1/0001220.pdf (accessed 8 March 2007).

National Institute for Health and Clinical Excellence (NICE). *Obesity: guidance on the prevention, identification, assessment and management of overweight and obesity in adults and children.* Clinical Guideline 43. London: National Institute for Health and Clinical Excellence; 2006. www.nice.org.uk/guidance/CG43/guidance (accessed 8 March 2007).

National Obesity Forum. *General Medical Contract: obesity and primary care.* 2005. http://nationalobesityforumorguk.pre-dns-change.com/images/stories/Healthcare_Professionals/NOF_GMS_contract_backgrounder.pdf (accessed April 2006).

O'Brien O, White AK. *Gender and Health: the case for gender-sensitive health policy and health care delivery.* Briefing Paper. London: King's Fund; 2003.

Office for National Statistics (ONS). Children's expenditure: by gender and type of purchase, 2000–1. *Social Trends 32.* London: Office for National Statistics; 2002.

Prentice A. Storing up problems: the medical case for a slimmer nation. Editorial. *Clinical Medicine.* 2004; 4: 991–1001.

Reeves R. How fat became a political issue. *New Statesman.* 2003; 18 August: 161–8.

Royal College of Physicians. *Storing Up Problems: the medical case for a slimmer nation.* Report of a working party of the Royal College of Physicians, Royal College of Paediatrics and Child Health and the Faculty of Public Health Medicine. London: Royal College of Physicians; 2004.

UK Public Health Association (UKPHA). *Choosing Health or Losing Health?* Response to the White Paper *Choosing Health – making healthy choices easier.* 2005. www.ukpha.org.uk/media/choosing%20health%20or%20losing%20health.pdf (accessed 8 March 2007).

Ulrich C. The economics of obesity: costs, causes and controls. *Human Ecology.* 2005; **33**(3): 101–3.

White AK, Lockyer L. Tackling coronary heart disease: a gender sensitive approach is needed. Editorial. *British Medical Journal.* 2001; **323**: 1016–17.

World Health Organization (WHO). *Gender and Health: a technical paper.* Geneva: WHO; 1998.

World Health Organization (WHO). *Obesity: preventing and managing the global epidemic.* Geneva: WHO; 2000.

World Health Organization (WHO). *The World Health Report 2002: reducing risks, promoting healthy life.* Geneva: WHO; 2002.

World Health Organization (WHO). *Controlling the Global Obesity Epidemic.* 2003. www.who.int/nutrition/topics/obesity/en/ (accessed 8 March 2007).

World Health Organization (WHO). *Global Strategy on Diet, Physical Activity and Health.* Geneva: WHO; 2004.

CHAPTER 4

Using body image to help men manage weight problems

Ewan Gillon and Kerri McPherson

In this chapter we will explore an important, yet often neglected, area of work relating to our understanding of male obesity; namely, men's body image. Since the mid-1990s, an increasing amount of attention has been paid to men's relationship with their bodies, highlighting what is often seen as their increased level of interest with regards to bodily appearance. Body image, which Cash (2004, p.1) defines as 'the multifaceted psychological experience of embodiment, especially but not exclusively one's physical appearance', may easily be seen as a useful mechanism to encourage men to reduce obesity and being overweight. However, men's body image, and its relationship to behaviour, is more complex than often assumed and there are a number of issues that present some very real challenges for those working with obese and overweight men to improve health.

In this chapter we will outline some of the key areas of research linked to men's body image, and consider the implications these have for working with men to manage weight-related health. In doing so, we shall highlight the many differences between men and women in relation to body, and stress the importance of a gender-sensitive approach to policy and practice in this area.

Background

The assumption that, on the whole, men pay little attention to the aesthetic appearance of their bodies is an absolute falsehood, yet one that permeates the beliefs of the general public and, until very recently, has acted as the fundamental underpinning of much academic research in the area. This viewpoint is highly problematic for it is enmeshed with the paucity of gender-specific research on how men view, and relate to, their bodies. Although men's approach to body image has been indirectly addressed in much work, the understandings produced by this have been highly feminised, often utilising gender as an *explanatory variable* for women's many difficulties with body (e.g. Orbach, 1978). From the vantage point of such studies, men, by virtue of their gendered identity, experience a disinterested, trouble-free approach to their bodies.

However, as we shall explain, this perspective may be questioned both in terms of its underpinning research base as well as its applicability to contemporary men's health.

The social context

Without a doubt, most of the research undertaken in the area of body image has focused upon women and the problems many women experience in living up to idealised femininities, stressing an ultra-thin physique that is both unattainable and unhealthy (Halliwell and Dittmar, 2004). The cultural pressure on women to live up to such ideals has been highlighted by many theorists (e.g. Wolf, 1991) as a significant factor in the high rates of body (dis)satisfaction and eating distress within the female population (EDA, 2000). This pressure is promulgated through media images drawing on traditional conceptualisations of women as objects of cultural gaze. As Berger (1972) suggests, 'men act and women appear', a process that feminist theorists (Bruch, 1974; Orbach, 1978) have located within patriarchal power dynamics and the consequent 'objectification' of the female body for the pleasure of men.

Such a perspective means that men have been traditionally seen as maintaining a far less problematic relationship to body as a result of their privileged social position and status as consumers of feminine objectification (Bordo, 1992). Body (dis)satisfaction is seen as a social phenomenon, a product of socio-political constructs that formulate femininity in subjugated, aesthetic terms not relevant to men. It is women, as a product of their lesser social status and power, who must 'look good', while men, due to their status as producers and closer relationship to the 'rational mind, not body' (Seidler, 1989), are 'looked after' sexually, emotionally and physically. This gender-based differential in body image provides an important insight into the many difficulties women experience in managing an embodied identity, and in particular, the prevalence of eating disorders such as anorexia and bulimia. However, we would argue that this has been at the expense of our understandings of body image in men.

The disordered eating paradigm

Until the mid-1990s much of the research exploring the concept of body image was located within the disordered eating paradigm, such that body image was investigated for its role in the onset and maintenance of eating disorders, including obesity. This research was comparative in nature, looking for differences between predefined groups of individuals; anorexic compared with normal weight; normal weight compared with obese; and men compared with women (Friedman and Brownell, 1995).

Implicit in these comparative studies are two fundamental assumptions. First, it is assumed that one of the groups of individuals represents the benchmark of optimal psychological functioning; a control group, against which others can be usefully compared. Second, it is assumed that body image is a simple, uni-dimensional construct that can explain differences between groups divided on other variables such as weight status or gender.

Indeed, as we allude to above, much of the early work in the area of body image supported the assumption that body image *concerns* were firmly located within the realm of the female. An immeasurable number of gender comparison studies reported no body image dissatisfaction in men in contrast to statistics showing the majority of women to be unhappy with the aesthetic appearance of their bodies (e.g. Fallon and Rozin, 1985; Pliner *et al.*, 1990). However, more recent advances in the field of body image have resulted in an outright rejection of this notion of 'aesthetic apathy' in men. The failure of previous studies to find body image dissatisfaction in samples of men does not reflect the lived experience of the majority of men, but instead may be seen as an artefact of inappropriate statistical calculation of the data collected from men, coupled with the employment of inappropriate data collection instruments (cf. Cafri and Thompson, 2004).

Feminised data collection measures

Due to the historical focus of body image research on women, the majority of measures for investigating body image (dis)satisfaction were derived from research on women and later used with men, either in their original form or simply adapted without being subject to the appropriate psychometric testing. The most frequently used measures of body image (dis)satisfaction are pen and paper schematic drawing scales, which display gendered images of varying body size. However, reflecting the centrality of fat in women's body image evaluations, the unit of variability is normally only adiposity; the scales show men or women getting incrementally fatter and thinner. The standard method of calculating body image (dis)satisfaction using one of these scales is to ask participants to rate the image that best represents their current body shape and the one that they aspire to. The discrepancy between these two values is used as a relative index of body image (dis)satisfaction.

As mentioned previously, the majority of women report dissatisfaction with their current body shape and these evaluations are normally always uni-directional. That is, women almost always aspire to be thinner than they currently are. This is not the case in men, who tend to evaluate themselves as *either* too big or too small when expressing dissatisfaction with body image (e.g. Cafri *et al.*, 2002; McPherson and Turnbull, 2005). Hence the calculation of (dis)satisfaction discrepancy scores in samples of men will result in positive and negative values – indicating the direction of dissatisfaction – depending on whether the individual wishes to increase or decrease their size. Early comparative studies failed to take cognisance of these signed values and their statistical calculations resulted in zero, or near zero, (dis)satisfaction scores for the samples of men. These scores were interpreted as body image satisfaction that protected men from the onset of eating disorders such as anorexia nervosa but, evidently, these zero scores were a consequence of miscalculation rather than aesthetic apathy.

Neglect of muscularity

The research base is further compromised by the now growing recognition that measures simply employing adiposity as the unit of body image (dis)satisfaction fail to capture the full extent of body image evaluations in men. Authors such as McCreary (e.g. McCreary and Sasse, 2000), Cafri (Cafri *et al.*, 2002) and Pope (e.g. Pope *et al.*, 2000) have painted a much more complex picture of the system of evaluation in men whereby the significance of *muscularity* is highlighted. Their research shows that men not only use muscularity in their evaluations of their own bodies, and those of others, but that (dis)satisfaction associated with muscularity shares the most significant relationship with other psychological variables such as self-esteem (McCreary and Sasse, 2000). Indeed, some have reported that the inclusion of muscularity (dis)satisfaction scores in statistical analyses extinguishes the relationship between adiposity (dis)satisfaction and psychological well-being (Cafri *et al.*, 2002).

The important point to make here, therefore, is that the traditional assumption underpinning much research showing men's lack of interest, or satisfaction with body image, may distort the nature of men's actual view of body and any concerns being encountered. We certainly have no wish to argue against the many profound difficulties experienced by women that have been highlighted within the research base. These are of huge significance and intimately related to culturally dominant constructions of femininity. Yet we do wish to suggest that there exists more of an 'unknown' as to the historical status of men's relationship to body than is often assumed. Although it may be possible that, historically, men and women occupied 'oppositional' standpoints, with men experiencing little if any (dis)satisfaction with body, this argument cannot be maintained by the research base alone. It may be the case that men's body image is historically far more complex than often imagined. However, what is clear, and of greater relevance to our present focus, is that men's body (dis)satisfaction is prevalent and increasing in significance within our contemporary culture.

The changing social context

In recent years a range of social and economic changes, such as the move to a service-orientated economy and the loss of traditional 'male' occupations, and the growth of a 'consumer' culture (Featherstone, 1991) have accompanied (e.g. Gill *et al.*, 2000) an increased visibility of male bodily ideals stressing strength, muscularity and leanness (Yelland and Tiggemann, 2003). Such idealised male physiques are now presented in a range of media settings, with magazines orientated around bodily improvement (e.g. *Men's Health, Men's Fitness*) presenting associations between attractiveness and muscularity, success and physical appearance. Added to this is the rapid expansion of male-specific grooming and bodycare products (Gill *et al.*, 2005), a state once again pointing toward the significance of physical appearance as a growing feature of male self-experience. In other words, men too are now objects of cultural 'gaze', with particular male bodies increasingly objectified as aspirational, idealised entities.

Body ideals exist at an individual and a cultural level. To the individual they represent the entirely private image that is aspired to (Thompson, 1990). At a cultural level, body ideals are the agreed standards of attractiveness (cf. Thompson and Stice, 2001) that social-cultural theories view as shaping and moulding the private ideals of the individuals exposed to them (Duggan and McCreary, 2004; Fallon, 1990; Fisher *et al.*, 2002; Orbach, 1993). As the visual representations of the 'perfect' gendered body continue to increase, it may consequently be expected that greater numbers of men experience dissonance because of the perceived incongruity between their own body and the cultural ideal.

A similar point is captured by psychological perspectives. Social Comparison Theory (e.g. Brown *et al.*, 1992), for example, highlights the role of peer-group comparisons in establishing and maintaining positive self-identity. When body becomes a legitimate basis for social comparison, the psychological pressure to adhere to physical ideals is heightened and the consequences of failure magnified, resulting in greater levels of body dissatisfaction among those to whom it is relevant, such as many men.

An evolutionary perspective

A further approach through which men's ongoing relationship to body may be understood is that of evolutionary psychology theory. This perspective highlights the psychological mechanisms which have evolved to drive male behaviour toward maintaining particular 'male' physiques that would seem to have much in common with the idealised bodies commonplace within contemporary culture.

Across evolutionary history our ancestors were faced with a variety of problems that threatened their survival and, through the processes of natural selection, modern-day humans have inherited those psychological mechanisms that facilitated the 'solving' of these problems (cf. Cosmides and Tooby, 2005). Mate selection is an important adaptive problem for both men and women and research evidence has supported the existence of evolved psychological mechanisms designed for this purpose in modern-day humans, namely the ability to rate the attractiveness of both ourselves and others (Buss, 1989; Buss and Schmitt, 1993).

The process of sexual selection (cf. Darwin, 1859) is such that body image is inextricably linked to evaluations of reproductive fitness. Individuals make, in many instances non-conscious, judgements about their own and other people's bodies based on whether or not they display features that are relevant to parental investment and/or 'good genes' (Buss and Schmitt, 1993; Gangestad, 1993; Kenrick et al., 1994; Trivers, 1972; Wade and Cooper, 1999). Being a sexually dimorphic species, Homo sapiens sapiens differentially assess attractiveness in men and women. Where women tend to be evaluated on their physical attractiveness and physical representations of fecundity (Buss, 1988, 1989, 1992; Kenrick et al., 1994; Trivers, 1972), men are evaluated on indices of masculinity, dominance and status (Brodie et al., 1991; Buss, 1989; Buss and Schmitt, 1993; Davis et al., 1991; Ellis, 1992; Mintz and Betz, 1986; Pope et al., 1999; Trivers, 1972; Wade, 2000).

Evidently, the modern environment is far removed from the one in which our species evolved. However, evolutionary psychologists argue that the same is not true of the human psychological architecture (Duchaine et al., 2001). Rather it is assumed that the same mechanisms that drove mate selection in our prehistory drive sexual behaviour in a modern environment (Buss, 1989; Buss and Schmitt, 1993). Furthermore, there is no reason to assume that the mechanisms that guide our preferences when seeking a sexual partner do not represent a fundamental categorisation of attractiveness per se. Indeed, the data collected in socio-cultural investigations of attractiveness and evolutionary investigations of mate preferences all point to the same pattern of behaviour. It is the lean, muscular men with masculinised features – the cultural ideal – who are rated as being most attractive.

Men's body (dis)satisfaction

So far, we have proposed that male bodily ideas are *different* to those of female ideals (i.e. stressing muscularity over slimness, etc.), that research in the area of body image has historically failed to account for these differences leading to a distinct lack of accurate research on how men actually relate to body, and finally that the increasing cultural visibility of male bodily ideals is likely to result in many men experiencing greater dissatisfaction with their bodily appearance.

Certainly, the increased visibility of idealised male bodies has been accompanied by a greater interest among health professionals and researchers in the issue of men's body image (Cafri and Thompson, 2004), and this has produced a number of strands of work focusing on men's changing relationship to their bodies as a site of concern (e.g. Levine and Harrison, 2004). Much of this confirms that the increased visibility of the male body has resulted in men experiencing greater levels of body dissatisfaction as well as a range of related difficulties. Work in the area of eating distress (e.g. Hospers and Jansen, 2005), for example, has described how eating disordered symptoms are closely related to a high level of body dissatisfaction among both gay and straight men. Similarly, a negative view of body has been identified by Pope *et al.* (2000) as a significant basis for obsessive exercise and muscle dysmorphia (i.e. extreme body change behaviours aimed at increasing muscularity).

Outwith clinical samples, general work within the male population equally points to significant levels of body (dis)satisfaction among men, again in a bi-directional fashion with the proportions of men wishing to be larger (i.e. to gain size) and smaller (i.e. to become slimmer) roughly equivalent (Cafri *et al.*, 2005). Furthermore, the issue of muscularity must also be highlighted, for much research has indicated many men's desire to accomplish a more muscular physique. Yet it is not as simple as suggesting that where women are concerned with adiposity, men are concerned with muscularity. Those studies that have moved away from the gender comparison approach, to investigating body image in men-only samples, are highlighting a more complex picture. This, albeit nascent, field of research suggests a need to define body image as both a multi-dimensional and a bi-directional concept. Men use both muscularity and adiposity in their body image evaluations (Cafri *et al.*, 2002); they incorporate body weight as well as body shape (McPherson and Turnbull, 2005); they make clear distinctions between aesthetic ideals and healthy ideals (McPherson and Turnbull, 2001); and the sharp reality is that not all men want to reduce their body size, even those who are medically overweight (McPherson and Turnbull, 2005). This is surely as far removed as you can get from the picture of aesthetic apathy that dominated our consciousness until the late 1990s.

What we do know is certain groups of men seem more prone to higher levels of body dissatisfaction than others. Younger men seem particularly vulnerable in this regard (e.g. McCabe and Ricciardelli, 2003), a finding which seems strongly inter-related with levels of self-esteem (Tiggemann and Wilson-Barrett, 1998). Such dissatisfaction with body among younger men may partly be explained by age-related identity concerns (Lee and Owens, 2002), such as the need to impress peers and appear 'attractive' to potential partners. Certainly, a study by Lynch and Zellner (1999) indicated that college students tended to overestimate the body size that women would find attractive in a male, a finding that may also reflect the high degree of media exposure given to muscularity in younger male role models. A qualitative study by Watson (2000) also provides some interesting evidence in this light, showing how older men tend to evaluate body less in terms of aesthetics and more on functionality, linked to the body's capacity to manage everyday tasks and family/work responsibilities.

Homosexual men, too, have been shown to have a higher level of body dissatisfaction than their heterosexual peers (Russell and Keel, 2002), a finding that has been linked to the close relationship between a masculine identity and a muscular, slender body within the gay community (Drummond, 2002). For some, however, the important factor here is not sexual orientation but of gender role identity (Lakkis *et al.*, 1999), with the higher levels of feminine role orientation seen in homosexual men (Strong *et al.*, 2000) viewed as predisposing a greater awareness of appearance-related issues. However, whatever the causal factor may be, the fact remains that gay men are far more likely to express body dissatisfaction than straight men, and as a result may be far more vulnerable to a range of unhealthy or high-risk behaviours, such as those associated with disordered eating or obsessive exercise.

Implications of men's body image for practitioners

Undoubtedly, research linked to body image in men highlights a number of key challenges for practitioners working with issues of weight problems in men. The youth and complexity of the area coupled with the enduring influence of historical assumptions regarding men's lack of interest in body make it difficult to establish exactly how to translate theory into practice and to work effectively with men. In order to explore these challenges, which are not discrete, we wish to identify two core themes which we feel underpin many of the dilemmas likely to be encountered. These are as follows.

The historical feminisation of body image concerns

As we have seen, the arena of body image is highly loaded with feminised meanings and suppositions that may conflict with those relevant to many men in contemporary western society. The notion of meaning is vitally important here, for both socio-cultural theories (cf. Drummond, 2005) and evolutionary psychology theories highlight the extent to which transmission of bodily ideals through media and other public forums influence both men's and women's view of their own bodies and those around them. Enmeshed within this process is a whole range of assumptions about gender, and the ways in which gendered identities are occupied and maintained through bodily practices and attitudes. Historically, concerns regarding body have been defined in highly gendered terms, as issues relevant only to women. Hence, despite the growing visibility of male bodily ideals within western culture, it is important to recognise that many men, particularly older men, are primarily accustomed to the arena of bodily awareness and body management practices such as weight reduction being associated with women (Ogden, 1992). This construction undoubtedly contributes to the continued paucity of male participants on commercial weight-loss programmes, and has thus given rise to male-specific programmes such as Garry Egger's 'GutBusters' in Australia (*see* Chapter 21).

The challenge for practitioners is thus how to negotiate the tricky dilemmas thrown up for many men in acknowledging body as a site of concern when such a process is traditionally associated with women and thus infused with feminine meanings implying that men do not experience concerns over how they look, or with their bodies in general. Acknowledging (dis)satisfaction with body image, or indeed body for any other reason, may thus be deeply shameful and embarrassing for some men, raising questions linked to gender identity and self-management. Yet recognising and handling such male experiences may be alien to many health practitioners, particularly women, who are entirely accustomed to issues of bodily (dis)satisfaction deriving from their gendered status as well as equally familiar with historical constructions of body concerns as primarily located within the female domain. Hence the necessary gender-sensitive approach may be, in actuality, more difficult to find than it first appears.

The multi-dimensional, bi-directional basis of men's body (dis)satisfaction

The second theme we wish to highlight is the differences between men and women in bodily ideals and the extent to which men are orientated toward muscularity as well as adiposity (multi-dimensionality), and toward gaining as well as losing body mass (bi-directionality). Unlike female body (dis)satisfaction, which centres very much around weight *loss* and slenderness, male aspirations are more complex and thus require some consideration in terms of how they meet with conventional messages regarding obesity and being overweight.

A particular issue here links to the fundamental aim of managing being overweight and obese by encouraging *weight loss*. As we have seen, much research has highlighted the desire of many men to appear 'big and strong', which presents somewhat of a challenge to those promoting the dangers of being overweight and obese. While such a message accords entirely with traditional constructions of ideal female bodies stressing slimness, it may be seen to conflict with commonplace notions of male bodies as physically dominant, strong and muscular. In such terms, asking men to *lose weight* may thus be heard as a request to become less masculine, in terms of such contemporary male ideals. As such, it may be the case that some men simply prefer to remain overweight or obese, due to the connotations of largeness signifying strength and power, over weight loss and its consequence – reduction in physical (and potentially social) stature. Similar conclusions may be relevant to men for whom the concept of *weight* (i.e. adiposity) is irrelevant. Being over*weight* for individuals in such circumstances presents little if any motivation for change, despite such terms being commonplace within health promotion literatures and strongly linked with raised adult morbidity.

The issue is thus how those working with men on issues of being overweight and obese manage the gendered meanings of body among men. These meanings are complex and often contradictory, as well as significantly different to those relevant to women.

An example: talking about body concerns

To exemplify the complexity of these themes and the challenge awaiting those in the field, we wish to present an extract from a small research study conducted by Gillon (1997, 2003), showing some of various meanings that are invoked and resisted by a male participant talking about his weight. The extract presented was part of an examination of the way men talk about food and body, an approach grounded within a discourse analytic framework (e.g. Edwards and Potter, 1992). Although this extract offers clearly one of innumerable possibilities in responding to a somewhat challenging question (discourse analytic work focuses on explanations and justifications and hence avoids the 'neutral' stance of much qualitative methodology), it demonstrates some of the possible concerns men may have in talking about a concern about being overweight or obese. It is important to add here that this research was with a non-clinical sample.

> I: Are you concerned with your weight?
> R: Errmm, mmm I wasn't until I got back after the summer holidays [laughs].
> I: [laughs]
> R: Ha ha ermm mm, no, when I was 22 up till I was 35 I was 11 and a ½ stone, and I ate masses, I ate loads. I used to play rugby and I think that's helped, but I was always a steady weight. errrr I've started doing weights at school and my weight's gone up, but I'm trying to convince myself it's cos I've put muscle on, but no not, I'm not con–. I'm not bothered about my weight if somebody said to me err you weigh 13 stone or 15 stone, weight's nothing to me, it doesn't make any difference. It's probably vanity, it's vanity with me. If I look, if I looked fat and awesome and I weighed 10 stone then I would try and get rid of it. If I was fat and awesome at 16 stone I would try to get rid of it. It's more to do with looks than actual weight.

In looking at this extract, it is clear that a number of different issues are addressed by the respondent. First, and importantly, he does disclose a concern over a recent increase in his weight, an outcome that he links both to his use of weights at school (he is a teacher) and also, but more implicitly, to the pleasures of his summer holidays. In couching his disclosure in such terms, as well as describing the stability of weight for a long period of his life at the same time, he diminishes any inference that he has a troublesome relationship to body. Such a relationship, we suggest, may both resonate with cultural meanings denoting worrying about weight as a 'feminine' activity, and the possibility that he has failed to manage his body effectively. While he could easily have simply answered 'yes' to the question, the fact that he doesn't do so illustrates that the meanings of acknowledging a 'concern' about weight are potentially uncomfortable. So much so, in fact, that as the account progresses the respondent shifts what he is saying to *deny* that he would ever feel concerned about his weight, and instead formulates the basis of interest in terms of how he looks. A concern over his body image thus seems to be a more acceptable motivation for changing things than how much he weighs. Such a construction certainly fits with socio-cultural ideas proposing that men too are now subject to aspirational images of male bodily ideals, and thus that the language of aesthetics is more enmeshed with dominant masculinities than that of weight, or indeed health. However, this language is used with great caution in this extract, for the speaker seems very aware of the implications of appearing preoccupied with how he looks (again, a notion that implies a 'feminised' approach to body), counteracting this by indicating both that he is aware of, and even agrees with, this interpretation ('it's vanity with me') and that concern would arise only in the most extreme of circumstances (i.e. if he looked 'fat and awesome') rather than being part of his day-to-day experiences.

Conclusions

There is little doubt that the culturally agreed, evolutionary defined standards of attractiveness for men play a significant role in the way men think about, and manage, their bodies. If this were not the case the association of body image (dis)satisfaction with both muscularity and weight loss/gain would not exist. Unfortunately, current public health policy and health education fails to take much cognisance of this with current campaigns aimed at reducing obesity and being overweight still framed in feminised language prioritising *weight loss* above all else. As we have argued, this premise fails to capture the complex meanings of body for men, ignoring the aesthetic importance of muscularity as well as failing to recognise the bi-directional nature of many men's aspirations to lose *or* gain weight (i.e. get bigger). Without a doubt, the historical legacy of feminised body image research still remains, informing much research (e.g. through the use of body-size measures for comparative purposes: cf. Markey and Markey, 2005) and practice. It is our contention that to develop a wholly effective method for working with overweight and obese men, a sophisticated and gender-sensitive approach is required that more fully accounts for the complex differences between (and among) men and women in relationship to body and the body ideals to which they aspire.

References

Berger J. *Ways of Seeing*. Harmondsworth: Penguin; 1972.

Bordo S. *Unbearable Weight: feminism, western culture, and the body*. Berkeley: University of California Press; 1992.

Brodie DA, Slade PD, Riley VJ. Sex differences in body-image perceptions. *Percept Mot Skills*. 1991; 72: 73–4.

Brown JD, Novick NJ, Kelley A. When Gulliver travels: social context, psychological closeness and self-appraisals. *J Pers Soc Psychol*. 1992; 62: 717–27.

Bruch H. *Eating Disorders, Obesity, Anorexia Nervosa and the Person Within*. London: Routledge and Kegan Paul; 1974.

Buss D. Sex difference in human mate preferences: evolutionary hypotheses tested in 37 cultures. *Behavioural and Brain Sciences*. 1989; 12: 1–49.

Buss DM. The evolution of human intrasexual competition: tactics of male attraction. *J Pers Soc Psychol*. 1988; 54: 616–28.

Buss DM. Mate preference mechanisms: consequences for partner choice and intrasexual competition. In: Barkow JH, Cosmides L, Tooby J, editors. *The Adapted Mind: evolutionary psychology and the generation of culture*. New York: Oxford University Press; 1992.

Buss DM, Schmitt DP. Sexual strategies theory: an evolutionary perspective on human mating. *Psychol Rev.* 1993; **100**: 204–32.

Cafri G, Strauss J, Thompson JK. Male body image: satisfaction and its relationship to well-being using the somatomorphic matrix. *International Journal of Men's Health.* 2002; **1**(2): 215–31.

Cafri G, Thompson JK. Measuring male body image: a review of current methodology. *Psychology of Men & Masculinity.* 2004; **5**(1): 18–29.

Cafri G, Thompson JK, Ricciardelli L *et al.* Pursuit of the muscular ideal: physical and psychological consequences and putative risk factors. *Clin Psychol Rev.* 2005; **25**: 215–39.

Cash TF. Body image: past, present, and future. *Body Image.* 2004; **1**: 1–5.

Cosmides L, Tooby J. Conceptual foundations of evolutionary psychology. In: Buss DM, editor. *The Handbook of Evolutionary Psychology.* Hoboken, NJ: John Wiley & Sons, Inc.; 2005.

Darwin C. *On the Origin of Species.* London: Murray; 1859.

Davis C, Elliott S, Dionne M, Mitchell I. The relationship of personality factors and physical activity to body satisfaction in men. *Pers Individ Dif.* 1991; **12**: 689–94.

Drummond M. Men, body image and eating disorders. *International Journal of Men's Health.* 2002; **1**: 79–93.

Drummond MJN. Men's bodies: listening to the voices of young gay men. *Men and Masculinities.* 2005; **7**: 270–90.

Duchaine B, Cosmides L, Tooby J. Evolutionary psychology and the brain. *Curr Opin Neurobiol.* 2001; **11**(2): 225–30.

Duggan SJ, McCreary DR. Body image, eating disorders, and drive for muscularity in gay and heterosexual men: the influence of media images. *J Homosex.* 2004; **47**: 45–58.

Eating Disorders Association (EDA). *The Hidden Cost of Eating Disorders: the need for action.* Norwich UK: Eating Disorders Association; 2000.

Edwards D, Potter J. *Discursive Psychology.* London: Sage; 1992.

Ellis BJ. The evolution of sexual attraction: evaluative mechanisms in women. In: Barkow JH, Cosmides L, Tooby J, editors. *The Adapted Mind: evolutionary psychology and the generation of culture.* New York: Oxford University Press; 1992. p. 267–88.

Fallon A. Culture in the mirror: sociocultural determinants of body image. In: Cash T, Pruzinsky T, editors. *Body Images: development, deviance and change.* New York: Guilford Press; 1990.

Fallon AE, Rozin P. Sex differences in perceptions of desirable body shape. *J Abnorm Psychol.* 1985; **94**: 102–5.

Featherstone M. The body in consumer culture. In: Featherstone M, Hepworth M and Turner BS, editors. *The Body: Social Process and Cultural Theory.* London: Sage; 1991.

Fisher E, Thompson JK, Dunn ME. Social comparison and body image: an investigation of body comparison process using multidimensional scaling. *J Soc Clin Psychol.* 2002; **21**: 566–79.

Friedman MA, Brownell KD. Psychological correlates of obesity: moving to the next research generation. *Psychol Bull.* 1995; **117**(1): 3–20.

Gangestad SW. Sexual selection and physical attractiveness: implications for mating dynamics. *Hum Nat.* 1993; **4**: 205–35.

Gill R, Henwood K, Mclean C. The tyranny of the six-pack: Understanding men's responses to representations of the male body in popular culture. In: Squire C, editor. *Culture in Psychology.* London: Routledge; 2000.

Gill R, Henwood K, McLean C. Body projects and regulation of normative masculinity. *Body and Society.* 2005; **11**: 37–62.

Gillon E. Men's Talk About Food: A discourse analysis. Unpublished PhD Thesis. The Open University. Milton Keynes. 1997.

Gillon E. Can men talk about problems with weight: the therapeutic implications of a discourse analytic study. *Journal of Counselling and Psychotherapy Research.* 2003; **3**(1): 25–32.

Halliwell E, Dittmar H. Does size matter? The impact of model's body size on advertising effectiveness and women's body-focused anxiety. *J Soc Clin Psychol.* 2004; **23**: 105–132.

Hospers HJ, Jansen A. Why homosexuality is a risk factor for eating disorders in males. *J Soc Clin Psychol.* 2005; **24**: 1188–1201.

Kenrick DT, Neuberg SL, Zierk KL, Krones, JM. Evolution and social cognition: contrast effects as a function of sex, dominance, and physical attractiveness. *Pers Soc Psychol Bull.* 1994; **20**: 210–17.

Lakkis J, Ricciardelli LA, Williams RJ. Role of sexual orientation and gender-related traits in disordered eating. *Sex Roles.* 1999; **41**: 1–16.

Lee C, Owens RG. Issues for a psychology of men's health. *J Health Psychol.* 2002; **7**: 209–17.

Levine MP, Harrison K. The role of mass media in the perpetuation and prevention of negative body image and disordered eating. In: Thompson JK, editor. *Handbook of Eating Disorders and Obesity.* New York: Wiley; 2004.

Lynch S, Zellner D. Figure preferences in two generations of men: the use of figure drawings illustrating differences in muscle mass. *Sex Roles.* 1999; **40**: 9–10.

Markey CN, Markey PM. Relations between body image and dieting behaviours: an examination of gender differences. *Sex Roles.* 2005; **53**: 519–30.

McCabe MP, Ricciardelli LA. A longitudinal study of body change strategies among adolescent males. *J Youth Adolesc.* 2003; **32**: 105–13.

McCreary DR, Sasse DK. An exploration of the drive for muscularity in adolescent boys and girls. *J Am Coll Health.* 2000; **48**: 297–304.

McPherson KE, Turnbull JD. Is there a difference between an aesthetic-ideal and a healthy-ideal body image? *Proceedings of The British Psychological Society.* 2001; **9**(2): 224.

McPherson KE, Turnbull JD. Body image satisfaction in Scottish men and its implications for promoting healthy behaviours. *International Journal of Men's Health.* 2005; **4**(1): 3–12.

Mintz LB, Betz NE. Sex differences in the nature, realism, and correlates of body image. *Sex Roles.* 1986; **15**: 185–95.

Ogden J. *Fat Chance! The Myth of Dieting Explained.* London: Routledge; 1992.

Orbach S. *Fat is a Feminist Issue – the Anti-diet Guide to Weight Loss.* New York: Paddington Press; 1978.

Orbach S. *Hunger Strike: the anorectic's struggle as a metaphor for our age.* London: Penguin; 1993.

Pliner P, Chaiken S, Flett GL. Gender differences in concern with body weight and physical appearance over the life span. *Pers Soc Psychol Bull.* 1990; **16**: 263–73.

Pope HG, Gruber A, Magwth B *et al.* Body image perception among men in three countries. *Am J Psychiatry.* 2000; **157**: 1297–301.

Pope HG, Olivardia R, Gruber A, Borowiecki J. Evolving ideals of male body image as seen through action toys. *Int J Eat Disord.* 1999; **26**: 65–72.

Russell CJ, Keel PK. Homosexuality as a specific risk factor for eating disorders in men. *Int J Eat Disord.* 2002; **31**: 300–6.

Seidler V. *Rediscovering Masculinity.* London: Routledge & Kegan Paul; 1989.

Strong SM, Singh D, Randall PK. Childhood gender non-conformity and body dissatisfaction in gay and heterosexual men. *Sex Roles.* 2000; **43**: 427–39.

Thompson JK. *Body Image Disturbance: assessment and treatment.* Elmsford: Pergamon Press; 1990.

Thompson JK, Stice E. Thin-ideal internalization: mounting evidence for a new risk factor for body-image disturbance and eating pathology. *Current Directions in Psychological Science.* 2001; **10**(5): 181–3.

Tiggemann M, Wilson-Barrett E. Children's figure ratings: relationship to self-esteem and negative stereotyping. *Int J Eat Disord.* 1998; **23**: 83–8.

Trivers RL. Parental investment and sexual selection. In: Campbell B, editor. *Sexual Selection and the Descent of Man.* Chicago: Aldine; 1972.

Wade TJ. Evolutionary theory and self-perception: sex differences in body esteem predictors of self-perceived physical and sexual attractiveness and self-esteem. *Int J Psychol.* 2000; **35**: 36–45.

Wade TJ, Cooper M. Sex differences in the links between attractiveness, self-esteem and the body. *Pers Individ Dif.* 1999; **27**: 1047–56.

Watson J. *Male Bodies: health, culture and identity.* Buckingham: Open University Press; 2000.

Wolf N. *The Beauty Myth: how images of beauty are used against women.* London: Vintage Books; 1991.

Yelland C, Tiggemann M. Muscularity and the gay ideal. Body dissatisfaction and disordered eating in homosexual men. *Eat Behav.* 2003; **4**: 107–116.

CHAPTER 5

Men, obesity and the media

Claire Mac Evilly

The problem of obesity is multi-dimensional and there are gender issues to be considered in the battle against weight gain. Levels of obesity in men have risen faster than those in women. In men, obesity has almost doubled in the last 10 years and there are a number of health risks, which men face specifically, as outlined in Chapter 2.

Media activity is overwhelmingly focused on women where weight is concerned, and the food industry is now more than ever engaged in making the greatest use of mass media to improve the health of society. Are the increase in weight gain by men and the role of the media related? Are men being let down by sex discrimination in the media? The answer to these questions lies in the fact that simply informing men about risk factors is not sufficient to stimulate the type of change that is necessary to facilitate weight loss. As the prevalence of obesity increases in men, and the lack of real behaviour change become apparent, there is a real need to rethink communication strategies and speak to men in such a way that they will listen to the advice and act on it.

Gender communication

One of the greatest social changes since World War II has been in the roles of men and women. Members of both genders have lived multiple roles, but some were firmly entrenched, such as men being the wage earners and women the caregivers. Communication has followed largely defined cultural and societal norms. In recent years many of the roles have remained the same, but are now occupied by members of either gender. So, for example, women may have careers in engineering or sports, and a growing number of men may have full-time care of the home, children, and the disabled. Both men and women have a variety of jobs in the workplace and positions in the hierarchy of management.

Communication between the genders has become more prevalent and pervasive in society, as norms have changed. When we add the mobility of our population and the differences among the cultures they represent, both the importance and difficulty of effective communication increase. Health communication can markedly affect the understanding and acceptance of new health behaviours and revised gender perspectives. Including gender-specific concerns in health communication can make health messages more effective in eliciting behaviour change (Zaman and Underwood, 2003).

Over the last few decades, both health professionals and food marketers have made systematic efforts to understand why people choose to eat the foods they do and how to communicate food choices. Marketing professionals have two main reasons to be interested. First, they can develop food products that consumers will buy, and second, they can create successful advertising and promotional campaigns to generate higher sales of the branded food products they are selling. Health professionals, on the other hand, want to understand the determinants of food choice as a foundation for effective nutrition education and advice.

Consumer behaviour is one area in which the differences between men and women are evident. The marketing professional identifies the consumer's recognised or latent needs and links these to his product or service through an identified brand, using skilful advertising and promotion. Marketing is a set of activities and business processes that comprise the so-called marketing mix, or 'four Ps': product (what it looks and feels like, its features and benefits), price, place (how it is distributed and purchased) and promotion.

The market is 'segmented' on the basis of demographic variables such as age, family size, family life, gender, income or occupation. Demographic variables are the most popular basis for distinguishing consumer groups. Gender segmentation has long been applied to clothing, hairstyling, cosmetics and magazines. Sex and/or gender identity are potential individual variables that may impact on the extent to which a marketing effort will be successful.

Opportunities for marketing health to men

In recent years the food industry has recognised the opportunity for marketing health to women. Women, after all, are responsible for 82% of consumer goods spending (Business Insights, 2005). They are also involved more in food selection and choice than men (Guthrie et al., 1995).

It has been argued that certain products are 'gendered'. While some products are linked to biological sex (e.g. feminine hygiene products), others have a feminine or masculine image that is not necessarily connected to biological sex (for example, dieting products) (Gainer, 1994). Most commercial diets and weight loss services are designed for women (see Chapter 10). Top gender-targeted weight loss products such as meal replacements and diet foods, health drinks and energy drinks reveal that gender targeting tends to fit with products with health benefits.

Gender does have a role to play in food choice. In a study by Glanz et al. (1998) women rated the importance of taste, nutritional value, cost and weight control impact in food products more highly than men.

While food products are marketed to men, the range of products aimed at men is quite different. This could be due to the fact that overweight men think they are healthier, more attractive and report higher levels of satisfaction than overweight women (McCreary and Sadava, 2001).

The food industry capitalises on gender differences and attempts to build our loyalty to specific brands through skilful advertising and promotion. In the area of sport and fitness-based foods and drinks the industry directs more of its targeting at male consumers. Sports drinks, for example, are aimed more at men, with campaigns using attractive, male celebrity sports professionals, the impression being that men are physically active more for their appearance than their health.

Other strategies for targeting consumers include gender exclusion strategies. One specific product aimed at men was the 2001 Yorkie *'It's Not For Girls'* campaign. The rationale behind the campaign was that there are not many things a man can look at and say that it is for him. The 'Not For Girls' campaign theme used humour, which the company felt appealed to the British male, and positioned Yorkie as a chocolate bar for men who need a satisfying hunger buster. With five solid chunks of chocolate, it's man sized!

Different attitudes towards health between the genders can equally lead to gender inclusion strategies. In one example Pepsi attempted to overcome the stigma attached to men dieting by formulating diet drinks which did not have the word 'diet' in the brand name, such as Pepsi Max and Pepsi One.

In today's consumer world, food brands are perhaps one of the most powerful forces in shaping what we eat. The appeal of brands is far stronger than the influence of a nutrition label, health promotion tool or government guideline. The advertising of these brands offers a compelling array of desirable consumer goals and advantages, often in a gender-specific way: achievement and recognition (a male drinking a sports drink imitating celebrity professional athletes), status (the latest sports car) and social acceptance (a member of a Pepsi generation). Today's successful brands form a strong psychological bond between the food product and the consumer, strongly motivating purchase and brand loyalty.

Advertising and public relations executives are experts in utilising mass media to achieve a product's sales and profit objectives. Though public health specialists are often critical of the influence of these commercial messages they might benefit from borrowing some of the business practices of these advertisers and PR professionals.

One such approach is social marketing. The Department of Health is adopting a new social marketing campaign on obesity in 2007. But what is social marketing? It is *the application of commercial marketing techniques to the solution of social problems where the bottom line is behaviour change (see* the National Social Marketing website: www.nsms.org.uk/public/default.aspx). It involves *the analysis, planning, execution and evaluation of programmes designed to influence the voluntary behaviour of target audiences to improve their personal welfare and that of society.*

Social marketing can be used to soften public, corporation or government attitudes prior to legislation. While commercial marketing is typically trying to encourage people to do something, social marketing often discourages behaviours (e.g. smoking, overeating, child abuse). As with commercial marketing, social marketing requires a great deal of planning and sensitivity, and an in-depth knowledge of the target audience.

Social marketing campaigns need to be ethical, effective and of high quality. In developing these programmes, a comprehensive public health brief with clear goals and messages should be developed, and it is vital that all communications are pre-tested with the audience.

Knowledge of the audience is essential in encouraging weight loss in men. The

Centers for Disease Control and Prevention in the USA have found that segmenting the audience for obesity prevention means that you can design effective and efficient strategies tailored to the needs of each target segment. In a sample population of almost 4,000 men and women, they clustered their behaviour, media use, shopping habits and weight status. Men predominately fell into the group that has low motivation and little interest in change, with no behavioural intentions (Riehman, 2005).

Media and gender issues

Global communications are expanding and newspapers and television are no longer the sole sources of information. Competition in the media has increased dramatically over the past 30 years. Television has moved from terrestrial-based stations to satellite and now into digital. Before the 1980s most television advertising was mass marketed to a broadly diverse audience through a relatively small number of media outlets. Since then, advertisers and media firms have emphasised divisions between subpopulations. By partitioning consumers and speaking to them differently, advertisers hope to market more of their products. Products in turn have begun to take on a more direct association with what marketing professionals like to call 'lifestyle' differences.

The content of global communications has also evolved, particularly where diet and health stories are concerned. The last 10 years has seen an explosion in coverage. Patients no longer get all their medical knowledge from their doctors. Dieting advice is given out regularly in magazines, newspapers, TV, radio and via the internet. There are complex issues about the portrayal of obesity in the media which apply across genders.

Scientists themselves have become part of the media machine and are now more than ever encouraged to promote the results of their research. Journalists want attention-grabbing headlines and consumers want a quick fix for their excess weight. When it comes to diet and health research, research results are often not as straightforward as they appear in the press. Published studies on the same topic can vary enormously in terms of sample size (small, medium, large), demographics (age, gender), data (self-reported versus objectively measured information) and length (weeks, months, years). Study design is another critical factor. The gold standard – a randomised, double-blind, placebo-controlled trial – is considered the most reliable because neither the researchers nor participants know who is on the diet or taking the medication or taking the placebo. Nevertheless the population is also becoming more sceptical, especially when successive trials give conflicting messages; the public perception is that scientists keep changing their minds.

While men are receiving more targeted media attention than ever before, this has not been optimised for diet and health messages. When *Loaded*, the original British lads' magazine, was launched in 1994 by IPC Magazines, now part of AOL Time Warner, it disproved the publishing dictum that there was no mainstream market for a general men's magazine. *Loaded*'s success spawned a gaggle of imitators: *FHM*, *Maxim* and *Men's Health*. *FHM*'s sales far outstripped those of *Cosmopolitan*, the leading British women's monthly. More recently the men's weekly magazine market has developed with the launch of *Nuts* and *Zoo*.

Research carried out by IPC showed that men wanted girls, football, conspiracy theories, jokes and reviews in their weekly magazines, leaving health and weight issues to the likes of dedicated titles such as *Men's Health* and *Men's Fitness*. Women's magazine, whether they focus on cookery, celebrity lifestyles or fashion, regularly include diet and health information. Men are losing out as the opportunity for gender-specific health messages in all publications, male-targeted or not, is being missed.

What can health professionals learn?

Few gender-specific campaigns are currently being run in obesity. However, with the interest in social marketing developing in the health and nutrition fields a number of case studies highlight how key concepts could be adapted to new campaigns on male obesity. The case studies demonstrate the range of issues that health professionals should be aware of in developing programmes to combat male obesity.

The US National Institute of Mental Health ran a campaign to educate the public about depression in men (http://menanddepression.nimh.nih.gov). The target audience was male depression sufferers and their families. The objectives were to increase public awareness of depression in men, to educate men to recognise, acknowledge, and seek treatment for their depression, and to encourage their families to detect depressive symptoms.

Taking a new approach of men talking directly to other men, the Institute worked with a distinguished documentary film-maker, Leslie Wiener. He filmed men as they spoke candidly about their experiences with depression (including a retired US Air Force First Sergeant, a firefighter, a writer, a publisher, a national diving champion, a lawyer, a police officer, a student, and others) to produce public service announcements for television, radio and print. A fact sheet for healthcare providers with information on screening for depression in primary care settings, including co-occurring conditions, as well as treatment options, was developed. The fact sheet gave details on how to use the two new screening questions from the US Preventive Services Task Force in conjunction with additional symptoms of depression.

This campaign was a good example of a government-led campaign that was effective in changing behaviour and improving health. In particular it shows how successful campaigns have secured the buy-in of health professionals by providing them with resources and materials to support their work.

Stop Aids is one of the longest running and most carefully evaluated social marketing programmes for AIDS prevention in the world. Based in Switzerland, the campaign was aimed at homosexual men. Its objectives were to increase condom use among Switzerland's at-risk groups, decrease discrimination against individuals with HIV/AIDS, and increase solidarity among the infected, and between those infected and the general population. The mechanics of the campaign included organising community groups. A special 'Hot Rubber' condom brand was created for gay men and new distribution points opened throughout the country for condoms, for counselling and for testing. Advertising appeared on billboards, in printed ads (newspapers, tabloids, magazines, student newspapers), on television, on radio, in movie theatre commercials and at sporting events. The campaign used a positive message promoting individual awareness and self-determination and avoided imposing a judgemental or moralistic view on any particular behaviour. This was seen as an effective way to address the socially sensitive subjects of sexuality and illicit drug use, while encouraging safe prevention habits.

The results demonstrated changes in the market for condoms. This was the central focus of the campaign and one of the key factors used to measure the programme's impact on the population. The sales of manufacturers supplying at least 80% of condoms in Switzerland were monitored and showed that between 1986 and 1990 condom sales increased by 80%, from 7.6 million to 15 million units (Dubois-Arber *et al.*, 2003).

This example shows how a campaign can be used to target specific health messages at men. It also illustrates that there is a role for industry in health-related social marketing programmes and that they can influence the supply chain.

The final case study concerns a UK-based initiative to encourage waist loss in men. The target audience was overweight and obese males and the objective was to encourage men to reduce their waistline by signing up to a 12-week programme at www.fatmanslim.com.

The initiative involved the development of a waist-loss kit on the internet, which featured downloadable advice from a male GP, talking the participant through the plan, which largely consisted of dietary and exercise advice. Media support throughout consisted of feature articles in mainstream and regional press.

This initiative was not overly commercial, was sensitive to the needs of the audience and was goal orientated. Because it was co-ordinated by a health professional, it supports the view that health-related social marketing programmes should be developed by credible, independent influencers who have expertise and public trust.

A new social marketing campaign looking at healthy living was launched by the Department of Health in 2007. It aims to provide a backdrop for initiatives that will improve the healthiness of people's lifestyles in the areas of diet and physical activity. It is being delivered in partnership with a wide range of organisations, including the food and leisure industries. The team responsible is currently developing a 10-year programme of national activity which began in early 2007. The first three years, 2007–10, will focus on children aged between 2 and 10 and importantly their parents and carers. The period 2010–13 will use the platform of the 2012 Olympics to provide inspiration for a fitter Britain. Details of the final stage, 2013–16, have not yet been released.

Summary

Obesity and being overweight continues to be a serious public health problem, rooted in three main areas: excess food, absences of controlling food behaviour and lack of physical activity (Jebb, 2005). This problem cannot be resolved by any single cause-and-effect solution. There is a real need for co-operation between the mass media, the food industry and health professionals to communicate appropriate messages to the general public. We need to find ways of talking to men about their weight in a way that men can hear. Health professionals need to consider the implications of their work with men as individuals but also to exploit media opportunities to get appropriate health messages across to men. Our aim should be a better understanding of the issues and challenges that have to be overcome in order to communicate the information men need to change their behaviour.

References

Business Insights. *Gender Marketing Strategies in Food and Drinks. Future opportunities, best practice innovation and NPD.* London: Business Insights; 2005.

Dubois-Arber F, Jeannin A, Meystre-Agustoni G *et al. Evaluation of the AIDS-prevention Strategy in Switzerland. Seventh summary report 1999–2003.* Lausanne: IUMSP; 2003. p. 21.

Gainer B. An empirical investigation of the role of involvement with a gendered product. *Psychology & Marketing.* 1994; **11**(2): 163–82.

Glanz K, Basil M, Maibach E *et al.* Why Americans eat what they do: taste, nutrition, cost, convenience, and weight control concerns as influences on food consumption. *Journal of the American Dietetic Association.* 1998; **98**: 1118–26.

Guthrie JF, Fox JJ, Cleveland LE, Welsh S. Who uses nutrition labelling, and what effect does label use have on diet quality? *Journal of Nutrition Education.* 1995; **27**: 163–72.

Jebb SA. Dietary strategies for the prevention of obesity. *Proceedings of the Nutrition Society.* 2005; **64**(2): 217–27.

McCreary DR, Sadava SW. Gender differences in relationships among perceived attractiveness, life satisfaction, and health in adults as a function of body mass index and perceived weight. *Psychology of Men and Masculinity.* 2001; **2**: 108–16.

Riehman K. Identification of audience segments for obesity prevention: results from a national market research database. Proceedings of the 15th Annual Social Marketing in Public Health Conference; 2005 June 15–18; Clearwater Beach, Florida.

Zaman F, Underwood C. *The Gender Guide for Health Communication Programs.* Baltimore, MD: John Hopkins Bloomberg School of Public Health/Centre for Communication Programs; 2003.

CHAPTER 6

Men, masculinities and health

Brendan Gough

In light of the concern about rising obesity in men, and about the men's health 'crisis' more generally, it seems reasonable to posit a role for 'masculinity'. In other words, there must be something about the way men are, or the way men are expected to behave, which makes men adopt unhealthy practices and remain fairly disinterested in their health. For example, men's diets traditionally centre around red meat, bulk, and large portions (Gough and Conner, 2006), and when the male propensity to consume alcohol is factored in, along with contemporary trends such as increasingly sedentary lifestyles, then it is small wonder that more men are becoming fat. And when men suffer health problems such as obesity, a masculine reluctance to admit vulnerability means that few men will seek professional help and/or will be deterred by the feminised healthcare system – in a recent survey of male patients the GP's surgery was likened to a 'woman's hairdressing salon' (see Gough, 2006).

However, it is argued here that masculinity cannot simply be reduced to a set of attributes or practices which all men adhere to, as if hardwired by biological entities such as hormones, genetics or brain composition. Instead, this chapter presents masculinity as socially constructed, multifaceted and complex, and argues against a facile relationship between masculinity and men's relatively poor health. I hope to show that masculinity is defined and enacted in various ways across different contexts, and that other factors such as social class, race and age influence the construction of masculinity and, in turn, men's health practices. What follows then is a review of the key contributions and debates around masculinity within recent social science literature. The implications for men's health, including the problem of obesity in men, are also discussed.

Multiple masculinities

Perhaps the first and obvious point to make is that 'masculinity' cannot be distilled into one all-encompassing dimension. If one were to ask a group of people for definitions of masculinity, no doubt several different aspects would be identified. This is what psychologists actually do when constructing questionnaires so that the full range of meanings around a given object can be gleaned and then clustered into 'factors'. For example, a classic measure of gender identity is the Bem Sex Role Inventory (BSRI – Bem, 1974), which contains several items and subscales which load on to the masculinity factor. Here are some of the items designated 'masculine' in the BSRI:

- acts as a leader
- aggressive
- ambitious
- analytical
- assertive
- athletic
- competitive
- dominant
- independent
- makes decisions
- willing to take risks.

Although some of these items are related, it is clear that 'masculinity' is considered to be multi-dimensional. Moreover, since women as well as men can score on 'masculinity' with this scale, 'masculinity' becomes divorced from biological sex. Indeed, Bem advocated that an 'androgynous' orientation was optimal for both men and women, i.e. exhibiting both 'masculine' and 'feminine' attributes was beneficial for psychological health. Although this work has been criticised on several grounds, such as its individualism and failure to account for the differential status accorded to masculine and feminine attributes within wider society, it has made an important historical contribution to the social psychology of gender. More recent work by feminist and social science scholars has developed our understanding of the social construction of masculinity and has illustrated how masculinity is conceived and practised by different groups across time and place, including research on working class masculinity (Tolson, 1977), managerial masculinity (Collinson and Hearn, 1996), female masculinity (Halberstam, 1998), and gay masculinity (Nardi, 2000).

The social science literature on 'men's studies', which has mushroomed in the last 20 years or more (Connell, 1995; Connell and Messerschmidt, 2005; Edley and Wetherell, 1995; Kimmel, 1987), rejects the biologistic notion that all men possess an 'essential' or 'natural' masculinity, in favour of a conceptualisation of masculinity as pluralistic (hence 'masculinities') and complex, whereby discrete masculinities exist in an intricate and sometimes conflictual relationship. To illustrate, a distinction can be drawn between traditional or conventional masculinities (e.g. the male breadwinner) and 'new' or 'contemporary' masculinities (e.g. the modern involved father) (see Pleck, 1987).

Both models of masculinity, old and recent, co-exist and impact on the lives of men by increasing the choices – and pressures – associated with being a working father. Another example: men are now targeted as consumers of beauty products and services, something unthinkable even 20 years ago, although the advertising of moisturiser and related items for men panders to 'masculine' values by featuring muscular torsos and/or male icons such as famous sportsmen. In this way, both old and new masculinities are co-presented, and to be a man today often involves attending to and incorporating aspects of both conventional and current ideals of masculinity (see Gill *et al.*, 2005).

With this in mind, the overweight or obese man occupies a vexed masculine position, since a large appetite and physical stature have long been regarded as masculine, but then again a lean but muscular physique is now favoured, as are sporting or physical activities (e.g. weight training) and image-consciousness. Arguably, in the current health- and beauty-aware consumerist climate, heavy men are increasingly pathologised and ostracised – and under increasing pressure from health promotion agencies and society generally to lose weight. Let us now turn to the theoretical literature on masculinities to develop our understanding and contextualise the debates about men's health and obesity.

'Hegemonic masculinities'

The seminal sociological work of Bob (now Raewyn) Connell (e.g. 1995) emphasises that one cannot simply choose and adopt those masculine ideals and activities which appear attractive. Just as our choice of products in the supermarket is limited by finances and product availability, our choices as men are constrained by social and cultural context, by the particular versions of masculinity which prevail locally. For example, academic achievement may be more valued in boys and men from affluent, professional backgrounds while sporting prowess may be more prized within working-class communities. Clearly this is a somewhat stereotypical claim, and we must take care to avoid generalisations about masculinity based on class or group membership. Moreover, that social class location does not determine one's masculinity is manifest by the influence of other intersecting identities, whether pertaining to race, sexual orientation, age or dis/ability. Fathers and sons, for example, may well look to different sources for constructing masculine identities.

Another layer of complexity is contributed by institutionally based ideologies, not least within the feminised culture of health, but also within other institutional locales such as education, work, law and sport. But it would be shortsighted to assume that institutions are monolithic and homogeneous, since complexity and contradictions are apparent. For example, medicine and health, despite being saturated with feminised ideals such as care and support at ground level, nonetheless prizes masculinised norms such as competitiveness, autonomy and job immersion in definitions of successful medical careers. Of course such gendered hierarchies have serious implications for the progression of women in medicine (see Kilminster *et al.*, 2007).

Notwithstanding myriad influences on masculinity, it is likely that in any given social context one definition of masculinity will prevail – what Connell terms 'hegemonic masculinity'. For example, men who identify as heterosexual generally occupy a privileged position relative to other (homosexual) men and women. In turn, heterosexuality is traditionally defined in masculinised ways, with an emphasis on phallocentric sex (culminating in male penetration), male activity and female passivity, male promiscuity and female fidelity (see Hollway, 1989). Of course, not all heterosexual men would identify with or enact such norms, and it should be possible for men and women to negotiate more egalitarian sexual interactions, or indeed for women to take up more dominant and assertive sexual stances, depending on the context.

Arguably, however, conventionally gendered heterosexual scripts continue to dominate media and popular culture and influence how men (and women) engage in sexual interactions and relationships. Indeed, various studies have shown how men (and women) continue to reproduce notions of sex difference which position men more favourably, whether as more rational, physically stronger, or as having more rights to public consumption. For example, Gough (1998) showed how male university students positioned women as biologically weaker and less fit for certain occupations such as aviation and the military. Similarly, a study by Willott and Griffin (1997) showed how long-term unemployed men, by earning money through 'unofficial' work, continued to define themselves as breadwinners and beer drinkers while construing childcare and domestic tasks as women's work.

The insults that boys and men hurl at each other whether at school, in work, on the sports ground or in the pub also serve to illustrate the tight policing of masculinity and its reliance on a (negative) relationship to the feminine. Thus males who profess disinterest in sport or who perform badly are routinely ridiculed as 'girls' (Messner, 1992) while men who do not drink (much) or, say, prefer gin to beer may be satirised as women (Gough and Edwards, 1998). This casual sexism is often overlayed with homophobic language, since gay men are constructed as effeminate within popular culture. So, males who reject sport and beer, or who take up feminised practices such as cooking or sewing, run the risk of being labelled as 'queers' or 'poofs', as well as girls (Gough, 2002). Hegemonic masculinities then are in part predicated on, and serve to reinforce, the oppression of women and gay men (and other men). It is also worth emphasising that hegemonic masculinities cannot be reduced to language, since a whole range of practices are implied, including 'wage labour, violence, sexuality, domestic labour and childcare, as well as unreflective routinised actions' (Connell and Messerschmidt, 2005, p. 842).

The ability to take up and/or re-vision hegemonic masculinities will however be constrained by one's relative status, as determined by the social capital one enjoys, indicated by occupation, wealth, achievements, etc. Additionally, Connell asserts that hegemonic masculinities will be difficult for those men who are inscribed within 'marginalised' and 'subordinated' masculinities (Connell, 1995). Marginalised masculinities refer to those identities on the periphery, distant from the white, middle-class, heterosexual triplex which historically has defined and legitimised hegemonic masculinities. Thus men from minority ethnic backgrounds, from working-class communities and those identifying as gay may encounter barriers to accessing resources which enable the uptake of hegemonic masculinities. Moreover, there are men whose experiences and identity are marked out as unmasculine within hegemonic discourse, notably gay men. The homophobia and heterosexism which informs most versions of hegemonic masculinities actively renders gay men unacceptable and invisible. The oppression of such 'subordinated masculinities' operates on many levels, from physical violence to under-representation in high-status occupations and in popular culture.

In the arena of men's health, it is imperative that power and status differentials between men are recognised, and that variability between (and within) groups of men is taken into account when designing and targeting health promotion interventions. It comes as no surprise, for example, that gay men are more susceptible to mental health problems such as depression and suicide (Bagley and Tremblay, 2000). Equally, it is well established that working-class men are over-represented in statistics relating to serious illnesses such as heart disease and cancer, or that life expectancy varies markedly by class location – a 15-year difference between the poorest and most affluent parts of London (Department of Health, 2004). Clearly, one must consider economic and lifestyle factors here, and how practices such as heavy drinking, smoking and restricted diets function as locally valued indicators of masculine and class-based identities.

At the same time, it must also be recognised that the field of health, along with health promotion and self-help discourse, can be perceived as foreign and patronising by clients from deprived backgrounds. For example, an interesting analysis of self-help books on men's health (Singleton, 2003) identified a neo-conservative ideology which constructs individual men as responsible for attaining good health and well-being. Singleton argues that this individualist rhetoric favours middle-class men and neglects the influence of social factors such as class and race on health status. More generally, the health promotion model of individuals as autonomous rational information processors who simply need to be educated to change their unhealthy ways must be challenged in order to facilitate collective, community-based interventions which take into account the social contexts in which people live (see Crossley, 2000; Murray, 2004).

Redefining masculinities

However, we must be careful not to lapse into a view of power and powerlessness as group or class-based. As Foucault (1980) has amply demonstrated, power is not possessed by individuals or groups; rather it is fluid, negotiable and dynamic. Hegemony is open to critique, and Foucault also emphasised resistance to power and social change. Whether a man has access to greater wealth, seniority or physical stature relative to other men will not always guarantee the upper hand. While men in professional occupations can enjoy numerous material and cultural benefits associated with their status, men who are plumbers, joiners and electricians attain hegemony in their particular spheres, and increasingly can compete with professional men with respect to income and investments.

The same point applies to other categories of difference such as age and sexual orientation. For example, while younger staff may well feel intimidated by senior staff in the working environment, older men may feel more alienated at the company Christmas party in a dance club. Similarly, some gay men may feel vulnerable at a company event where partners are invited, whereas some heterosexual men may feel uncomfortable in a 'gay' pub. So, it would be churlish to locate power once and for all with particular men or forms of masculinity, or to separate out masculinity from the other social identities that men subscribe to, or from the particular social context where masculinity is enacted.

And yet, hegemonic masculinities can be difficult to challenge because although sometimes reinforced by brute force, as in the violent oppression of women and men deemed unmasculine, power is more often retained through ideological domination – in other words, through the construction of favoured masculinities as normal or natural and the (often subtle) depiction of women and other men as inferior or il-legitimate. In my own work, for example, I have drawn attention to the discursive othering of women and gay men by male middle-class heterosexual university students (Gough, 1998, 2002). A classic formulation, originally identified in studies of racism (see Billig, 1988), is to preface a hearably prejudiced statement with a disclaimer, as in 'I'm not sexist but ... women should not be allowed to fly planes'. This discursive work by male research participants is clearly designed to manage potential accusations of prejudice and present the speaker as liberal and tolerant. Variations on this theme include citing evidence of 'insider' knowledge, as in 'Some of my best friends are gay' and disclaiming personal stake, as in 'Personally I'm not bothered but ... others will be offended'. For more discussion of prejudiced discourse see Wetherell and Potter (1992) and Speer and Potter (2000). So, this manner of demonising others upholds hegemonic masculinities in indirect, and arguably more effective, ways. With the focus on 'others' such as women and gay men, hegemonic masculinities remain unmarked and unproblematic.

This analysis ties in with Connell's notion of 'complicity', which suggests that men do not have to actively adopt crude or aggressive hegemonic practices, especially if they enjoy high status positions, since authority can be retained without resorting to blatant power plays. Indeed, in contemporary culture there has been something of a rejection of straightforwardly macho performances, aligned with concessions towards the feminine – a hero is now permitted to display vulnerability (as long as he saves the day and gets the girl), a footballer may cry after a crucial defeat (or victory), and men can wear hairbands with relative impunity (that is, if they are suitably macho in other departments). In the context of men's health, Gough (2007) notes that men are increasingly included in media features on diet and health, but in ways which critique 'fad' (read 'feminine') diets and recuperate cooking and food as masculine domains à la Gordon Ramsay.

Paradoxically, Wetherell and Edley (1999) have suggested that citing distance from hegemonic ideals, such as macho masculinity, can work to reinforce other hegemonic ideals such as male autonomy and choice. Most men in their study referred to themselves as 'ordinary' or 'average' rather than macho, while some additionally construed themselves as 'rebellious' through reference to feminised practices such as sewing. However, both ordinary and rebellious positions draw upon recognisably masculinised ideals: the independent rational thinker in the first case, and the romantic non-conformist in the second. In a similar vein, feminists have long argued that men have not really changed much at all, and that masculinity has simply been repackaged rather than radically reinvented. For example, men may be more involved in parenting, but their involvement constitutes baby entertainment more than the serious business of childcare (Sunderland, 2000).

In other contexts, it would appear that hegemonic masculinities deliberately reject any semblance of femininity, but these masculinities are not played straight; instead, they are vividly overblown and framed 'ironically'. The exaggerated masculinity of 'new laddism' encapsulated in mass-market male-targeted magazines (most recently *Nuts* and *Zoo*), and comprising a strict diet of beer, football and semi-naked women, is routinely defended on grounds of 'fun' and 'irony', i.e. the features are not meant to be taken seriously (see Benwell, 2004). From a men's health perspective, the tragedy here is that such magazines could easily run articles on health issues relevant to their young male readership, including the dangers of unsafe sex, binge drinking and poor diet. Even magazines ostensibly concerned with the health of men, such as *Men's Health*, proffer a different agenda on close inspection based around strength training, muscularity and restricted diet (Labre, 2005; Stibbe, 2004).

It has also been argued that attempts at men's health promotion in the media also rely on stereotypes of masculinity (e.g. Gough, 2006; Lyons and Willott, 1999). For example, Gough's (2006) analysis of a men's health supplement (2005) provided by the *Observer* newspaper highlighted a tendency to present men and masculinity as homogenous, implying that all men were unhealthy and naive, while announcing 'male-friendly' initiatives such as work-based programmes as the solution to the men's health 'crisis', thereby reinforcing hegemonic masculinities and absolving men from proactively changing themselves. So, across a range of contexts from men's health to men's magazines it would seem that hegemonic masculinities, whether reworked to incorporate feminised practices, performed ironically, or reproduced 'straight', remain powerful. Whatever the content of a particular version of hegemonic masculinity, it is a construct which can be flexibly and creatively mobilised in different situations to fulfil different functions.

Masculine biographies

From a psychological perspective, however, it is not enough to appreciate the social location of men and the social construction of masculinities. What is also required is insight into the life histories and lifestyles of *individual* men. A psychosocial approach (Hollway and Jefferson, 2000) can help us to understand why two men from similar social backgrounds may differ markedly in terms of masculine identities and health practices. Why does one man like to drink beer and fight on a Saturday night while his neighbour and peer prefers to drink wine and watch a film? A psychosocial approach therefore cautions against social determinism, i.e. reading masculinity off social categories such as class and race.

Conversely, a slide into psychological reductionism must be avoided, since individuals do not simply choose their identities, at least not freely, but are embedded in particular personal, interpersonal, social and cultural contexts which will influence and constrain any choices made. For example, it is likely that, regardless of similarities in class or race, a man raised without a father will adopt different masculine practices to a man whose father was distant, or compared to another whose father was aggressive, or another whose father was loving. So, masculine identities and practices are in part shaped by a man's personal biography, including early family relationships, peer interactions, school experiences and leisure choices.

Using psychoanalytic concepts, it can also be argued that the uptake of hegemonic masculinities fundamentally involves psychic division and conflict, since hegemonic masculinities are predicated on an unconscious repression and suppression of the feminine (see Gough, 2004; Segal, 1990). So, not only is the social construction of masculinity based (partly) on a rejection of the feminine, but at the level of the individual there is an emotional disinvestment in the maternal and feminine from an early age and a concerted effort to emulate the masculine father figure. Whether one accepts Freud's Oedipal story or not, it is undeniable that social institutions, including the family, perpetuate conventional gender relations and place taboos on 'gender-inappropriate' behaviour.

Essentially, the psychoanalytic perspective reminds us that a preoccupation with only the masculine (or feminine) is an irrational, defensive posture which can entail difficult choices, regrets and personal costs. For example, in a fascinating case study of the former world heavyweight boxing champion Mike Tyson, Jefferson (1998) draws attention to the psychosocial environment which facilitated Tyson's transformation from 'fairy boy' to 'destroyer', citing bullying, father absence and a defensive desire to locate and banish weakness outside of himself. Jefferson uses Kleinian concepts such as splitting and projection to explain Tyson's aggressive response to extreme psychic anxiety engendered by a harsh childhood. By splitting off 'weakness' from himself and placing it elsewhere, Tyson is able to contain the problem through violent suppression. But, as is well known, Tyson's violence spilled over to other arenas, resulting in assorted violent crimes including rape, all pointing to a desperate, ongoing, and unresolved conflict about masculine identity.

Although the example of Mike Tyson is a rather dramatic instance of male insecurity despite (or because of) hegemonic masculinities adopted, it can be argued that the difficulty many men have with expressing emotion (other than anger) and communicating openly about vulnerability stems from a similar obsession with maintaining masculinity and avoiding any semblance of femininity. Since perceived invulnerability, pain endurance and hardness are bound up in most definitions of hegemonic masculinity, the obvious costs in terms of men's health are obvious. To publicly declare oneself as suffering pain and proceeding to seek help is, for many men, an admission of weakness, which is why so many men report symptoms at advanced stages of a disease or do not present until a serious medical emergency ensues (Kapur *et al.*, 2004).

Conclusion

It should be clear that masculinity is a complex social construct, mediated by a range of cultural, situational and personal influences. It also follows that the relationship between hegemonic masculinities and men's health practices is complicated, and that much more research is required to unravel links between men's identities and health-related activities. In considering this relationship, we must take care not to lump all men together and assume that men as a group always and everywhere remain disinterested in their health. Although the evidence base is sparse (Lee and Owens, 2002), there are some examples of men taking care of themselves, especially in dedicated environments such as anonymous helplines and male-only clinics (see White and Cash, 2005). Nor must we presume that masculinity is inherently health-defeating, since masculinised practices such as sports participation and manual labour convey tangible health benefits, including tackling obesity, in an age of indolence. As I have argued, masculinity is a convoluted construct which may be deployed flexibly to fulfil a range of goals, often to the detriment of men's health – but not always. More research is required to investigate the relationship between masculinities and health-relevant practices and outcomes so that more effective health promotion interventions can be designed for men.

References

Bagley C, Tremblay P. Elevated rates of suicide behaviour in gay, lesbian and bisexual youth. *Crisis*. 2000; **21**(3): 111–17.

Bem SL. The measurement of psychological androgyny. *Journal of Consulting and Clinical Psychology*. 1974; **42**: 155–62.

Benwell B. Ironic discourse. Evasive masculinity in men's lifestyle magazines. *Men & Masculinities*. 2004; **7**(1): 3–21.

Billig M. The notion of prejudice: some rhetorical and ideological aspects. *Text*. 1988; **8**: 91–110.

Collinson DL, Hearn J, editors. *Men as Managers, Managers as Men: critical perspectives on men, masculinities and managements*. London: Sage; 1996.

Connell RW. *Masculinities*. Cambridge: Polity; 1995.

Connell RW, Messerschmidt JW. Hegemonic masculinity: rethinking the concept. *Gender & Society*. 2005; **19**(6): 829–59.

Crossley ML. *Rethinking Health Psychology*. Buckingham: Open University Press; 2000.

Department of Health. *Choosing Health: making healthier choices easier*. London: Department of Health; 2004.

Edley N, Wetherell N. *Men in Perspective. Practice, power and identity*. Hemel Hempstead: Prentice Hall/ Harvester Wheatsheaf; 1995.

Foucault M. *Power/Knowledge*. Sussex: Harvester Press; 1980.

Gill R, Henwood K, McLean C. Body projects and the regulation of normative masculinity. *Body & Society*. 2005; **11**(1): 37–62.

Gough B. Men and the discursive reproduction of sexism: repertoires of difference and equality. *Feminism & Psychology*. 1998; **8**(1): 25–49.

Gough B. 'I've always tolerated it but …': heterosexual masculinity and the discursive reproduction of homophobia. In: Coyle A, Kitzinger C, editors. *Lesbian and Gay Psychology*. Oxford: BPS Books/ Blackwell; 2002.

Gough B. Psychoanalysis as a resource for understanding emotional ruptures in the text: the case of defensive masculinities, *British Journal of Social Psychology*. 2004; **43**(2): 245–67.

Gough B. Try to be healthy, but don't forgo your masculinity: deconstructing men's health discourse in the media. *Social Science & Medicine*. 2006; **63**: 2476–88.

Gough B. 'Real men don't diet': an analysis of contemporary newspaper representations of men, food and health. *Social Science & Medicine*. 2007; **64**(2): 326–37.

Gough B, Conner MT. Barriers to healthy eating among men: a qualitative analysis. *Social Science & Medicine*. 2006; **62**(1): 387–95.

Gough B, Edwards G. The beer talking: four lads, a carry out and the reproduction of masculinities. *The Sociological Review*. 1998; **46**(3): 409–35.

Halberstam J. *Female Masculinity*. Durham, NC: Duke University Press; 1998.

Hollway W. *Subjectivity and Method in Psychology: gender, meaning and science*. London: Sage; 1989.

Hollway W, Jefferson T. *Doing Qualitative Research Differently. Free association, narrative and the interview method*. London: Sage; 2000.

Jefferson T. Muscle, 'hard men' and 'iron' Mike Tyson: reflections on desire, anxiety and the embodiment of masculinity. *Body & Society*. 1998; **4**(1): 103–18.

Kapur N, Hunt I, Lunt M *et al.* Psychosocial and illness related predictors of consultation rates in primary care – a cohort study. *Psychological Medicine.* 2004; **34**: 719–28.

Kilminster S, Downes J, Gough B, Murdoch-Eaton D, Roberts T. Women in medicine – is there a problem? A literature review of the changing gender composition, structures and occupational cultures in medicine. *Medical Education;* 2007; **41**: 39–48.

Kimmel M, editor. *Changing Men: new directions in research on men and masculinity.* Beverly Hills, CA: Sage; 1987.

Labre MP. Burn fat, build muscle: a content analysis of *Men's Health* and *Men's Fitness. International Journal of Men's Health.* 2005; **4**(2): 187–200.

Lee C, Owens RG. *The Psychology of Men's Health.* Buckingham: Open University Press; 2002.

Lyons A, Willott S. From suet pudding to superhero: representations of men's health for women. *Health.* 1999; **3**(3): 283–302.

Messner M. *Power at Play: sports and the problem of masculinity.* Boston, MA: Beacon; 1992.

Murray M, editor. *Critical Health Psychology.* Basingstoke: Palgrave; 2004.

Nardi PM, editor. *Gay Masculinities.* Thousand Oaks, CA: Sage; 2000.

Pleck J. American fathering in historical perspective. In: Kimmel MS, editor. *New Directions in Research on Men and Masculinities.* Englewood Cliffs, NJ: Prentice Hall; 1987.

Segal L. *Slow Motion: changing masculinities, changing men.* London: Virago; 1990.

Singleton A. 'Men's bodies, men's selves': men's health self-help books and the promotion of health care. *International Journal of Men's Health.* 2003; **2**(1): 57–73.

Speer S, Potter J. The management of heterosexist talk: conversational resources and prejudiced claims. *Discourse & Society.* 2000; **11**(4): 543–72.

Stibbe A. Health and the social construction of masculinity in *Men's Health* magazine. *Men and Masculinities.* 2004; 7(1): 31–51.

Sunderland J. Baby entertainer, bumbling assistant and line manager: discourses of fatherhood in parentcraft texts. *Discourse & Society.* 2000; **11**: 249–74.

Tolson A. *The Limits of Masculinity.* London: Tavistock; 1977.

Wetherell M, Edley N. Negotiating hegemonic masculinity: imaginary positions and psycho-discursive practices. *Feminism & Psychology.* 1999; **9**(3): 335–57.

Wetherell M, Potter J. *Mapping the Language of Racism: discourse and the legitimation of exploitation.* Hemel Hempstead: Harvester Wheatsheaf; 1992.

White A, Cash K. *Report on the First Phase of a Study on Men's Usage of the Bradford Health of Men Services.* Leeds: Leeds Metropolitan University; 2005.

Willott S, Griffin C. 'Wham, bam, am I a man?' Unemployed men talk about masculinities. *Feminism & Psychology.* 1997; **7**(1): 107–28.

PART 2

Tackling male weight problems

CHAPTER 7

Managing male obesity in primary care

Caroline Gunnell

As I write this chapter all primary care trusts (PCTs) in England are experiencing the largest organisational change in the history of the National Health Service. 'Commissioning a Patient Led Service' was introduced by the Department of Health in 2005 and its aim is to ensure that GPs deliver better local services for patients.

In 2004 the Quality and Outcomes Framework (QOF) was introduced as part of the new General Medical Services contract for general practice. The QOF provides financial rewards to general practices for the provision of high quality care. This is intended to benefit both patients and the NHS. For example, PCTs should see a reduction in the number of avoidable hospital admissions through improved chronic disease management. The QOF rewards practices for the provision of quality care, and helps to fund further improvements in the delivery of clinical care.

Participation by practices in the QOF is voluntary, but many practices with Personal Medical Services (PMS) contracts, as well as most practices on General Medical Services (GMS) contracts, are participating in the QOF. For participating practices, the QOF measures practice achievement against a range of evidence-based clinical indicators and against a range of indicators covering practice organisation and management. Practices score points according to their levels of achievement against these indicators, and practice payments are calculated from points achieved.

Obesity is not addressed specifically in the QOF and at present all that is required is that practices collect BMIs on new registration adult patients. At the moment measurements on children are not required; waist:hip ratios are not requested; and there is nothing in place to encourage obesity prevention work for long-term conditions management. It really is quite worrying to see how far we still have to go in general practice. It might be more beneficial if a GP's payment package were related more sensibly to public health priorities, either linked to the QOF or some other funding system.

These organisational changes – and many others in recent years – have not deterred primary care clinicians from developing strategies to address the growing obesity concern. The long-awaited obesity guidelines from the National Institute for Health and Clinical Excellence (NICE) were published late in 2006 and are available from

NICE (www.nice.org.uk). They require practitioners to work in a far more co-ordinated fashion to tackle the obesity epidemic.

In relation to men and obesity the introduction of the Gender Equality Duty for all public services in 2007 will be an opportunity to address the lack of male-centred services more closely. The PCTs of the future will have immense potential to develop services which reduce the impact of obesity on men's health. It is now up to primary care practitioners to take the lead and provide services, specialist or generalist, which meet the need of the male populations they serve. Working as a team has never been more important.

It is true that there is a paucity of evidence relating to male obesity, but there is a wealth of evidence for the treatment of men and women, and children, with obesity in the primary care setting, especially so since the launch of the National Service Frameworks for diabetes (DoH, 1999), coronary heart disease (DoH, 2000) and children (DoH, 2004).

Some PCTs have developed their own strategies for tackling obesity; others have developed enhanced service agreements with GPs. Since the launch of *Commissioning a Patient Led Service* (DoH, 2005), PCTs have opportunities to fund 'contestable' services, which are set up slightly differently from the practice itself, or within a practice as a separate service. PCTs from now on will be commissioning services from a range of potentially innovative providers.

All this means that patients will have more and more opportunities to choose who they see for their weight problem. We need to ensure that the range of services, and point of service, on offer are configured in a way that meets men's needs.

Opportunities for men in primary care

Working in an evidence-based way, we should be listening to, and working alongside, public health practitioners to address the environmental factors that are influencing the obesity epidemic in men, and then developing new ways of engaging with men in the workplace, home, community and leisure environment. General practice could be the best place to initiate this exciting work, but not necessarily using the medical model of care. Nurses, pharmacists, dieticians and even members of the local community are well placed to be leading these services, within a carefully thought-out care pathway.

In this relatively new way of working, the responsibility for weight management should be owned by the man who wants to lose weight, and not, as has been historically the case, a paternalistic position taken by healthcare professionals, or a commercial one taken by a slimming clinic or weight loss service.

In no area is innovation needed more than in accessing those men who are obese due to poverty, mental health, and other environmental and social difficulties. We know it is always the more articulate men who manage to access services. Where are the others?

Overcoming barriers to men in primary care

The health behaviour of men has been discussed in Chapters 4 and 6. What is clear is that men's attitudes to their health and well-being influence if, when, and how men access and use primary healthcare. There are many fine examples of successful health promotion campaigns directed at men. Chapter 20 includes a range of projects which were set up in the community by a practice nurse, Jane DeVille-Almond. They ranged from a health clinic for men in a barber's shop to a weight loss mobile clinic at the Goodwood Festival of Speed.

However, projects like these are not necessarily known about or acknowledged within primary care, perhaps because they have been set up in the community, or in occupational health departments, industry or in private healthcare organisations. Because there are so few examples of successful campaigns for overweight men within general practices, the NHS does not record this valuable work or share it in a useful way. Perhaps it is now time to develop a forum for considering male weight problems in primary care, fostering new ways of thinking and new research projects in this setting.

The gender balance in healthcare practitioners has changed beyond recognition in the last 20 to 30 years. The medical profession in the 'old' Health Service was dominated by men. Did it hamper men coming forward, afraid of looking weak in front of another, powerful, man? Now that there are many female GPs, do they feel confident and well equipped to be addressing male health issues and engaging with men? What will the new breed of healthcare practitioner receive by way of training in gender-sensitive healthcare now that, within the 'duty of care' all clinicians by registration abide by, there will be a need to promote and practise gender-specific care?

Recently opening hours at most surgeries have become shorter and many practices are closed at weekends. This may mean that men with a weight issue have to take time off work to see their GP, and at the same time are forced into admitting to someone else, perhaps a boss or colleague, that the weight is a problem. This may seem acceptable to many women, but for men it may present a problem. We know that women are more used to having time out of work for medical reasons, are also more likely to share these with a friend or family member, and are used to seeking help from their local practice.

A further point is that obese men, as many authors in this book attest, seldom seem to see themselves as health risks. Thus they are not likely to see themselves as patients, even though their general practice will probably refer to them as such. Why would they want to be labelled as patients when, in their eyes, they are only 'slightly overweight', have been so for some time and they are not ill (yet). But as Kate Davidson explains in Chapter 13, it is unusual to see an obese 75-year-old in primary care. Obese men simply do not live to this age.

Management of obesity in primary care – recent studies

A report published by the Dr Foster organisation in 2005 identified that 49% of primary care organisations (PCOs) have not been involved in setting up weight management programmes and 69% of general practices have not established weight management clinics. As obesity is a primary threat to health in the UK, this is a worrying statistic. Furthermore, 76% of PCOs do not monitor the prevalence of obesity. PCO funding for obesity management services remains very low, on average just 0.33% of the annual baseline budget. A small percentage of PCOs still do not adhere to guidelines produced by NICE for drug therapy (3%) and surgery (19%) for the treatment of obesity.

Despite this gloomy picture there is no shortage of reports and guidelines focusing on the management of obesity in primary care. Much has been written about the treatment of childhood obesity in primary care, though not with a gender-specific outlook. For treating children, Jain's systematic review (2005) concludes that no interventions are really effective, although strategies that reduce sedentary behaviour (particularly television watching) and activities that involve parents show the most encouraging results (Campbell *et al.*, 2001; Centre for Reviews and Dissemination, 2002; Summerbell *et al.*, 2003).

The National Obesity Forum (NOF, 2004) has published guidelines on the management of adult weight problems in primary care, which clearly set out the groups to be treated, the first-line approach, dietary changes, other dietary options, drug treatment, and other therapies, which include behavioural therapy, referral to hospital obesity clinics and bariatric surgery. But these guidelines do not offer guidance on how to engage with men and manage male obesity.

One of the questions raised in the systematic review by Jain (2005) was whether any treatments worked. The review concluded that even with dietary and exercise treatments for adult obesity only modest weight loss is achieved (about 3.5 kg) compared with no treatment or usual care (Glenny *et al.*, 1997; Katz *et al.*, 2003; McTigue *et al.*, 2003). Weight loss drugs such as Sibutramine and Orlistat, used in conjunction with diet or exercise programmes, also produced 3–5 kg weight loss, but the effects did not often last after the drug was stopped (Haddock *et al.*, 2002; Lenz and Hamilton, 2004; McTigue *et al.*, 2003; Padwal *et al.*, 2003). Although the weight loss of 3–5 kg was statistically significant and had some health benefits (Kolotkin *et al.*, 2001) its clinical significance was not shown, i.e. it may not have been enough to improve the health or quality of life of patients. In most studies with long-term follow-up, the weight loss gradually came back. For patients with severe obesity, surgery was effective. Gastric surgery resulted in 25–44 kg weight loss up to two years after the operation, and 20 kg loss up to eight years later (Clegg *et al.*, 2003; Colquitt *et al.*, 2003).

The drug treatment of obesity has always been difficult to manage in primary care, due to some historic misuse of the early medications and therefore some hesitancy in prescribing at all for this condition. There is also the added barrier of lack of guidance and protocols for drug treatment, and the expense of the treatments to the primary care organisations.

With the help of the NICE guidelines on obesity (2006) some of these difficulties may be resolved, and with the strengthening of the medicine management depart-ments in PCTs, protocols for using anti-obesity drugs in primary care may become more widespread.

Only a few studies have assessed attempts to prevent obesity among adults, children or communities (Katz *et al.*, 2003). These were mostly educational campaigns aimed at individuals, sometimes including environmental changes such as altering food options in grocery stores or schools. None resulted in weight loss.

Another research project (Moore *et al.*, 2003) concluded that a training package promoting a brief, prescriptive approach to the treatment of obesity through lifestyle modification, intended to be incorporated in routine clinical practice, did not reduce the weight of this at-risk cohort of patients.

Determining if a man is overweight or obese

We already collect the body mass index of all our adult patients, though not necessarily very accurately. If we ask the patient how much they weigh and how tall they are, the accuracy of the data is questionable. In some practices this is what happens, with the pressures of time and 'hot-desking', and not locating where the scales and height chart are. In other practices there are excellent weight management clinics. The lack of equity of these services should be addressed by commissioners in the future. In the future it should be possible for all practices to have access to excellent weight management facilities.

But where exactly is the waist circumference? I recently overheard a conversation in which a GP maintained the waist measurement was the same as the trouser size! For men, trousers are often worn well below the fattest part of the waistline – the bit we should be measuring.

Some research by Canoy *et al.* (2004) on abdominal obesity and respiratory function shows that waist:hip ratio is a better indicator than body mass index in determining the role of obesity in predicting lung function. This research was carried out on white British men and women, and therefore this work may be less generalisable to other populations or ethnic groups.

How we monitor overweight men in our practice populations continues to be debated. What is clear is that we do need to gain agreement on the best way to measure men's weight, adopt the same method universally, and then provide facilities in every practice for these measurements to be taken accurately.

How can we engage with men on weight issues?

We need to be far more innovative and accessible in the way we engage with men. More and more men have access to computers, though this is by no means universally the case. The computer interface between the practice and its male population could be central to primary care communication strategies of the future. So many men nowadays would like to ask a simple, or what they may feel 'silly', question of a practitioner without having to leave their work environment, take time off, or tell their boss where they are going. There is a great opportunity for local primary care services to be able to chat to their male patients via email, and then use the appointments system and visiting time for those who need it. Further opportunities exist for practice websites to feature healthy men sections, discussion groups on obesity issues, and so forth.

The opportunities for school nurses, health visitors, pharmacists and other primary care practitioners to start addressing the male population have never been so numerous. As an example, a PMS scheme could be set up and nurse led, working alongside the local pharmacist and dietetics service, linking with educational packages, school dinner services and leisure centre facilities, all aiming their care at overweight and obese men and boys. A good model to refer to is the smoking cessation service in primary care. There may be lessons to learn from this. An audit of how many men this programme reached would be useful and how staff addressed the gender differences.

Overweight boys and teenagers present a special challenge. To identify those with high-risk obese parents is the first step. They could then be alerted, via an electronic alert system within the practice, at birth by health visitors/midwives, and school nurses for the family input. Practice nurses could pick this up at immunisation appointments and give lifestyle support.

The health and lifestyle of GPs and nurses may not provide a great role model for male patients and may need to be addressed by the practice themselves. The lack of occupational health for healthcare workers in the practice may also need to be addressed.

Setting up a new obesity service for men in primary care

Getting started
- Define the gender profile of patients in the practice (how many males to females) and the number of men in each age group.
- Search for males with a high BMI (overweight BMI 25–30, obese 30–40, morbidly obese over 40) and those who have never had any BMI measurements taken.
- Search for waist measurements in males – if recorded. Table 7.1 shows how waist measurement may indicate increased health risks.
- Implement waist measurement and BMI into new patient check templates and place an alert on those records that have not been done to ensure they are done at the next patient visit.
- Where possible record waist:hip measurements for male patients and locate those with a health risk (see Table 7.2).
- Search for men at particular risk of being overweight or obese: those with cancer in family, diabetes in family, cardiovascular disease (CVD). Develop a strategy within the practice to reach this group and monitor them.

Staff skills
- Identify level of interest in men and obesity within the practice team.
- Identify those who have had specific training in this area.
- Identify a lead for developing this service.
- Identify recognition for the lead and professional development needs.
- Develop multidisciplinary steering group with terms of reference.

Nurses are ideally placed to look after men with obesity and encourage them to make lifestyle changes through motivational support. Dieticians are the best people to provide dietary advice. Pharmacists can play a significant role in identifying men with a weight

TABLE 7.1 Waist measurements indicating increased health risks.

	Waist measurement larger than:	
Caucasian men	40 inches	101.6 centimetres
Asian men	36 inches	91.4 centimetres
Caucasian women	35 inches	88.9 centimetres
Asian women	32 inches	81.3 centimetres

TABLE 7.2 Waist:hip measurements indicating increased health risks.

Waist:hip ratio (WHR) for males	Health risk based solely on WHR
0.95 or less	Low risk
0.96 to 1.0	Moderate risk
1.0 or higher	High risk

problem who visit a pharmacy, perhaps for their medication or for other products they may purchase.

Develop a business case

- Identify the extent of male obesity locally by looking at national and local public health data.
- Map services already in place in the local area and investigate what is on offer. These could be NHS services, private or charitable organisations, commercial organisations.
- Look at the literature available on setting up obesity management services and identify which model would suit your practice population.
- Conduct a feasibility study of how you would set up a service, who would staff it, who would be targeted, where it would be located, what the service would offer, and what the desired outcomes are before you put a business case to the PCT for funding.
- Remember you must be offering something new, efficient and different, but feasible. Do not bite off more than you can chew. Start with a very simple service. It can develop over time with care and experience.

Evaluation and improvement of the service

The potential for evaluating the service should be in place from the start, using the initial audit as a baseline against which to measure achievements. Further audits of the service should be conducted at six-monthly intervals. The results of these audits should be shared with staff and lead into a planned approach to improve the service. This may mean further training, education of patients, relocation of premises, equipment monitoring and more.

References

Campbell K, Waters E, O'Meara S, Summerbell C. Interventions for preventing obesity in childhood. A systematic review. *Obes Rev.* 2001; **2**: 149–57.

Canoy D, Luben R, Welch A *et al.* Abdominal obesity and respiratory function in men and women in the EPIC-Norfolk Study, United Kingdom. *Am J Epidemiol.* 2004; **159**: 1140–9.

Centre for Reviews and Dissemination, University of York. The prevention and treatment of childhood obesity. *Eff Health Care.* 2002; **7**(6): 1–12.

Clegg A, Colquitt J, Sidhu M, Royle P, Walker A. Clinical and cost effectiveness of surgery for morbid obesity: a systematic review and economic evaluation. *Int J Obes Relat Metab Disord.* 2003; **27**: 1167–77.

Colquitt J, Clegg A, Sidhu M, Royle P. Surgery for morbid obesity. *Cochrane Database Syst Rev.* 2003; **2**: CD003641.

Department of Health. *National Service Framework for Diabetes.* 1999. www.dh.gov.uk/PolicyAndGuidance/HealthAndSocialCareTopics/Diabetes/fs/en (accessed 8 March 2007).

Department of Health. *National Service Framework for Coronary Heart Disease.* 2000. www.dh.gov.uk/PolicyAndGuidance/HealthAndSocialCareTopics/CoronaryHeartDisease/CoronaryArticle/fs/en?CONTENT_ID=4108602&chk=nf93gd (accessed 8 March 2007).

Department of Health. *National Service Framework for Children, Young People and Maternity Services.* 2004. www.dh.gov.uk/PolicyAndGuidance/HealthAndSocialCareTopics/ChildrenServices/ChildrenServicesInformation/fs/en (accessed 8 March 2007).

Department of Health. *Commissioning a Patient Led Service.* 2005. www.dh.gov.uk/PublicationsAndStatistics/Publications/PublicationsPolicyAndGuidance/PublicationsPolicyAndGuidance Article/fs/en?CONTENT_ID=4116716&chk=/%2Bb2QD (accessed 8 March 2007).

Dr Foster. *Primary Care Management of Adult Obesity.* 2005. www.drfoster.co.uk/library/reports/obesityManagement.pdf (accessed 8 March 2007).

Glenny AM, O'Meara S, Melville A, Sheldon TA, Wilson C. The treatment and prevention of obesity: a systematic review of the literature. *Int J Obes Relat Metab Disord.* 1997; **21**: 715–37.

Haddock CK, Poston WS, Dill PL, Foreyt JP, Ericsson M. Pharmacotherapy for obesity: a quantitative analysis of four decades of published randomised clinical trials. *Inst J Obes Relat Metab Disord.* 2002; **26**: 262–73.

Jain A. Treating obesity in individuals and populations. *BMJ.* 2005; **331**: 1387–90.

Katz DL, O'Connell ML, Yeh MC, Nawaz H. *Evidence-based Guidelines: obesity prevention and control.* Atlanta, GA: Centers for Disease Control and Prevention; 2003. GrantU48-CCU115802;10/00–8/03. Part of the study published as: Public health strategies for preventing and controlling obesity and overweight in school and worksite settings. *MMWR.* 2005; **54**(RR-10). The rest is available from the authors at www.yalegriffinprc.org (accessed 8 March 2007).

Kolotkin RL, Meter K, Williams GR. Quality of life and obesity. *Obes Rev.* 2001; **2**: 219–29.

Lenz TL, Hamilton WR. Supplemental products used for weight loss. *J Am Pharma Assoc (Wash DC).* 2004; **44**: 59–67.

McTigue KM, Harris R, Hemphill B *et al.* Screening and interventions for obesity in adults: summary of the evidence for the US Preventative Task Force. *Ann Intern Med.* 2003; **139**: 933–49.

Moore H, Summerbell CD, Greenwood DC *et al.* Improving management of obesity in primary care: cluster randomised trial. *BMJ.* 2003; **327**(7423): 1085.

National Institute for Health and Clinical Excellence (NICE). *Obesity: the prevention, identification, assessment and management of overweight and obesity in adults and children.* 2006. www.nice.org.uk (accessed 8 March 2007).

National Obesity Forum (NOF). www.nationalobesityforum.org.uk (accessed 8 March 2007).

Padwal R, Li SK, Lau DC. Long term pharmacotherapy for overweight and obesity: as systematic review and meta-analysis of randomised controlled trials. *Int J Obes Rel Metab Disord.* 2003; **27**: 1437–46.

Summerbell CD, Ashton V, Campell KJ, Edmunds L, Kelly S, Waters E. Interventions for treating obesity in children. *Cochrane Database Syst Rev.* 2003; **3**: CD001872.

CHAPTER 8

Working with men in groups – experience from a weight management programme in Scotland

Jim Leishman

Scotland has gained a reputation for having one of the poorest health records in Europe with a life expectancy for both men and women consistently lower than the rest of the UK and most of Europe. To compound this misery even further, Scotland – in common with other western nations – is facing a burgeoning of the problems associated with obesity. According to recent statistics Scottish children are getting larger and are now among the fattest in the western world, more overweight even, in some age groups, than our transatlantic cousins in America (NHS Quality Improvement Scotland, 2003).

In the home of the deep-fried Mars Bar, eating a healthy balanced diet full of fresh fruit and vegetables has never been a priority. In Scotland we have local chip shops meeting Scottish tastes by deep frying everything from the aforementioned Mars Bars to pizza and meat pies, always served with a generous portion of chips and washed down with sugary, gassy drinks. On the surface it appears that Scotland has a hard task ahead to shake off its reputation as the 'sick man of Europe'.

However, Scotland is awake to the problem, having introduced a range of initiatives aimed at turning the tide of physical inactivity and poor diet. Free fruit is provided for the very youngest school children and new nutritional standards have been set for school meals. In an attempt to get children physically fitter, activity co-ordinators have been introduced in schools and safer routes to schools developed to encourage children to walk or cycle more.

An investment of £4 million has also been made to support the development of men's health initiatives across the country. The aim of these was to promote healthier lifestyle choices among Scottish men, as well as to identify health problems at an early stage. In these initiatives men were encouraged to participate in a health and lifestyle assessment and offered advice and support to meet their individual needs. A major challenge was to identify ways to engage more effectively with men, especially those men who had in the past proved to be the hardest to reach due to social exclusion.

The Camelon Centre

Each of these initiatives differed slightly in how it interacted with men and in the services it provided. However, all the initiatives had in common a model of assessment and service delivery developed in the Forth Valley by the Camelon Centre for Men's Health. The Camelon Centre was the brainchild of community nurses Jim Leishman and Alison Dalziel. They envisaged a centre dedicated to improving the health of local men. The Centre opened in September 2001, offering health assessments designed specifically for men. This was then followed by a range of services to improve the health of the local men who attended.

The Centre is situated in one of the most deprived areas of Scotland – an area where attracting men to services aimed at preventing health problems had previously proved difficult. Recognising that this would be a major obstacle, much thought was given to how best to attract men. Jim and Alison came up with an idea that, in addition to the usual means of promoting a new service such as advertising in local newspapers and radio, as well as through posters and leaflets, letters would also be sent out from GP surgeries inviting men to make an appointment. The basic assumption was that men would be more likely to respond to a personal invitation, especially if the invitation was formal and on GP letter-headed paper.

With a response rate of one in six to these letters this proved to be a significant step in getting men to attend the service. Having the service available in the evening, and therefore more accessible to a larger number of men, was another important factor in the success of the Centre.

Initially available just one day a week, the service proved extremely popular with almost full attendance in the first two years of opening. This led to a further centre opening in 2003 and three more in 2005 to cover the rest of the Forth Valley area.

Expanding the work via the five centres

In each centre a small nursing team, all trained in aspects of men's health, provides individual assessments lasting approximately 45 minutes. Physical checks such as blood pressure and cholesterol are provided, but an emphasis has also been placed on lifestyle and behavioural issues.

An audit of the first 1,000 men who attended the service showed that 80% of them had risk factors associated with disease or were showing symptoms of illness, the majority of which were unknown to them prior to the assessment taking place. This included 28% who were found to be either depressed or suffering from stress, 42% who had raised blood pressure, 45% who were either unable to exercise or did very little physical activity and 12% who reported sexual health problems such as erectile dysfunction. Of the men who attended, one in four had had no previous contact with a health professional for over a year.

The feedback from the men was extremely encouraging, with the majority describing the experience as an extremely positive one. They particularly welcomed the time and opportunity to sit down and talk to someone about their own health and well-being – something that most of them had never done before.

Assessment method

A specific style of assessment was adopted at the Centres, one which encouraged men to be fully engaged in the process. Typically, the nurse explores with each man his general understanding of the area of health being assessed, clarifying what the normal or recommended levels are as well as the risks of being outside these levels. Each man's own status within each area is then assessed and a comparison made with the 'normal' or recommended ranges. The possible health benefits of making changes to habits and lifestyle are then discussed as well as exploring ways in which this can be achieved. Emphasis is placed on each man recognising that change is required rather than being told what to do.

Perhaps, while discussing lifestyle issues with a man, the assessment reveals that a man is drinking excessive amounts of alcohol – a problem that is acknowledged by the man and more importantly a problem that he wants to do something about. Possible ways to reduce his alcohol intake would be explored. If, however, he does not consider his drinking habits to be a problem or is simply not interested in making changes, then the assessment moves on with an open invitation to re-contact the Centre should he wish to seek help at a future date. While the assessment will highlight areas of concern it acknowledges that change in behaviour or lifestyle will only take place if the individual feels it is important to do so and that change is achievable. It is rare for change to take place in an individual because someone else feels it should happen.

At the end of the full assessment, findings are summarised and each man encouraged to identify, as well as prioritise, actions that would help maintain or improve his health. If a man presents with symptoms that require medical attention then he is referred to his GP.

Support programmes are offered, often building on services already established in the community, such as smoking cessation and couples counselling. Where services are lacking, new ones are developed in the Centre itself to deal with issues identified through the assessment process. A weight management programme was the first of these services to be developed.

Weight management programme

With the vast majority of the men presenting at the Centre found to be overweight, and one in every three men obese, helping men manage their weight became a clear priority. The initial approach was to give advice and self-help literature on how to lose weight. However, it was clear early on that for most men this was just not good enough. What men continually asked for was more direct support to help them lose weight.

The level of demand for this service was surprising and seemed to go against commonly held assumptions that men are much less concerned about weight issues than women. It is also presumed that men are more accepting of being overweight and are considered to be reluctant to attend weight management programmes, especially if this involved them being in a group.

Surprisingly this proved not to be the case in Camelon with overweight men not only consistently asking for more help but also more than willing to sign up to a weight management programme even if this involved being in a group. This was particularly true for men identified as being in the obese category.

Men who were identified as being obese were offered a place on a weight management programme that would be available in the evening at the Centre.

The need to redesign services for overweight patients had been recognised as a priority following the publication of the *SIGN Guidelines for Obesity in Scotland* (SIGN, 1996) and a subsequent audit of practice in the area. This meant that services were already being developed locally that could be adopted by the men's health centre. This model included a staged process of assessment, recruitment and treatment and was designed especially to target overweight people at high risk of disease. Part of this new model was the introduction of a 12-week programme of weight management. Although it had not been used with a group of men before, having previously been piloted with groups that were almost entirely made up of women, it was decided to offer this programme.

Many people involved were sceptical about the decision to develop a weight management programme for groups of men. The national Counterweight programme suggested that men were difficult to recruit into initiatives aimed at addressing weight problems. A strongly held belief was that men would be particularly reluctant to attend if this involved them being in a group. While it was agreed that men would probably opt for a one-to-one programme if offered this option, it was considered expensive and time consuming. These assumptions, however, proved misplaced with men snapping up the places offered for the group programme. At one time almost 100 men were on a waiting list to attend. This seemed to prove that if men are treated with understanding and honesty regarding their weight they will respond positively to offers of help.

During the initial general health and lifestyle assessment all men irrespective of their size had the health risks associated with being overweight explained to them. Particular emphasis was placed on problems associated with central obesity.

Working with men within the weight loss programme
Height and waist size are recorded and each man is asked what he thinks the results will show, a common response being that 'I'm a bit overweight' or that 'I'm not too bad apart from my belly'.

The normal and at-risk range of waist measurements are described and a comparison made with the man's own measurements. Using a BMI chart each man is shown how to calculate his BMI. At this point men can often be startled at the results, particularly if their measurement falls within the obese category. The response from men at first is typically one of disbelief, then dismay that they have put on so much weight as to be classified as obese. A common quote from men at this stage is: 'I knew I was fat but never obese'.

Negative connotations associated with the word obese have been described (*see* Box 8.1).

BOX 8.1 Negative connotations of the word 'obese'.

'Obese sounds like "beast".'

'Obese, I hate obese. I hate the word obese.'

'It's a cruel world ... It's giving an image of a huge person, way over the top.'

'If you're having a laugh with somebody you'll turn around and say, "hey, you fat bastard", things like that, but if you turned around and say to them "you're obese", that's a more derogatory way of saying it.'

Source: Andrew Irving Associates. *Just a Name? The experience of obese people.* HEBS overweight and obesity qualitative research - presentation report, London. 1997.

The word 'obese' appears to have invoked negative images for many of the men who attended the Camelon Centre. Clearly having this word associated with them during their assessment proved to be an unsettling revelation. However, it was also cited by many of the men who went on to attend a weight management programme as the main motivating factor for them joining.

John, 42, was typical of these men:

> *It really hit me like a ton of bricks, I mean I knew I had been putting on weight over the years and thought the tests would show that I was a bit fat, but finding out I was obese really knocked me for six. The facts were there staring me in the face. I had to do something about it.*

Michael, 38, similarly described:

> *The word obese, that's what got to me. Where I work most of the guys are on the big side. My size just seemed normal. When the girl [assessing nurse] showed me the chart I was really shocked to see that I was clinically obese. If it had showed me as being fat it wouldn't have got to me as much and I probably wouldn't have done anything about it.*

It was also apparent that most men either underestimated their body size or had a poor understanding of how weight is classified. If they were overweight they would typically describe themselves prior to the assessment as being normal weight. Similarly men who were found to be obese would often describe themselves as being 'probably overweight' prior to their assessment.

Considering most men in the UK are overweight, it is hardly surprising that most men who are overweight consider themselves to be of normal weight, with obese men often regarding themselves as being just overweight compared to the norm. This uncertainty about healthy body size, evidenced by the men attending the Camelon Centre, appears to reinforce studies that suggest that men often underestimate their body size (McCreary, 2002). With a propensity for men to underestimate their weight, along with the negative stereotypes that many people associate with obesity, such as gluttony and laziness, it is hardly surprising that, for many men, finding out they are in the obese range of weight classification evokes a strong emotional reaction. It is therefore important that these men are treated with compassion and understanding and that a non-judgemental attitude is adopted, one that is unbiased and sympathetic to their individual situation. Unconstructive attitudes by health professionals towards obese people have been shown to reinforce negative stereotypes and deter them from seeking help (Waine, 2002).

Offering support that has been proven to help men, and remaining optimistic regarding their situation, can help men view the assessment as a positive step towards a healthier future. Men will often ask how much weight they need to lose to meet their ideal body weight. However, for many men to achieve this using the BMI classification would require them to lose a large amount of weight. For many this is unachievable, and if given as their goal would diminish confidence and cause them to withdraw from the change process. Men should therefore be encouraged to focus less on achieving their ideal body weight and instead their attention should be directed towards smaller, more realistic goals. A 5–10% weight loss has been shown to reduce the risk of developing type 2 diabetes, cardiovascular disease and other obesity-related conditions (Goldstein, 1992). This can be seen as a much more achievable weight loss to aim for.

The challenge that a diagnosis of obesity can have on self-image, as well as the implications that it has on health, mean that a sensitive and understanding approach needs to be adopted. The approach should be one that is non-judgemental and allows men time to ask questions and express their feelings. Information and support should be relevant to their individual circumstances and needs, for example by offering a weight management programme at a time suitable to them. That the service provided in Camelon was exclusively for men and was available in the evening have been described as important factors in men deciding to attend. However, the most important factor seemed to be the knowledge that men similar to themselves had benefited from the programme. This led to the majority of men who were offered a place on the weight management programme agreeing to attend.

Prior to commencing a programme of weight management the following baseline information should be gathered. It can also be helpful to repeat some of these assessments at the end of the programme.

- **Motivation and confidence** are key to successful weight management and any programme designed to help men should attempt to improve and build on these factors. How confident the men are in losing weight, as well as their level of motivation, are evaluated prior to commencing the programme by asking each man to consider how confident he is that he can lose weight by indicating a score between 1 and 10, with 1 being not at all confident and 10 extremely confident. Similarly each man should consider and score how motivated they are. It can be helpful to repeat this at the end of the programme and compare the scores given.
- **Body weight, BMI and waist circumference.** Although this information would have been recorded during previous assessments, the men may have gained or lost weight during the time spent waiting to join a programme.
- **Blood pressure.** Raised blood pressure is strongly associated with weight gain and especially with abdominal obesity, which is more prevalent in men. A relatively small weight loss of 2.5 kg has been shown to reduce mean blood pressure by 10–13 mm Hg (Stamler *et al.*, 1980).
- **Current medication,** both prescribed and self-prescribed, may affect a man's weight.

- **Blood tests** such as plasma lipids, blood glucose and thyroid-stimulating hormone.
- **Exercise and activity levels.** A progressive decrease in physical activity with age is a major reason for weight gain (Prentice and Jebb, 1995). Activity levels for each man should be assessed prior to them commencing a weight management programme. This can be explained as any activity or exercise that is prolonged for half an hour each day or for two periods of 15 minutes. It should be at a level that makes the man breathe slightly harder and makes him feel an increase in his body temperature. Assessment should include whether he:
  1 rarely participates in activity at this level.
  2 is unable due to poor health or disability
  3 has this level of activity on a maximum of three days per week
  4 maintains this level of activity on five or more days of the week.
  This assessment should take into account work-related activity as well as non-work-related episodes of exercise.

Choice of venue and staff training issues

A commonly held assumption is that men are particularly reluctant to attend health premises and that such venues should be avoided in preference for social or non-health community venues. This assumption seems to be based on the general poor attendance by men of health promotion services that are based in clinics or health centres as well as the well-documented fact that men are less likely to visit their general practitioner than women.

Discussions with men in the Camelon Centre seemed to challenge these assumptions. These focus groups were made up of local men, many of whom admitted to visiting their GP only rarely. They were quite strongly dismissive of the suggestion of using a pub or social club for a health-related activity. Using the local clinic or health centre seemed to them to be the logical choice of venue for services aimed at improving their health. They seemed confused at the suggestion that men view health centres and GP surgeries as predominantly women's places. Moreover, they described their reluctance to visit services in the past as a tendency they shared in only using services when they had a problem they could not deal with themselves.

Evidence suggests that staff trained specifically in weight management produce better results than untrained staff involved in routine medical management (SIGN, 1996). It is therefore important to consider the training needs of individuals who are facilitating a weight management programme. As well as providing training on the basic principles of weight management and nutrition, training should focus on group facilitation skills.

The Camelon Centre's 12-week weight management programme

The US Institute of Medicine recommend that the avoidance of weight gain needs to be the principal aim of the medical care of an obesity-prone patient (Thomas, 1995). Obesity management is moving towards weight maintenance, avoiding further weight gain and encouraging modest weight loss rather than the goal of a return to normal weight levels. This approach is in keeping with guidelines suggesting that weight management should comprise a 12-week structured programme for weight loss followed by a programme of weight maintenance (SIGN, 1996).

Often weight loss programmes are centred on a calorie reduction eating plan or are based for the most part on setting and planning goals. The 12-week programme adopted at Camelon used both these methods. However, it concentrated on reinforcing two simple messages: eat a healthier, more balanced diet and lead a more active lifestyle.

Adopting healthier eating was a consistent message throughout the 12-week programme. Men were encouraged to eat more starchy carbohydrates, include more fruit and vegetables in their diet and reduce the amounts of fat, salt and sugar.

As a starting point they were encouraged to reflect on their current eating habits by completing a diary of all the food and drink they had consumed over a two- to three-day period. Reflecting on the types and amounts of food and drink they regularly have is an excellent starting point to gain an understanding of why they have gained weight.

A model of healthy eating that illustrates the different food groups and the recommended intake is introduced. Comparing this model of eating with their recently completed diaries helps men understand some of the changes they need to make in order for them to move towards a healthier, more balanced, diet.

Taking the time to prepare and present a variety of foods in their recommended portion sizes can be a powerful way to illustrate a major reason why many men gain weight – overeating on large portions of food. Men would describe how their meals consisted of eating food that was heaped onto their plate. Reducing portion sizes, particularly with regard to the meat, potatoes and dairy products they ate, and replacing these with more fruit and vegetables to fill them up, was the major change to eating habits that many men made.

Similarly, asking men to keep a diary recording how active they were (for example, how much physical work they do, how much they walk, gardening, or how much sport and exercise they do) is for many an eye-opener on how inactive they have become, especially when this is compared to the recommended levels of activity for men.

Men were asked to reflect on their activity diary and look for ways that they could add some exercise to their daily routine, such as walking to work, always using the stairs instead of a lift, a daily bike run or a walk every lunch time.

Often men were shocked at how inactive they had become and would talk about a time when they were fitter and slimmer. They described a time when they exercised more and played more sport and thought a return to this amount of activity would be key to them losing weight. These men, and in particular younger men, often viewed suggestions based around them gently increasing their activity by walking more as too sedentary for them and what they wanted was a return to more vigorous forms of exercise.

In Camelon free passes to local sports centres were provided for all the men attending the programme. An exercise referral system was set up, allowing men a safe return to exercise as well as a tailored programme for each man wishing to participate. It is also helpful to explore the opportunities that are available locally for men, such as walking groups, cycle runs and sports activities and asking representatives from these groups along to talk to the men so they know that opportunities exist for them to be more active.

A successful weight management programme encourages men to make changes that become a part of their everyday life and are therefore long enduring. This can be achieved by asking them to consider setting themselves small goals throughout the programme. It is important that any goals set are SMART (Specific, Measurable, Achievable, Realistic, and Time limited). Examples of SMART goals written by men on the programme include:

> *As from Monday I will eat healthier at lunchtimes by taking my lunch with me and avoid eating in the work's canteen on Mondays, Tuesdays and Wednesdays. On these days my lunch will always contain two pieces of fruit. I will review this in two weeks time.*

> *When I get home from work and I'm waiting for my wife to come in to cook my dinner, instead of having tea and biscuits like I usually do I will take the dog for a walk for half an hour.*

This last example illustrates a problem that many men seemed to share in that they rarely prepared meals. They also had very little involvement in planning their weekly grocery list and rarely shopped for food, never mind actually cooking a meal. Often for these men their only involvement was to sit down and eat. It was therefore important to encourage these men to be more active in their food choice and to be more aware of food generally. Information was given throughout the programme to help increase their knowledge of food, for example how to understand food labels and how to cook more healthily.

The effect alcohol has on weight gain played a small part in the initial programme. However, it was clearly a major factor for many of the men gaining weight. Describing the relationship that alcohol has with weight and exploring ways for men to moderate their intake should be an important part of any weight management programme for men.

The benefits of the group approach

At the beginning of the programme men cited their family as being their main means of support in their attempt to lose weight. Interestingly, however, at the end of the programme men described the support they received from the group as the main reason they had lost weight. Early on in the programme group support can be nurtured by placing men in small teams of two or three. Introducing a competitive element into the programme by offering a small prize to the team that manages to lose the most weight by the end of the 12 weeks can foster closer working between group members. Using male traits such as competitiveness and team spirit can motivate some men into achieving their individual goals. As the programme progresses it is important to focus less on the small teams and more on the group as a whole.

Inviting men from a previous weight management group to tell their story to a new group can help inspire newcomers. Hearing the achievements of men similar to themselves who have been through the programme and achieved their goals can be hugely motivating. While helping to illustrate the rewards that can be achieved it can also help to bring the group together. The competitive nature of men, especially when in a group, often takes over with them voicing a desire to emulate or better the success of previous groups.

Weight loss achieved by men was illustrated in real weight. Bags of sand representing actual weight loss were made up for each man. This proved to be an extremely powerful way to demonstrate their success and one that the men appreciated. They liked feeling the tactile evidence of their loss and would often take their bags of sand away with them to show off to their family and friends.

During the 12 weeks the camaraderie between the group members grows. They start to share information and tips that have helped them as individuals to meet their goals. They often plan to get together to do an activity such as visit a gym, plan walks or to go swimming. Quotes from men illustrate these feelings of camaraderie:

> *The support we got from each other was one of the most important elements of our success. It was really great to talk to other men with similar programmes.*

> *We had a good laugh, everyone was in the same boat. The team, that's what helped me.*

Group weight management programmes have been shown to provide better outcomes than individual programmes, even in those people who had expressed a preference for individual treatment (Renjilian *et al.*, 2001).

A further positive outcome from a men's weight management programme is the effect it can have on their wives, partners and children, with men influencing the family's lifestyle by adopting a healthier diet and having a more active lifestyle.

Box 8.2 shows the results from the first 45 men in the Camelon 12-week programme.

BOX 8.2 Results from the first 83 men in the Camelon 12-week programme

40%	(33)	lost < 5%
35%	(29)	lost > 5%
11%	(9)	lost > 10% (highest weight loss was 15.4 kg)
9%	(7)	lost nothing
5%	(4 men)	gained a small amount of weight

Counterweight (see page 78) were expecting 16% of all patients entering their programme to achieve weight loss of > or = to 5% at 12 months. At Camelon 46% achieved weight loss greater than 5% at three months.

Average weight loss from the 12-week Camelon programme = 5.4%.

Men were reviewed at various stages *after* attending the 12-week group sessions: 75% were still lower than their start weight and 15% were the same as their start weight. Feedback from 32 returned questionnaires:
100% had changed their eating habits to become healthier.
100% of the men felt confident in their ability to maintain the changes they had made.

Men say how they feel

Martin was one of the men who attended the Camelon programme. Here he describes his experience.

> I attended the Centre last year just to see what my blood pressure was but the thing that shocked me was finding out how fat I was. My weight then was 113 kilograms and because I'm not that big the result showed that I was not just fat but actually obese. Most of this fat was around my belly which they said was especially dangerous for my health. The guy [assessing nurse] asked if I would be interested in attending a weight management programme. I agreed to attend but was a wee bit worried that it was going to be some sort of diet programme where you starve. I wasn't that keen in attending a group neither but they said it worked well and is usually a good laugh so I agreed to give it a try.
>
> I was pleasantly surprised to find out that this was not a diet I was on but actually a course to educate us men on eating healthier, the need to be more active and to control our portions. At first I didn't think it would work for me because I felt I was eating the same amount of food I always had, just more fruit and veg. However, when I was given a bag of sand at the half way stage of the programme (the weight I had lost at that time) it felt really heavy. I was surprised and pleased I was no longer carrying this weight: 10 kg and 9 cm from my waist. I was really proud of myself and it spurred me on to keep going.
>
> Through the programme my wife and I now eat healthier than we ever did before and our portions have decreased considerably. At times I was probably eating the equivalent of two main meals at one sitting. I am sweet toothed and enjoy chocolate, gums and crisps. I have not stopped eating what I like, just reduced how often I have them.
>
> Recently I have been unable to work through an injury to my back and due to an appendectomy. This has resulted in my exercise being nil at the moment, but through eating healthy I have maintained what weight I have lost and currently weigh around 94.5 kg.
>
> Without what I learned on this programme I am sure my weight would have gone up considerably as the years passed by. I now regularly meet up with the guys from our group but instead of going to the pub we always plan to do something active.

Conclusions

Weight management groups clearly work well for men. Being in a group with other men with similar problems and goals can undoubtedly be an important means of helping men to lose weight. It is also evident that if health messages are kept real and relevant to their individual circumstances men will respond to them.

The real challenge remains the same, and that is to find ways to engage with men more effectively regarding their health. Advantage needs to be taken of all the opportunities that exist to engage with men, especially on a one-to-one basis, during which the risks associated with their weight need to be explained with honesty and perhaps a degree of blunt frankness, tempered with empathy and consideration towards their individual circumstances.

References

Andrew Irving Associates. *Just a Name? The experience of obese people*. HEBS overweight and obesity qualitative research - presentation report, London. 1997.

Goldstein DJ. Beneficial health effects of modest weight loss. *International Journal of Obesity*. 1992; 16: 397–415.

McCreary DR. Gender and age differences in the relationship between body mass index and perceived weight: exploring the paradox. *International Journal of Men's Health*. 2002; 1: 31–42.

NHS Quality Improvement Scotland. *Clinical Outcomes Report*. Edinburgh. November, 2003.

Prentice AM, Jebb SA. Obesity in Britain: gluttony or sloth? *BMJ*. 1995; 311: 437–9.

Renjilian DR, Nezu A, Shermer R *et al*. Individual versus group therapy for obesity: effects of matching participants to their treatment preferences. *Journal of Consulting and Clinical Psychology*. 2001; 69(4): 707–21.

Scottish Intercollegiate Guidelines Network (SIGN). *SIGN Guidelines for Obesity in Scotland. Integrating prevention with weight management*. SIGN Publication Number 8. Edinburgh: SIGN; 1996.

Stamler J, Farinaro E, Mojonnier LM *et al*. Prevention and control of hypertension by nutritional-hygienic means. Long term experience of the Chicago Coronary Prevention Evaluation Program. *JAMA*. 1980; 243(18): 1819–23.

Thomas PR, editor. *Weighing the Options. Criteria for evaluating weight-management programs*. Inst of Med. Washington, DC: Nat Acad Press; 1995.

Waine C. *Obesity and Weight Management in Primary Care*. Blackwell Science, Oxford; 2002.

CHAPTER 9

Weight management in men – community pharmacy approaches

Kurt Ramsden and Julie Hunter

The background, aetiology and scale of the obesity epidemic in western acculturated countries need no explanation in a book of this kind. As community pharmacists we see many of the complications of obesity through the medium of medicines. Obesity plays a role in the physical and mental health of a significant proportion of the patients we see every day and is seen as an inevitable consequence of life by many people. Suffice to say it is a huge problem requiring a broad range of measures and the widest possible outlook if we are to make significant inroads into what many now regard as the most important single issue influencing western healthcare.

Changing public perceptions of the pharmacist

Community pharmacy, and pharmacists, are, to many if not most people, places for medicines and shopping. The public perception of the pharmacist has changed little since the birth of the NHS over 60 years ago. There is, however, change in the air. For many years community pharmacy has argued that it is capable of delivering much more than the basics of dispensing prescriptions, selling over-the-counter medicines, and stacking shelves with toothpaste and shampoo. In April 2005, a new NHS Contract for Community Pharmacy came into force. This contract formally recognised many of the additional services that had been available for many years as well as setting out a framework for new services, making the future for pharmacy and the public it serves look more exciting. One of the areas where pharmacists can contribute is the promotion of healthy lifestyles, and in particular the prevention and management of obesity.

Pharmacies and men's health

There is a large volume of anecdotal evidence that men currently are reluctant users of pharmacy services and certainly use them far less than women. A study by the Community Pharmacy Research Consortium (CPRC) published in 1999 supports this. It found that:

Women make more use of pharmacies than men. In particular, women with small children are more likely to consult pharmacy staff. Individuals with chronic illnesses (e.g. diabetics, coeliacs) are also frequent users of pharmacy services. On the other hand, men use pharmacies infrequently, especially those in full-time employment, and those aged 16 to 24. (CPRC, 1999)

This was recognised within the 2005 report, *Choosing Health Through Pharmacy: a programme for pharmaceutical public health 2005–2015*, accessed via www.dh.gov.uk/ en/PublicationsandStatistics/Publications/PublicationsPolicyAndGuidance/ DH_4107494 which had a section on men's health and had as its action points:

- pharmacy services should be promoted and developed as a source of advice, information and support for self-care for men
- pharmacies should consider how they could make their services and premises more attractive to men.

What these action points do is to formally recognise the central importance of pharmacists in making our services accessible to men and that we have a clear mandate to consider new ways of targeting the men in our communities.

Origins of our weight management service

The story of our weight management services goes back a number of years, and was initially pursued as much for commercial gain as it was for meeting a health need. In the mid-1990s we were asked to become stockists of a well-known Ultra Low Calorie Diet (ULCD) which was at the time only available via general practitioners who ran 'clinics'. This evolved in the late 1990s into pharmacy-led clinics, which opened the market to a wider audience. At its height we were helping around 15 patients per week to lose weight rapidly with this strict 'Total Food Replacement' programme. Both men and women enjoyed the simplicity and speedy results that followed. Indeed, men seemed particularly keen. This was despite the significant cost, side effects (such as bad breath, constipation) and poor palatability of the product.

As time went by, the early successes many people experienced were hard to sustain. We began to see the same individuals return for further supplies, having gained all previously lost weight, and in some cases put on more. The evidence we gathered on ULCDs was beginning to suggest that they rarely produced sustainable results, so we began to investigate better ways of delivering weight management services.

One of the ironies of obesity is that it is a 'disease' of the poor. While this may be a simplification of the causes of obesity, there is no doubt that those belonging to socio-economic groups D and E are more prone to weight problems. So not only did ULCDs fail regularly, but they were also out of reach of those in most need. Our PCT had already identified this as an issue, so we began to look at ways of reducing economic barriers to inclusion in our service.

Developing the service

Traditionally, the problem with innovative thinking in the pharmacy slice of the NHS cake is that it is rarely accompanied by funding. The ULCD option was self-funding, but to move to a service which was free at the point of contact would require a source of revenue. Knowing that our chances of NHS monies were initially very limited, we approached the pharmaceutical industry. A major player in the anti-obesity drug market expressed an interest in facilitating a pilot by provision of training, support materials and (crucially) a grant to deliver the service.

Keen to ensure we were following best practice and thus increasing our chances of future sustainability, we discussed our plans with our local PCT (Langbaurgh) through the health promotion team and the director of public health. We were particularly keen to ensure that our service was consistent with that offered by other NHS providers in the area, as obesity services had been established for some time as a result of an established local obesity strategy. NHS services were focused on lifestyle change, with no formal referral pathways for pharmacotherapy or special diets. This took us outside our traditional areas of expertise, so training was undertaken to ensure we were 'on message'.

Harnessing the benefits of pharmacy-led services

As already mentioned, pharmacy has not been associated with this type of service. However, we believed we had a few 'unique selling points' which would enable us to complement existing services and make pharmacy a bigger player in the drive to improve public health. Our key strength has always been accessibility, and the recent changes to the NHS Pharmacy Contract mean that we now have a private consultation room – essential for us to deliver this, and other, new NHS services, such as medicines use reviews and supply of emergency hormonal contraception. This enabled us to be accessible to a wider audience than before.

Another advantage of community pharmacy over general practice was how the mindset of people differed in the two environments. Traditionally, people are in a 'self-care' mode when they visit a pharmacy for healthcare products and advice, whereas when they visit a surgery they are 'handing over' responsibility for their health to a doctor or nurse. Ownership of their weight management issues therefore seems more likely with pharmacy and other community-led services. At the time of writing, self-care is very much a key part of the drive towards a patient-led NHS, and it is not hard to see why. By fostering self-care, we encourage people to take more responsibility for their own health which benefits the individuals themselves and the taxpayer.

One of the other gaps in existing service provision in weight management was for those people who were not comfortable in a group setting and wanted (or needed) a one-to-one consultation. With our consultation room we were able to offer this, adding another option.

Training the staff

We had originally envisaged using the pharmacist directly to deliver the weight management service. It became clear that while this might be attractive in some respects, there were advantages to training an enthusiastic pharmacy assistant, Julie Hunter. The PCT had a ready-made training 'TROCN 3' package which was aimed at motivated health workers who might or might not have other medical qualifications.

Similar in standard to an 'A' level, it represented a comprehensive tool for anyone who wished to deliver a service. By training a non-authority figure, we felt that service users would find them easier to identify with, communicate with, and confide in. All this came with the professional back-up of a pharmacist, who was available for advice on anything beyond the scope of our expert. Queries around weight gain as a result of medication, for example, could be dealt with (and, in most cases, eliminated).

Marketing

The service itself was marketed via posters in public places, word of mouth, in the pharmacy itself, and some local GP practices. We also received some press coverage in the local paper. As already stated, it was built around lifestyle modification, and looked at eating habits, levels of exercise, and psychological barriers for change. We made no conscious effort to target either gender, and had no preconceived ideas about uptake from men and women.

Men and weight loss: a pharmacy perspective

Our weight management clinic has been running successfully now for seven months, and with excellent results, but what is interesting is that out of all the people that have attended, only 15% are men.

Women, it seems, have been watching their weight and appearance for as long as we can remember, and there are constant reminders of how we should look every time we turn on the television or open a magazine, but all of these articles or adverts are aimed at females, which would lead us to believe that men do not have concerns about their weight. But this is not true.

In our experience men's attitudes to weight issues differ from those of women in many ways. Men in the main tend only to approach the problem if advised to do so by a doctor or medical practitioner, e.g. high cholesterol, blood pressure, diabetes, etc. Given the choice they would prefer to try and correct this through diet rather than medication. Another noticeable difference is that men do not generally use food to replace emotion. Unlike women, they do not comfort eat or snack. Because of this one might think that a regular healthy eating plan might come easily to them, but that is not always the case. We must take into account reducing portion sizes, regular meals and making time for physical activity.

A problem area within men's weight management is how best to target them. A poster in a clinic or pharmacy might not always get their attention or they might feel uncomfortable about making an inquiry. Although a pharmacist would discuss their worries in confidence and give them the best advice possible, the matter should always be approached with care and consideration. In the past, obesity and diet issues were seen to be a feminine issue; dare we say 'real men' weren't seen to watch their weight or appearance.

A good approach would be to try to reach men in their own surroundings, within the workplace, somewhere they could attend on their own or with work colleagues, combining weight management with blood pressure or cholesterol checks. This would take the emphasis off being just about their weight problem. Some men may prefer to keep it to themselves, away from work and home life, so running clinics in pharmacies on certain days and times, dedicated just to men's health, would make them realise that this is not a problem they suffer alone. This would make them feel more at ease. We also feel that we will only reach certain men through the women in their lives – a partner or mother – but the decision to change has to be their own.

We are well aware of how overweight and obesity levels have risen over the last 20 years, but once men get over the stigma that is attached to weight problems and watching their appearance, and are made to feel that it is not something they need to be embarrassed about, the subjects of healthy eating and weight management can be approached confidently, and hopefully this will go towards helping the statistics to improve.

Pharmacy is going to play a larger role in health matters in both men and women in the future, having the training and equipment to carry out different health checks, whether it be blood pressure, cholesterol or weight management. These clinics will be more accessible, with a pharmacist on hand and regular communication with GPs, if needed. It will also give men and women peace of mind about the matters that are concerning them.

The future of our pharmacy-led service

Julie's experiences and opinions on weight management will form a critical part of future service development for us. While we have enjoyed unprecedented success in attracting women to a pharmacy-based weight management service, it seems clear that in order to attract men we will need to be more creative, particularly with respect to marketing. Perhaps many men see pharmacies as 'too feminine', and this adds to the list of barriers they can erect to continue to lead unhealthy lifestyles. We are considering a campaign which specifically targets men under the banner of a 'Men's MOT', which will initially incorporate blood pressure measurement, cholesterol testing, blood glucose testing, and of course a check on obesity levels. The chances of this becoming a reality depend upon the continued enthusiasm (and funding) by the PCT as much as it does on our own commitment. Time will tell.

So what have we learnt about men and their weight? We have a long way to go before men devote as much thought and effort to weight management as women. Indeed, it seems easy to extend this gulf in attention between the sexes to many other areas of health. The challenge is therefore to raise the awareness among men of the need for self-care, and (critically) to reduce any associated stigma. This cannot be achieved overnight, or by any single group of professionals. It will continue to require a multidisciplinary approach, which will need to extend into the general male psyche. We look forward to the contribution pharmacy can make towards this vital goal.

References

Community Pharmacy Research Consortium (CPRC). *The Public's Use of Community Pharmacies as a Primary Health Care Resource.* January 1999. www.rpsgb.org.uk/pdfs/cprc.pdf (accessed 9 March 2007).

Department of Health. *Choosing Health Through Pharmacy.* London: DoH; 2005.

CHAPTER 10

Commercial slimming groups in the management of weight problems in men

Amanda Avery

Traditionally commercial slimming groups are attended by overweight and obese female members and thus perceived as having a small role to play in supporting men to lose weight. The commercial sector is very aware of the concerns men may have about joining a group that is traditionally viewed as a female environment. Hence resources have been deployed to make the groups more accessible to men. These include more men running groups – both mixed-sex and men-only groups – as well as more marketing aimed at men, and the formation of web-based programmes.

When men overcome the barriers to attend they generally do very well in terms of weight loss, and thus health status, and improve their self-esteem and well-being.

As the commercial slimming sector has an extensive, well-established infrastructure of slimming groups across the UK, it is being recognised as a potential partner, through referral from the NHS, in halting the current rise in obesity. Hence it is of paramount importance that the commercial sector continues to open its doors to more men.

This chapter will look at what the commercial slimming sector can offer, evidence of male involvement, a search of the literature to ascertain what research has been undertaken to date, and presentation of some male success stories. It will conclude with future strategies for a more gender-sensitive approach towards clients from the commercial slimming sector.

The commercial slimming sector

Choosing Health (Department of Health, 2004) recommended that obesity services be upgraded across England and Wales to include regular monitoring and personalised advice on diet, physical activity and behavioural strategies to tackle the causes of over-eating and under-exercising. Offering free or reduced-cost attendance at commercial weight management groups was recognised in this document and others as a means of expanding PCO capacity.

The three major commercial slimming organisations in the UK are Slimming World, Weight Watchers and Rosemary Conley. All three organisations run weekly groups to support their members both to lose weight and maintain weight loss. Generally speaking it is the member's choice to seek the help of such a group, and it follows that they have already identified the need for, and made some commitment to, weight management. It is possible that the requirement to pay a joining, and then a weekly, fee adds to the impetus to succeed.

People joining a commercially run group know that they will be joining other people who are also struggling to lose weight. For some people the weight will have crept on gradually over a number of years and it may be for a health reason that they now need to lose weight. Whatever an individual's personal struggles, there will be others in the group experiencing very similar life issues. Furthermore, the group is facilitated by a person who has already chosen the same route to assist their own weight management, has wanted to help others, and has received additional training to do this.

While the content of the different organisations' groups does vary, they all provide the resources to support the well-recognised evidence that more successful weight loss outcomes, and maintenance of weight loss as an outcome, are achieved when there is regular support (House of Commons Health Committee, 2004). Given the prevalence of being overweight and obese it is unlikely the current level of public sector resources will be able to provide the frequency of support required to address this evidence base.

The weekly groups are locally based and the content of the group discussion is flexible to meet the needs of the local community. All three organisations provide high quality literature, including a range of practical recipe books, to support the group sessions. To maintain their quality standards, all three companies seek the advice of eminent scientists working in disciplines related to weight management. Further independent research is conducted to ensure best practice.

Slimming World

Note: The author, being employed by Slimming World, has a greater knowledge of the contribution of this particular organisation than others in its mission to support people, of both genders, to maintain a healthy individual weight.

Slimming World was founded in 1969 and currently has over 250,000 members attending 5,500 weekly group sessions in the UK. Recognising that men need gender-sensitive weight management options, in 2002 the company made it their mission to be more male friendly, with emphasis not only on having more men running groups (both mixed and men-only), but also making the supporting literature and advertising material much more male-orientated. In 2003 the number of males attending the groups increased from 3 to 5% of total membership. While this is a small percentage, it does equate to 12,500 men.

The groups are held in a variety of local community venues, including public houses, social clubs and community centres across the UK, and the organisation has recently opened up a number of groups in Northern Ireland. The company's aim is to set up one group for every 5,000 population, and there is the capacity within the organisation to increase the number of groups available to meet the needs of the local population. This is supported by a comprehensive training programme which ensures there are always enough trained people to facilitate the groups.

The Slimming World dietary approach is known as Food Optimising, which is based on scientific principles ensuring a healthy balanced dietary intake for all population groups. Consideration is given to the energy density of different foods and the role of the different nutrients in appetite regulation. There is also an element of psychology in that members are able to choose one of two different eating plans on a daily basis, thus allowing for individual food preferences and tastes. In general the aim is to move away from counting, weighing and measuring foods and to satisfy individual appetites by unlimiting the intake of less-energy-dense food choices. On one of the choices, low-fat protein foods can be eaten without restriction to satisfy the appetite, and a certain amount of carbohydrate should still be eaten, while the other choice encourages unrestricted amounts of starchy carbohydrates and pulses and portion-controlled amounts of the low-fat protein foods. On both choices fruit and vegetables are eaten according to appetite but certain foods such as confectionery, crisps and alcohol are included in controlled amounts. Hence men attending a Slimming World group need never feel hungry and they can still enjoy a curry and a pint of lager or egg and chips (just cooked in a healthier way)! Indeed, through the group discussion and through the recipe books members learn how simple changes can make a big difference with respect to weight management.

Not only do people joining Slimming World improve their eating habits but they are also encouraged to become more physically active. Intrinsic to Slimming World groups is 'Body Magic', a programme which encourages members to increase their activity levels in a stepwise approach. The programme acknowledges that many people who are extremely overweight have probably not done any exercise for a long time and will feel quite self-conscious about exercising in public places. Realistic activity pathways are therefore encouraged. The groups welcome being informed about local activities, such as walking groups, so that members can be sign-posted to these activities. The Body Magic programme was introduced into the groups in 2002 after careful consideration as to how best to help members take a more positive approach to increasing their activity levels. More recently Slimming World have forged a partnership with one of the private fitness groups so that those members who wish to increase their activity levels can join this gym and Slimming World with a reduced membership fee.

Independent research has evaluated the effectiveness of the consultants running the Slimming World groups. Within their training programme, the consultants receive training in the basics of running a group, nutrition related to weight management, the importance of exercise, and behaviour modification techniques to ensure lifestyle changes are maintained.

Raising an individual's self-esteem, sense of self-worth and psychological well-being is of paramount importance. No-one is ever judged because of their weight, and indeed a person's weight is never discussed – only weight changes are shared. Members select their own personal weight-loss goals and are given support to ensure their own targets are realistic and achievable, with an emphasis on, and reward system for, achieving a 10% weight loss.

While it is appreciated that body mass index is not always the most appropriate measure of weight problems in men, weight remains predominantly the most recorded parameter in the groups and allows regular monitoring of success. However, the consultants are provided with tape measures and supporting literature, so an individual member could choose for changes in waist measurement to be their goal, resulting in associated health benefits. The use of waist measurement as an indicator of health is particularly important in men, where BMI may not be an appropriate measure. However, the fact that target weights are individually agreed upon, and also the emphasis on a 5–10% weight loss, which is then maintained, ensure that weight losses encouraged are realistic for both men and women.

Box 10.1 emphasises the key features of the support provided at Slimming World

---

BOX 10.1 Key features of Slimming World's approach to weight management.

- Locally recruited group consultants who have been members at a Slimming World group themselves and have needed to lose weight.
- Ongoing training and support for group consultants, via a structured training programme.
- 2,500 trained consultants support 5,500 groups across the UK each week. Each group is different according to the needs of the local community in which it is based, catering for vulnerable and disadvantaged groups of the population.
- A range of motivational and behaviour modification tools available to support members as they make lifestyle changes.
- Nutrition advice in line with the Balance of Good Health but which allows members an element of choice to suit their personal tastes and preferences. Fruit and vegetables are particularly encouraged. Advice is tailored to meet the needs of the individual.
- Group support with all members encouraged to take an active part with the social element also being seen as important.
- Weekly weighing and recognition of successful weight loss and lifestyle change, with support being offered in between weekly sessions as necessary.
- Special arrangements made for people employed in shift work, and those who may experience difficulty getting to the same group at the same time each week.
- Emphasis on the health benefits of a 10% weight loss and personally selected individual target weights.
- Incentives to encourage weight maintenance with the importance of weekly group attendance emphasised. Attendance is free when target weight is achieved and for as long as the member maintains their weight loss (within plus or minus 3 lb of their target weight).
- An approach to increasing members' levels of activity, over a period of time, that is sensitive to the fact that overweight people may not have done any exercise for many years. A synergistic effect between modifying diet and increasing activity levels is emphasised.
- The overall aim is to raise members' self-esteem, build members' confidence and to empower them with the skills to make lifestyle changes.

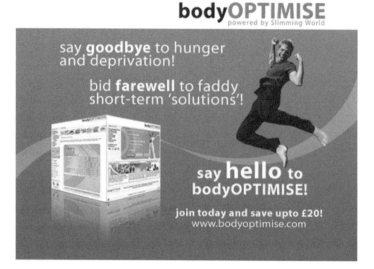

Figure 10.1 Body Optimise website.

groups. Of particular importance to men is the fact that shift workers may access more than one group in order to fit group visits round their different shift patterns.

For those people, both men and women, who do not wish to access weight management support within a group setting, Slimming World offers both a postal membership scheme and also a comprehensive website package known as Body Optimise (*see* Figure 10.1). Membership of both packages has increased substantially over the past year with the increase in membership across both genders. Interestingly the proportion of Body Optimise members is the same as group membership: 95% females and 5% males.

Further information about Slimming World is available at their website: www.slimming-world.com.

Weight Watchers

Weight Watchers is an internationally based company with over 40 years' experience of running weight management groups. A network of over 6,500 meetings per week is maintained.

Box 10.2 emphasises the key features of the Weight Watchers' approach to weight management.

Rosemary Conley Diet and Fitness clubs

Box 10.3 emphasises the key features of Rosemary Conley's approach to weight management.

BOX 10.2 Key features of the Weight Watchers' approach to weight management

- The diet plan is based on a points system where individuals are given a number of points to use throughout the day.
- Different foods are given different points, based on a healthy eating, balanced and flexible approach.
- Skills and strategies for behaviour change are an integral part of the programme.
- Regular physical activity is recommended as part of the plan.
- Ten per cent weight loss is recommended as an achievable and realistic first goal.
- Meetings are weekly and weigh-ins done in private. Confidentiality is guaranteed with no naming and shaming.
- Group leaders have successfully lost weight themselves and are carefully selected.
- The Weight Watchers points system is also available online: www.weightwatchers.co.uk.
- Weight Watchers have designed a home-based programme particularly to meet the needs of men. This is known as the MP5 programme.

BOX 10.3   Key features of Rosemary Conley's approach to weight management

- Members follow a healthy, low-fat diet plan called 'Eat Yourself Slim' combined with an optional exercise programme adapted for individual fitness levels, for an inclusive price.
- Weekly classes typically involve a private weigh-in and one-to-one consultation, followed by a five-minute motivational talk and a 45-minute exercise session to music with a qualified instructor.
- Promote a healthy rate of weight loss (0.5–1 kg or 1–2 lb per week) and set realistic weight loss targets.
- In addition, or as an alternative, to the classes, there are the Rosemary Conley Diet and Fitness videos, books and magazines which people can follow at home, plus a postal support system and a web-based package.
- For more information visit: www.rosemary-conley.co.uk.

Evidence

While there is a wealth of anecdotal evidence to support the effectiveness of commercial slimming organisations in the short term there is limited long-term published data. However, we must not lose sight of the fact that generally long-term results from weight management programmes are poorly reported. There is also the suggestion that weight loss is inevitably short-lived once 'treatment' has ended. For no particular reason the commercial slimming sector are more heavily criticised in this area.

It has been reported that generally between one-third and two-thirds of lost weight is regained within the first year and virtually all lost weight regained by the fifth year (Perri *et al.*, 1992). However, Lowe *et al.* (2001) suggest that most of the data on weight regain was from research conducted within university or hospital environments and hence the study population was not representative of a typical population. In their study of people achieving their target weight following a commercial weight loss programme (Weight Watchers), Lowe and colleagues found that long-term maintenance of weight loss was better than suggested by this earlier research. From a national sample of 1,002 target members (4% males) at five years after achieving their target weight, it was found that 19.4% were still within 5 lb of this weight, 18.8% maintained a loss of 10% or more, 42.6% had maintained a loss of 5% or more and 70.3% were still below their initial weight. Hence, we can conclude that long-term weight maintenance in participants who had reached their target weight in at least one commercial programme was better than suggested by earlier research.

More recently Heshka *et al.* (2003) reported greater weight loss in a population of overweight and obese people who received support to assist weight loss through commercial slimming groups than a clinically matched group who received two 20-minute counselling sessions with a dietitian plus supporting self-help materials. The 423 (15% males) overweight and obese people were randomly assigned to one of the two programmes and weight losses compared over a two-year period. While the self-help group lost 1.4 kg at one year, there was a return to baseline weight observed at two years. In contrast the commercial group lost 5.0 kg at one year and the weight loss was still 2.8 kg lower than baseline at two years. It was noted that those participants who attended 78% or more of the commercial group weekly sessions maintained a mean weight loss of 5 kg at the end of the two-year study. Waist circumference was also reduced in the commercial group by 4.5 cm at one year and 2.5 cm at two years.

To evaluate the benefits of setting up men-only groups in the commercial slimming sector, Bye *et al.* (2005) analysed data collected from members of seven men-only groups run by Slimming World six months after these groups had been established. At the point of data collection average BMI had decreased from 35.9 to 32.5 kg/m². At least 5% weight loss had been achieved by 90% of the sample since joining, and in those who had been members for 24 weeks, 69% achieved a 10% weight loss. The remaining 31% had all achieved at least 5% weight loss. Average weight loss at 12 weeks was 9.2%. Shift working did not affect weight loss success.

The results compared favourably with a study where patients were referred from primary care to Slimming World (Lavin *et al.*, 2006). The mean weight loss in males in this study was 7.8% at 12 weeks. Furthermore, once enrolled at the mixed-gender groups there was no difference in attrition rate between men and women. Indeed, in terms of attendance a group approach would seem to be the favoured approach to supporting weight loss. One-year studies report attrition rates of 40% for a dietary/behavioural programme (Tsai and Wadden, 2005), 22% for a group approach with men (Andersson and Rossner, 1997) and 41–67% for a self-help programme (Torgerson *et al.*, 1999).

Overweight and obese people, of both genders, need to be recognised as particularly vulnerable in that they generally have low self-esteem and self-confidence. Thus self-esteem and mental well-being are important outcome measures in any weight management programme. To sustain any behaviour change, such as adopting healthier eating habits and increasing physical activity levels, self-esteem needs to be addressed. Mental well-being was measured in the Greater Derby study reported earlier.

Compared with a Southern Derbyshire representative sample, the obese patients referred from primary care generally had low levels of well-being before enrolment. However, improvements in all aspects measured (feeling calm and peaceful, having a lot of energy, feeling downhearted and low) were seen in those completing both 12 weeks (calm P = 0.001, energy P = 0.001, downhearted P = 0.015) and 24 weeks at a commercial slimming group (calm P = 0.02, energy P = 0.001, downhearted P = 0.001). Qualitative data support these findings with patients viewing the referral to a commercial group very positively.

> *I was helped at a time when I had a very low self-esteem; the group consultant was excellent and very supportive.*
>
> *The other slimmers were brilliant, a good laugh was had by all and we lost weight.* (MALE ATTENDING MIXED GROUP)

'Real' evidence

With a BMI of over 40, Iain Hamill's weight problem was serious. Diagnosed with diabetes and high blood pressure, even doing the simplest tasks like tying his shoelaces left him breathless. Despite warnings from his GP about his health, it took the photographs of himself from his son's wedding for Iain to decide to make the change and join Slimming World (*see* Figure 10.2).

Not sure what to expect, Iain was initially embarrassed about walking through the doors of his local group. Being a man in what he perceived a woman's environment made things even harder. 'I was very embarrassed at first but I was made to feel very welcome once I'd got through the doors.'

Since joining in February 2001, Iain has lost 7 stone 6 lb, not to mention the 12 inches from his chest, 3½ inches from his neck and 10 inches from his waist (he has had to buy new trousers every couple of months). After years of being overweight, Iain can finally wear his wedding ring again (*see* Figure 10.3).

Health and diabetes

More quotes from Iain:

> *My diabetes was brought on by being overweight and as my weight increased my diabetes became out of control and so did my blood pressure. I had been in and out of hospital before I started going to the groups. I had my big toe amputated on my right foot and part of my left foot as well. I tried to make a joke about it being a drastic way to lose weight and my GP went mad at me. He told me that I would never feel well unless I lost weight.*
>
> *My GP was aware that I'd joined Slimming World and he monitored my progress. The last time I saw him was in July of last year and he was really pleased with what I had achieved – I haven't needed to see him since!*
>
> *Losing the weight has really helped my diabetes control as well as my blood pressure. My blood sugar levels are no longer erratic and I really do feel a lot healthier. I used to attend the Hospital Diabetic Clinic every three*

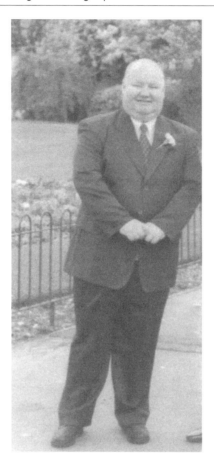

Figure 10.2 Iain Hamill before his weight loss.

months but now I only need to attend once a year. When I last saw my diabetes consultant he was really interested in how I lost the weight and now uses me as an example to patients who are struggling with their weight.

Family

One advantage of being a man is that I don't have to go near the kitchen – all my meals are cooked for me! Because of this I've never been tempted to 'pick' while meals are being cooked. Because we've shared the same meals, Julie, my wife, has also lost a stone.

My son joined Slimming World after being reassured by me that it was OK for men to attend the groups and that he would get all the help he needed. We never discussed recipes as it didn't seem like a manly thing to do when there was football to be talked about! We did, however, bring home recipes and tips from the group and passed them on to our wives as we relied on them to do the cooking for us.

There was friendly rivalry between us each week regarding our weight

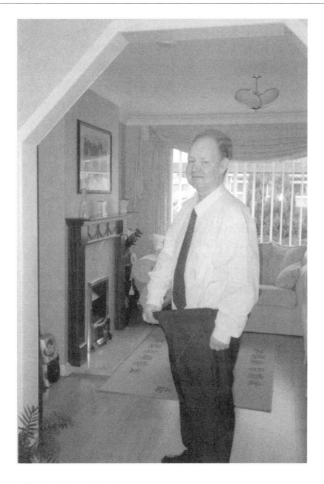

Figure 10.3 Iain Hamill after his weight loss.

> *losses and he was really chuffed when I became a semi-finalist in the 2002*
> *Man of the Year competition.*
>
> *My son lost 2 stones in total and since then my daughter-in-law has*
> *given birth to another baby girl so I will need to keep fit if I am going to*
> *run round after two lively granddaughters.*

Food

> *The only way I'd tried to lose weight before was with will-power alone –*
> *and that didn't last for very long. With Food Optimising I was never hungry.*

In 2002, 7½ stones lighter, Iain enjoyed all the things that his previous weight prevented, including having a holiday without being bothered by the heat, wearing shorts without embarrassment and getting through the turnstiles to support Everton Football Club from the terraces rather than the sofa.

Today he continues to enjoy these benefits having maintained the weight loss.

Conclusion

To conclude, men may be supported to lose weight by attending a commercial slimming organisation. They just need some persuasion to walk through the doors and attend a group!

Acknowledgement

The author is grateful to Iain Hamill, the Slimming World member described in the text, for permission to include his story, some of his quotations and two photographs of himself.

References

Andersson I, Rossner S. Weight development drop-out pattern and changes in obesity – related risk factors after two years of treatment in obese men. *Int J Obesity.* 1997; **21**: 211–16.

Bye C, Avery A, Lavin J. Tackling obesity in men – preliminary evaluation of men-only groups within a commercial slimming organisation. *J Hum Nutr and Diet.* 2005; **18**(5): 391–4.

Department of Health. *Choosing Health: making healthier choices easier.* Public Health White Paper. London: Department of Health; 2004.

Heshka S, Anderson JW, Atkinson RL *et al.* Weight loss with self-help compared with a structured commercial program. *JAMA.* 2003; **289**(14): 1792–8.

House of Commons Health Committee. *Obesity.* London: The Stationery Office; 2004.

Lavin JH, Avery A, Whitehead SM *et al.* Feasibility and benefits of implementing a Slimming on Referral service in primary care using a commercial weight management partner. *Public Health* 2006; **120**(9): 872–81.

Lowe MR, Miller-Kovach K, Phelan S. Weight maintenance in overweight individuals one to five years following successful completion of a commercial weight loss program. *Int J Obesity.* 2001; **25**(3): 325–31.

Perri MG, Nezu AM, Viegner BJ. *Improving the Long Term Management of Obesity.* New York: Wiley Bioscience; 1992.

Torgerson JS, Agren L, Sjostrom L. Effects on body weight of strict or liberal adherence to an initial period of VLCD treatment. A randomised, one year clinical trial of obese subjects. *Int J Obesity.* 1999; **23**: 190–7.

Tsai AG, Wadden TA. Systematic review: an evaluation of major commercial weight loss programs in the United States. *Ann Intern Med.* 2005; **142**: 56–66.

CHAPTER 11

Tackling weight problems in men in the workplace

Steve Deacon

Being overweight or obese has important implications for employment and work productivity due to the related consequences of reduced work suitability and fitness, disability-impaired productivity and increased costs for sickness absence and early retirement due to ill health. Obesity accounts for 18 million days of sickness absence each year and 30,000 deaths annually (National Audit Office, 2001). Many obesity-related deaths are premature and affect people of working age, shortening life by an average of nine years.

Other chapters in this book describe the factors causing the epidemic of obesity: declining physical activity and increased calorie consumption. Work and the workplace are major influences on these behaviours. The first 20 years of the adult obesity epidemic, from the 1970s to the 1990s, was explained mainly by declining physical activity, in part due to the reducing manual demands of work. Work has become less physical as we have moved from a manufacturing to a service economy. The knowledge worker sitting at a desk all day has replaced the manual worker who operated machinery and lifted loads. Further, amendments to employment and health and safety legislation have required that the manual content of work be made less demanding to avoid discriminating against women and older workers who are generally less strong or with lesser stamina than an average man. The resulting reduction in physical activity is associated with an increased tendency to being overweight or obese. Indeed, working men have become heavier over the years, reflecting lifestyle changes in the general population and also this reducing physical activity at work. Similarly, the change in eating habits that has fuelled the obesity epidemic since the 1990s, with increased snacking of high-calorie foods, is partly related to changing work patterns.

The ageing of the workforce compounds both these behaviours as the prevalence of obesity increases with age. About 5% of men aged 16 to 24 years are obese but by age 55 to 64 years the obesity rate has increased nearly five-fold to 23%. The percentage of older people in the workforce is increasing as the birth rate declines and people are working longer. Currently, about 40% of adults are aged over 50 years, but by 2030 this will have risen to more than 50%. This will increase the numbers of overweight and obese working people.

Thus there is a mutual benefit for employers and employees to take an active interest in measures to promote weight loss and thereby improve the quality of life and work productivity.

Obesity and access to work

Being overweight has important implications for access to work. Many organisations require job applicants to complete a health declaration and possibly undergo a medical examination. The purpose of these is to assist an employer's need to match an applicant's capability to those of the proposed job. This involves a general consideration of physical (and mental) health and also an assessment of any medical disability. Also some specific occupations require a high level of physical fitness, e.g. armed or emergency services. Exercise testing is sometimes used to see whether an applicant is fit enough to cope with a demanding job and obese persons may be at a major disadvantage in achieving the required fitness standards. Further, being obese may be a specific exclusion factor for some occupations. These include commercial diving or working on ships, mainly because obese workers are more likely to have medical problems and emergency rescue is much more difficult in these working environments.

Obese workers may be more prone to accidents resulting from impaired balance and agility and are at greater risk of physical injury from falls, etc., due to higher body weight. Indeed, safety considerations may exclude obese applicants from jobs that involve climbing ladders or accessing confined spaces. Also, obesity may interfere with the wearing of safety equipment for protection against accidents or harm to health at work. For example, unfit overweight people cope less well with tight clothing or wearing a mask. Further, some specific work-related conditions are more common in obese workers. For instance, carpal tunnel syndrome, a condition caused by a trapped nerve at the wrist resulting in hand and arm pain, is four times more common in obese workers.

Many occupations have expectations of stereotype images. Obese people are unlikely to be considered for some jobs, such as a dietician or fashion model. Similarly, impaired self-esteem resulting from obesity and poor body image may inhibit career advancement and promotion. Anecdotal evidence suggests that some men worry that they may be discriminated against for senior management positions if they are perceived as a health risk in a stressful role.

A literature review (Williams and Malik, 2005) reported that the impact of prejudice is highly relevant to employment. Research in the USA has shown that overweight people have difficulty in obtaining employment, and are also more likely to be selected for redundancy (Roehling, 1999). Also, healthcare staff, including doctors, have been reported to believe that obese people are less intelligent, less likely to have friends and likely to be more lazy (Price *et al.*, 1987).

Obesity and disability

Obesity may predispose to physical disability, due to the mechanical implications of a high body weight limiting activity, or medical disability, due to associated ill health arising from arthritis, cardiovascular complications, depression or diabetes mellitus. The law provides a measure of employment opportunity and protection for people with serious medical disability. The Disability Discrimination Act (DDA) 1995 and subsequent amendments require employers to make 'reasonable' work or workplace adjustments where:

■ an individual has a well-recognised medical condition
■ the condition has been present or is anticipated to be present for > 12 months
■ the disability affects their normal everyday activities.

Several categories of everyday activities are defined and in relation to obesity these might include mobility and lifting/carrying everyday objects. Employers often seek advice from their occupational health practitioners about the interpretation and application of the DDA but the final arbiter in such matters in the event of a claim of discrimination is always an Employment Tribunal. The test of 'reasonable' depends upon a consideration of the capability of the employing organisation to accommodate disability. This test is more demanding of large or profitable organisations that are considered to have greater resources.

The provision of adjustments is intended to tackle such issues as access to the workplace (e.g. wheelchair ramps, altered work hours) or amended work organisation (e.g. provision of special equipment aids or sharing work duties with other colleagues) to ensure that a disabled person is not at a disadvantage and can be engaged in productive employment.

General employment and occupational health practice does not regard being overweight or obese per se as a medical disability. However, it is likely that gross or morbid obesity could be managed as a disability under the criteria of the DDA. Unfortunately such a high degree of obesity would probably preclude many forms of common employment. This raises issues for termination of employment and possible retirement. There are no authoritative guidelines, and each employing organisation and pension fund will manage such issues according to their own specific circumstances. Again, in general terms, it is likely that simple obesity and any related physical disability would be managed as a work capability issue. Many employers have attendance standards and expectations of work capability. An obese person with frequent sickness absence due to many different causes for trivial ill health complaints would normally be managed differently to one for whom these absences were linked to an underlying associated serious medical disability.

Employment practice and case law indicate that it is possible to dismiss an employee with frequent absences for unrelated trivial absences. However, where there is a serious underlying medical disability the employer must seek to make 'reasonable' adjustment to accommodate this disability. Possible reasonable adjustments for an obese worker might include modified workplace equipment such as larger work clothing, a larger/stronger chair and/or modified duties to avoid physical activities that may be unsafe or outside the person's work capability.

This is a difficult area of employment law and the author is not aware of any well-established legal or professional guidelines to assist employers or health practitioners in advising in such situations. Also, it is pertinent to note that employees also have an implied obligation to co-operate with their employer to meet the obligations of their employment contract. This includes co-operating with medical treatment to promote their health and fitness for work. Thus an obese employee has a duty to manage their eating and lifestyle habits to reduce their obesity and thereby be available for work on a regular basis to undertake their required work duties to the expected standard.

Work factors promoting obesity

Automation and the move to a service economy have reduced the physical demands of work in industrialised countries. Jobs with a lot of regular physical exercise help to burn off the calories and keep down body weight. This effect of physical activity on body weight is seen when contrasting health status between occupational groups with different activity levels. A major study undertaken in the Royal Mail Group (Welch *et al.*, 2000) showed that obesity, arthritis, disability and GP consultations were more prevalent in lower occupational grades. These lower grades are characterised by greater physical activity. Indeed, a typical postman walks or cycles up to six miles each weekday. The overall obesity rate for postmen is about 9% and compares favourably with 21% for the UK male population. Other work observations have shown that bus conductors had less heart problems than the driver of the bus due to their different levels of physical activity.

A complex mix of work and personal lifestyle influences can also give rise to some important effects on body weight. Shift workers and those with sedentary jobs are reported to have higher body mass indices and waist to hip ratios (Ishizaki *et al.*, 2004). Indeed, waist to hip (W–H) measurement is sometimes suggested as a better marker for body fat distribution. Higher W–H ratios have been reported in male managers more than in other male workers and ascribed to the sedentary nature of their work, higher alcohol intake and lower leisure time physical activity. Work patterns such as shift work or longer hours often lead to changed eating habits and reduced leisure exercise time, encouraging increased body weight. Indeed, research has shown that the number of years of shift working is predictive for body mass index (Parkes, 1999).

Some jobs working with food and drink may encourage overindulgence and becoming overweight. The stereotype image of some jobs incorporates this such as the 'fat chef or publican' as against the thin ballerina or trapeze artiste. There is no evidence that psychological workload affects body weight. However, comfort eating is very common and many people snack during the day at work. Again overindulgence can lead to becoming overweight.

Workplace costs of obesity

Employers must balance their need for profitable operations with their obligations for the welfare of their employees. Unfortunately many employers regard overweight and obese workers as attracting higher costs at several stages in the employment process, including increased sickness absence, provision of larger sizes or custom safety clothing or personal protective equipment, increased travel costs, higher accident rates and higher healthcare costs (Williams and Malik, 2005).

Obese workers are also reported as having more difficulty in getting along with co-workers, and severe obesity may result in higher numbers of lost work days (Pronk *et al.*, 2003). Also, body mass index is predictive for annual healthcare costs where employers provide health insurance as part of the employment contract (Bungum *et al.*, 2002).

Some specific concerns relate to the health and safety effects of being overweight or obese. Higher rates of disordered breathing are reported in overweight and obese people (Borys and Boute, 1994). The syndrome of obstructive sleep apnoea is a significant factor in falling asleep at the wheel during driving and results in a higher accident rate.

Workplace food

The workplace meal is often the main meal of the day for many workers and meal provisions and choices are key influences for body weight. The increasing availability of food, and particularly snack foods, and increasing food consumption appears to have fuelled the obesity epidemic during the 1990s (Putnam *et al.*, 2002).

A poor diet and body weight affects how well people work, according to new research from health charity DPP (Developing Patient Partnerships) released in October 2005 (DPP, 2006). Results from interviews with 1,124 workers showed well over half (57%) admit to thinking that how heavy you are affects how well you work, while the majority (70%) think that the type of food you eat also has an impact on work quality.

The results show that 62% of workers blame eating badly at work for weight gain with 54% indicating that lack of time and work stress make it difficult to motivate healthy eating. Low energy levels cause 49% of people to struggle through their working day – that could explain why 26% think afternoon naps should be allowed.

However, this research suggests that educating people about healthy eating options and motivating them to become more active could have a significant impact on personal health and well-being as well as productivity levels.

Work as a setting for health promotion

The prevalence of obesity is now above the critical threshold of 15% set by the World Health Organization for epidemics needing intervention. The preferred national strategy to address this epidemic in the UK involves partnership between government, the healthcare professions and employers. Access to health services at work is a key component of any national programmes to promote the health of working people. In 2005 the Department for Work and Pensions, the Department of Health, and the Health and Safety Executive launched the National Charter for Health, Work and Well-being to improve the health of working people. This programme will encourage work-based health promotion activities.

Health promotion is optimised in settings with 'captive' populations. Some examples include schools, prisons and the workplace. The workplace offers a supportive setting to access workers to engage them through health education, specific programmes and enables tracking of progress. Further, success in health promotion is often achieved by joint engagement with colleagues and partnering with a 'buddy'.

Review of published literature shows that obesity research has been targeted mainly at individuals and that most interventions produce only small weight reductions with little impact on the obesity epidemic. Most experts agree that the obesity epidemic is environmental but research has largely ignored this factor (Swinburn and Egger, 2002). It is time to be realistic with individuals about the limited effectiveness of lifestyle interventions and obesity drugs and to focus on public health interventions. Both sides of the energy balance must be tackled, such that people can 'move a little more, eat a little less'. The necessary changes to eradicate 90% obesity require only walking an extra 2,000 steps/day (which equals expending an extra 0.418 MJ per day and eating 0.418 MJ less per day).

Early life physical fitness predicts later life physical fitness. Those in physically active occupations in early life have a better chance of maintaining body weight in later years. Men starting work will usually have participated in sport at school or in higher education, but regular leisure exercise often stops on taking up employment or beginning a family due to competing time pressures. The combination of reduced work and leisure time physical activity promotes increased body weight.

Higher education is associated with increased awareness of personal health, and research shows that people with higher qualifications tend to take better care of themselves by not smoking, eating a healthier diet and taking more exercise. Hence it is commonly observed that professionals and managers tend to be healthier and less overweight than less well-qualified workers.

The responsibility for leading health promotion in the workplace is often placed with the occupational health department. However, the issues and benefits affect the whole organisation. The author's experience suggests that a multidisciplinary approach to health promotion is essential for success. A steering group of senior managers, employees and employee representatives is most effective in gaining complete engagement and organisational support. Health promotion objectives should be aligned with organisational objectives and adequate budgets and resources provided as for other management objectives.

Work off the fat

There are many work-related opportunities to promote a healthy approach to encourage weight loss. These include the following.

- *Travelling to work* – walk or cycle to work, or park your car at the far side of the car park and walk to the work entrance.
- *Vary your job to include more activity* – standing while working expends more energy and helps burn off the calories.
- *Use the stairs* between floors rather than taking the lift.

- *Plan your work* and take the time to walk when you can.
- *Take a walk in your refreshment break* – going for a short walk is a great way to take a refreshment break.
- *Use a workplace fitness centre if available* – regular leisure exercise is very beneficial for those with sedentary jobs.
- *Join work challenges* – many groups undertake diet challenges, walks or fun runs for charity. A shared challenge to lose weight is likely to be more successful and rewarding.
- *Set up a workplace health club*:
  - obtain and distribute information on exercise and healthy eating
  - establish walking paths
  - lobby the canteen to provide healthier choices of foods
  - start a club for those wanting to lose weight
  - ask your employer about health checks at work
  - run competitions to encourage improved fitness and weight loss.

Anecdotal reports from the USA relate that some employers are now designing workplaces with services such as car parks and canteens at a distance from work areas to encourage/require their workers to exercise by walking to their workplace. Indeed, some employers provide designated walking paths around their work sites to encourage their employees to take walk exercise during refreshment breaks. It is easier to 'build in' rather than 'bolt on' and the design of new workplace premises offers an opportunity to consider the provision of kitchen/canteen facilities to promote healthy eating, health and fitness facilities, cycle racks and sports facilities.

Workplace case study: Royal Mail Group

Royal Mail Group (RMG) comprises three main businesses in the UK: Royal Mail Letters, Post Office Limited and Parcel Force Worldwide. These businesses have a combined workforce of nearly 200,000 people with a heritage of a predominantly male workforce of near 80%. This has been due to past self-selection towards men for post delivery work that forms the bulk of all employment in RMG. The business has an active diversity function promoting the employment of both sexes, all ethnic groups, disadvantaged social groups and the disabled.

A comprehensive occupational health service is provided to all employees at all locations. This covers health assessment at recruitment, specialist vocational assessment, advice and treatment for those absent from work due to injury or illness and an active approach to health promotion. In 2006 a Health Bus was launched to visit sites that did not have workplace health room facilities and to provide a flagship for the national well-being programme. The RMG well-being strategy involves partnerships with providers of specialist services. For instance, Quadrant Catering is working to develop healthier recipes and improved ways of presenting canteen food and promoting healthier food choices. Fitness centres are run at 37 sites throughout the UK and many other sites have associations with local sports facilities or participate in sporting events such as the Corporate Challenge. RMG actively sponsors individual employees in sports events for charity and in 2006 the RMG Chief Executive, Adam Crozier, with 30 other RMG colleagues, completed the London Marathon in support of charitable causes. The various employee and manager communications and journals publish regular articles on health and well-being matters.

In recognition of the large male workforce, RMG has developed close links with the Men's Health Forum (MHF) and has sponsored many MHF campaigns to promote men's health, especially in the workplace. In particular RMG were proactive in sponsoring the 2005 MHF campaign to reduce obesity in men. RMG men have a lower rate of obesity (9%) compared with men in the general population (22%) partly due to the regular physical activity involved in post delivery. A postman typically walks or cycles a distance of 6–8 miles each day carrying a mail sack of up to 16 kg weight. However, there is still scope for improvement and RMG ran workplace events at 40 major sites, held workplace learning and listening sessions in work time to promote men's health throughout the organisation and distributed 20,000 MHF manuals in support of the campaign.

Conclusion

Employers and their health advisers will increasingly need to address the issues of employing and supporting an increasingly overweight workforce. Individual men who are overweight or obese have a much higher risk of ill health and reduced quality of life. These problems affect their access to work, work capability and productivity. Employers need to control their operating costs and improve profitability through improved productivity. Thus it is in everyone's interests for collaborative workplace programmes to promote the achievement of ideal body weight.

References

Borys JM, Boute D. Obstructive sleep apnoea syndrome; a frequent complication of obesity. *Biomed Pharmacother.* 1994; **48**(3–4): 37–41.

Bungum T, Satterwhite M, Jackson AW, Morrow JR. The relationship of body mass index, medical costs and job absenteeism. *Scan J Work Environ Health.* 2002; **28**(1): 64–71.

Developing Patient Partnerships (DPP). Poor diet and how much a person weighs affects how well they work. *Medical News.* 31 Jan 2006.

Ishizaki M, Morikawa Y, Nakagawa H *et al.* The influence of work characteristics on body mass index and waist to hip ratios in Japanese employees. *Ind Health.* Jan 2004; **42**(1): 41–9.

National Audit Office (NAO). *Tackling Obesity in England.* London: NAO; 2001.

Parkes KR. Shift work and age as interactive predictors of body mass index among offshore workers. *Occ Med.* 1999; **49**: 491–7.

Price JH, Desmond SM, Krol RA. Family practice physician's beliefs, attitudes and practices regarding obesity. *Am J Prev Med.* 1987; **3**(6): 339–45.

Pronk NP, Martinson B, Kessler RC *et al.* The association between work performance and physical activity, cardiorespiratory fitness and obesity. *Am J Health Behav.* 2003; **27**(4): 456–62.

Putnam J, Allshouse J, Kantor LS. US per capita food supply trends: more calories, refined carbohydrates and fats. *Food Rev.* 2002; **25**: 2–15.

Roehling MV. Weight based discrimination in employment: psychological and legal aspects. *Personnel Psychology.* 1999; **52**: 969–1016.

Swinburn B, Egger G. Preventive strategies against weight gain and obesity. *Obes Rev.* 2002; **3**: 289–301.

Welch R, Boorman S, Golding JF *et al.* Variations in self-reported health by occupational grade in the British Post Office: the Q-Health Project. *Occ Med.* 2000; **50**(1): 3–10.

Williams N, Malik N. The big issue. *Occupational Health*. 2005; **57**(10): 20–2.

CHAPTER 12

Weight problems in boys and young men

Paul Gately and Duncan Radley

Obesity levels continue to increase across the globe despite high public awareness of the issue. There is strong evidence that obesity is associated with a range of physical and psychosocial co-morbidities (Reilly *et al.*, 2003). Given the scale of this public health problem and the likely outcomes it is imperative that prevention and treatment strategies are put in place to tackle the growing epidemic. Given that between 50 and 80% of overweight and obese children will become overweight or obese adults, action is required in the paediatric population (Freedman *et al.*, 2004). The context for this chapter is to identify obesity in boys and young men. However, there are limited data specifically focused on the male population, and most studies tend to report data on children as a whole group rather than males and females separately.

Assessment

Arguably one of the biggest difficulties with child and adolescent obesity is the challenge of measurement and identification. Similar to adults, children and adolescents are popularly classified using body mass index (BMI). However, in contrast to the generally accepted BMI classifications for overweight and obese adults (25 kg/m² and 30 kg/m², respectively), there are no universally established criteria for children and adolescents. In children stable cut-offs are inappropriate given the differences between genders and the natural occurrence of changes in height and weight as they grow and develop. Therefore, accounting for these factors, classification systems for children and adolescents use age- and gender-specific BMI values. The most common system in use consists of national BMI percentiles charts. However, at present there is no consensus on which percentiles should be used as the boundaries to define being overweight and obese. In the UK the Health Survey for England (Department of Health, 2004) defined being overweight above the 85th percentile and obese above the 95th percentile, whereas the Scottish Intercollegiate Guidelines Network (SIGN, 2003) recommend the 91st and 98th cut-offs.

An often used alternative to national percentile charts are the International Obesity

Task Force (IOTF) BMI standards for children and adolescents (Cole *et al.*, 2000). Devised from six nationally representative samples worldwide, the cut-offs for being overweight and obese are designed to coincide with the adult values of 25 kg/m² and 30 kg/m². While BMI is the most widely used method for classifying children and adolescents as overweight or obese, it does have its limitations. BMI is based on weight and height, which does not consider differences in fat mass (FM) and fat-free mass (FFM). The contribution of the FM and FFM compartments to BMI varies in the growing child. At certain stages children will tend to put on more fat and at other times lose it (Malina and Bouchard, 1991). In addition, FFM changes throughout growth with large increases in boys following puberty (Malina and Bouchard, 1991). It is important to note that at present classifying a child overweight or obese above any percentile is an arbitrary decision and not based on a known relationship with specific health indicators.

Prevalence

Similar to adults the increasing prevalence of weight problems in children and adolescents in the UK reflects a global trend, although comparisons between countries are difficult due to limited data and the use of varying classification criteria. Using the IOTF standards, it has been estimated, for children and adolescents aged 5 to 17 years, that the worldwide prevalence of being overweight is approximately 7.5%, with an additional 2.5% classified obese (Lobstein *et al.*, 2004). However, it can be seen from Table 12.1 that prevalence levels vary dramatically between continents (Lobstein *et al.*, 2004).

Table 12.2 summarises the recent surveys investigating the prevalence of weight problems in the UK. It is clear that the UK levels of being overweight and obese are high and they continue to increase irrespective of gender. These data not only highlight the variation in total prevalence when using different classification systems but interestingly estimate disparate prevalence values for different systems between genders. Using BMI at the 85th centile highlights boys as having a higher prevalence, while in the majority of studies BMI at 91st centile, or when using the IOTF standards, estimates girls as having a higher prevalence. In addition, using waist at the 91st

TABLE 12.1 World wide prevalence of child and adolescent overweight and obesity.

Country	Prevalence (%)	
	Overweight	Obese
Americas	25	7
Europe	15.5	4.5
Near/Middle East	9.5	6.5
Asia-Pacific	4.0	1.0
Sub-Sahara Africa	2.0	0

Source: Lobstein *et al.* (2004).

TABLE 12.2 The prevalence of overweight and obesity in the UK.

Author	Year	Measures	Age group (years)	Prevalence (%) of overweight (including obesity)			n =
				All	Boys	Girls	
Reilly et al. (1999)	1999	BMI (> 85th)	6	22			2,630
			15	31			
McCarthy et al. (2003)	1997	BMI (> 91st)	11–16		21	17	776
		Waist (> 91st)			28	38	776
Bundred et al. (2001)	1998	BMI (> 85th)	2.9–4	23.6			2,633
Chinn and Rona (2001)	1974	BMI (IOTF)	4–6		6.4	9.1	4,139 (B), 3,871 (G)
	1984		7–8		5.4	9.3	3,259 (B), 3,008 (G)
	1994		9–11		9.0	13.5	3,016 (B), 2,858 (G)
Rudolf et al. (2001)	1996–1997	BMI (> 85th)			22	22	787(B), 975(G)
Rudolf et al. (2004)	1996–2001	BMI (IOTF)	12–14		14	16	315
Health Survey of England (2003)	2003	BMI (> 85th)	2–10		29.6	25.9	≈ 4,000
Gately 2006 (unpublished report)	2004	BMI (> 85th)	11–12		35.7	34.1	4,150
		BMI (IOTF)	11–12		24.8	29.3	4,150
		Waist (> 85th)	11–12		37.4	48.3	4,150
		Per cent body fat (> 85th)	11–12		24.6	28.6	4,150

centile McCarthy *et al.* (2003) and Gately (unpublished report) report around 10% greater prevalence of weight problems in girls than boys. Worryingly, these data also suggest that BMI may substantially underestimate the prevalence of obesity compared to values derived using waist circumference as the classification system.

Health risk

Several reports have highlighted the physiological, psychological and social consequences of being overweight (Health Select Committee, 2004; National Audit Office, 2001; Wanless, 2002). Investigating the association of being overweight to cardiovascular risk factors, in a sample of 9,167 5–17 year olds, the Bogalusa Heart Study reported overweight children had increased odds ratios in a number of risk factors compared to their non-overweight peers, including elevated total cholesterol (2.4), triglycerides (7.1), low-density lipoprotein cholesterol (3.0), systolic blood pressure (4.5), diastolic blood pressure (2.4), fasting insulin (12.6) and decreased high-density lipoprotein cholesterol (3.4) (Freedman *et al.*,1999). In addition to cardiovascular disease risk factors childhood obesity is associated with increased prevalence and/or severity of orthopaedic conditions (e.g. slipped capital epiphyses), pulmonary conditions (e.g. sleep apnoea) and gastrointestinal conditions (e.g. hepatic steatosis) (Mullen and Shield, 2004). Finally, it is important to consider that the escalating prevalence and severity of childhood obesity coupled with the persistence into adulthood will undoubtedly lead to increased health risks in childhood and earlier onset and increased severity of adult obesity associated disorders.

While these data are of great concern, a particularly striking and more immediate consequence of childhood obesity is the high level of social exclusion and psychological morbidity, as they become targets of persistent and systematic discrimination from both adults and peers (Cramer and Steinwert, 1998; Staffieri, 1967). Such concerns are supported by our own work with overweight and obese children. A boy who attended our residential camp programme articulated that his PE teacher 'told his class that whoever finished last during the warm up would have to do a further ten laps of the field'. The child said, 'I thought I was doing okay until the rest of the class sprinted off just before the line and I had to do ten laps and missed football'. He was 24 stone!

Throughout adolescence prejudice and discrimination would appear to continue. Janssen *et al.* (2004) found positive associations between BMI category and verbal and relational victimisation in both boys and girls and physical victimisation in girls only. Furthermore, being overweight during adolescence has been shown to negatively affect self-esteem (Walker *et al.*, 2003), educational performance (Canning and Mayer, 1967), admission to college (Canning and Mayer, 1966) and apartment rental (Karris, 1977).

Obesity prevention programmes

There are a number of settings within a child's world where strategies for the prevention of obesity can be implemented. The local community and home environment, for instance, have potential for preventative strategies. Unfortunately, while increasing availability and accessibility of active recreational opportunities has been strongly recommended, this is extremely difficult within an existing urban environment. Furthermore, due to the sheer number and heterogeneity of homes and the limited options for access, it may be extremely difficult to successfully target the home as a setting for direct obesity prevention (Swinburn and Egger, 2002).

It has been suggested that schools are the most natural setting for affecting the energy balance of children (Resnicow and Robinson, 1997), consequently offering the opportunity to affect rates of being overweight and obese. In addition to a significant proportion of children's time over a period of the year, schools have the existing physical education facilities as well as control over the nutrition environment within one eating episode.

There are an abundance of reviews summarising worldwide childhood and adolescent overweight and obesity prevention strategies, including school-based interventions programmes (Campbell *et al.*, 2001; Doak *et al.*, 2006; Floodmark *et al.*, 2006; Fulton *et al.*, 2001; Resnicow and Robinson, 1997; Story, 1999; Summerbell *et al.*, 2005). Given the number and range of obesity prevention strategies we will not repeat these findings. Instead, the conclusions of three reviews that include a large proportion of interventions will be outlined, followed by more detailed description of two UK-based interventions. In addition, given that on average one in five children is obese to the extent that their health will already be negatively affected, consideration will also be given to more intensive inpatient treatment programmes.

Cochrane Reviews on prevention and treatment

Summerbell *et al.* (2003) reviewed 22 obesity prevention interventions in children, 19 of which were pre-school/school-based. Including controlled trials from 1990 to 2005, 10 long-term (at least 12 months) and 12 short-term (12 weeks to 12 months) were identified. Considering long-term interventions, six combined physical activity and nutrition/dietary education, two focused on physical activity alone and two focused on nutrition/dietary education alone. In eight of the studies there was no difference in overweight status between the group(s) who received the intervention and those who did not. One combined intervention resulted in improvements in girls only and one physical activity intervention resulted in minor reductions in overweight status. Considering short-term interventions, eight combined physical activity and nutrition/ dietary education and four focused on physical activity alone. In 10 of the studies there was no difference in overweight status between the group(s) who received the intervention and those who did not and in two physical activity interventions favourable minor reductions were found for the intervention group. In discussion the authors comment, 'The results of these studies indicate that the interventions employed to date have, largely, not impacted on weight status of children to any significant degree' (p. 16). Furthermore, the authors go on to state, 'The studies, overall, have largely been underpowered and/or poorly designed, given the complexity of the intervention and the outcomes sought' (p. 17).

Summerbell *et al.* (2003) also reviewed the literature on interventions for treating obesity in children. They outlined 18 randomised controlled trials that were accepted, having fulfilled the criteria for the review. The studies included investigations in physical activity and sedentary behaviours, behavioural therapy with varying degrees of family involvement or specific behavioural strategies. The reviewers concluded that there was little power in the studies, limiting the ability to make evidence-based recommendations. Summerbell also outlined within the results that 'results were not presented separately for each gender', which limits our ability to investigate the impact of interventions on boys specifically.

Cardiovascular disease interventions review

There have been several school-based studies that have assessed the effectiveness of strategies to reduce cardiovascular disease (CVD) risk in children. These are broad-based prevention programmes not specifically targeting obesity. However, such strategies warrant mention due to the behaviours they target being similar to those within obesity-specific prevention programmes.

Resnicow and Robinson (1997) reviewed 16 school-based CVD prevention programmes. Positive effects, i.e. reduction of CVD risk factors, were observed more frequently for the outcome measures of smoking (83%), cognitive (65%), fitness (36%), diet (34%) and lipid (31%), with blood pressure (18%) and overweight measures (16%) being observed infrequently. These results indicate that prevention programmes in schools that address obesity as one of several CVD risk factors have limited effectiveness in preventing obesity.

UK schools-based intervention programmes

Sahota et al. (2001a) reported findings from a multifaceted primary school-based intervention known as APPLES – Active Programme Promoting Lifestyle in Schools. Taking place over one school year the multidisciplinary programme aimed to influence diet and physical activity behaviours in children aged 7 to 11 years. The randomised controlled trial included 634 children from 10 primary schools (five intervention, five control) in Leeds, paired according to size, ethnicity and level of social disadvantage. The intervention concentrated on the whole school environment with teachers receiving training, modifications of school meals, and the development and implementation of school action plans which incorporated various health promotion activities. These included the integration of nutrition education in the curriculum, support for physical education lessons, healthy eating class sessions, and improved health resources.

The main outcome measures assessed included growth by BMI, dietary information using 24-hour recall and three-day food diaries, physical activity and sedentary behaviour by questionnaire, and psychological well-being. After one year Sahota et al. (2001a) reported there were no significant differences between intervention and control children in BMI, physical activity levels, psychological state or sedentary levels. Twenty-four-hour dietary recall showed there was a modest increase in the consumption of vegetables. Although results were disappointing, the authors note that the implementation of the programme was highly successful and process evaluation revealed positive changes at school level in terms of ethos and attitudes of the children (Sahota et al., 2001b).

James *et al.* (2004) reported findings from a cluster randomised controlled trial known as CHOPPS – the Christchurch Obesity Prevention Project in Schools. Undertaken in six primary schools in the South West of England, 644 children, aged 7 to 11 years, were randomised by class. The intervention lasting one school year was aimed at reducing the consumption of carbonated drinks (sweetened and unsweetened). At the end of the intervention, three-day diaries returned at both baseline and follow-up by 36% of the children revealed a reduction in self-reported soft drinks consumption by 0.6 glasses (250 ml per glass) in the intervention group compared with an increase of 0.2 glasses in the control group. At 12 months body mass index, measured in 89% of children, revealed no significant difference in change in BMI or BMI z scores between the intervention and control groups. However, it was reported the percentage of overweight and obese children decreased by 0.2% in the intervention group compared with a 7.5% increase in the control group.

Warren *et al.* (2003) reported findings in 213 children, aged 5 to 7 years, participating in a school- and family-based intervention known as Be Smart. Undertaken in three primary schools in Oxford, the intervention lasted 20 weeks over four school terms. During lunchtime clubs 25-minute behaviourally focused lessons were based upon Social Learning Theory. Intervention groups focused on either nutrition (Eat Smart), physical activity (Play Smart) or both (Eat Smart Play Smart) while the control group (Be Smart) learnt about food in a non-nutrition sense (e.g. food traditions) and about the human body.

The main outcome measures assessed either at school or through postal questionnaires to parents included: BMI, nutrition knowledge, physical activity and dietary information. At the end of the intervention, there was a significant improvement in nutrition knowledge in all groups and a significant increase in fruit consumption in the Eat Smart and Be Smart groups. There was no intervention effect on diet, physical activity or nutrition knowledge, no significant changes in the consumption of confectionery or crisps in any group and no significant changes in the rates of being overweight and obese. Undoubtedly the disappointing results were confounded by a poor parental response rate to postal questionnaires with 70% returned at baseline and only 45% at the final stage, and contamination of the control group.

School-based intervention programmes summary

There is a lack of UK school-based prevention programmes targeting obesity prevalence, and whether or not US programmes are transferable is unknown. Studies undertaken worldwide may share similar objectives but the differences they have in terms of study design and quality, target population, theoretical underpinning of intervention approach, intervention content and format, and evaluation and outcome measures, make it difficult to draw any conclusions regarding effectiveness in general of any single programme component. Considering all these factors and given the lack of intervention success it is extremely difficult to tease out the effective components. It is clear further research is required to establish the most appropriate components for an effective schools-based obesity prevention programme.

Another aspect concerning school-based programmes that has received little attention is the need for them to be cost-effective, sustainable and feasible.

Consideration must be given to the personnel responsible for implementing the programmes and whether regular classroom teachers can effectively implement all components of the programme, especially the education and behavioural modification components. Furthermore, the extent and suitability to which programmes can successfully be incorporated into the regular curriculum is unknown. Unfortunately, there are many additional barriers to developing and implementing obesity prevention programmes with schools, due to such things as lack of school commitment, lack of staff time, lack of funding and lack of classroom time (Stang *et al.*, 1997).

Inpatient treatment programmes

In children with significant levels of obesity or co-morbidities more intensive intervention approaches may be justified, especially if they have failed in previous attempts to lose weight. Specialist inpatient obesity treatment centres (including summer residential programmes) provide an alternative to more radical pharmacological and surgical approaches. Access to such programmes is limited, the high expense and the lack of centres around the world excluding many children. Further inspection of the range of treatment options available in such programmes also demonstrates that they have different objectives. Several of the long-term hospital-based programmes attempt to reduce children's body mass to within the normal weight range, while summer camp programmes or programmes of shorter duration attempt to initiate weight loss as well as educate participants and their families in behaviour modification techniques that can continue in the home environment.

A number of studies have utilised a variety of inpatient treatment programmes, varying considerably in their duration (18 days to 12 months) and content (Archibald *et al.*, 1981; Brown *et al.*, 1983; Dietz and Schoeller, 1982; Endo *et al.*, 1992; Pena *et al.*, 1989; Stallings *et al.*, 1988; Wabitsch *et al.*, 1996). Several early inpatient programmes were not holistic in their nature, few reporting the use of behaviour modification during treatment and the predominant focus being on dietary manipulation. More recent interventions have improved in content, to include dietary modification, physical activity and some form of behaviour modification, with significant contributions in the field coming from France (Dao *et al.*, 2004a, 2004b; Rolland-Cachera *et al.*, 2004) and Belgium (Braet, 2006; Braet *et al.*, 2004; Deforche *et al.*, 2003, 2005).

Dao (Dao *et al.*, 2004a, 2004b) reported the outcomes of a multidisciplinary programme where children, aged 9 to 17 years, were housed at a therapeutic unit for between 6 and 12 months except for weekends, which were spent at home. The programme, including dietary restriction of 1,600–1,800 kcal/day during the weight reduction phase and progressive submaximal physical activity, resulted in a significant reduction in BMI for both boys and girls by 9 kg/m^2 and 10 kg/m^2, respectively. A strength of the Dao *et al.* intervention (2004a, 2004b) was the measurement of changes in aerobic fitness (VO_{2max}) and body composition using Dual-Energy X-ray Absorptiometry (DXA). DXA revealed similar total fat mass reduction in boys and girls, both around 19.0 kg, coupled with a non-significant decrease in lean body mass (LBM) in girls, by 0.6 kg, and an increase in LBM in boys, by 0.7 kg. VO_{2max} when expressed per kg body weight increased significantly in boys and girls. However, when expressed as an absolute value LBM increased only in boys (from 2.60 ± 0.56 L/min to 2.96 ± 0.64 L/min).

Braet et al. (Braet, 2006; Braet et al., 2004) and Deforche et al. (2003, 2005) have both reported on interventions carried out at the Medical Pediatric Center Zeepreventorium, Belgium. This 10-month residential treatment programme for obese children and adolescents includes moderate dietary restriction, physical activity and psychological support. Braet et al. (2004) report a reduction in BMI by around 8.5 kg/m², and although BMI increased during a 14-month follow-up period, values remained reduced below baseline by 4.9 kg/m². In 2005, Deforche et al. reported results from a further cohort of children, aged 9 to 16 years, who underwent the 10-month intervention and at 1.5 year follow-up. Adjusted BMI was significantly reduced by 54 ± 18% from 175 ± 26% pre to 121 ± 17% post, while at 1.5 year follow-up although adjusted BMI increased to 155 ± 28%, there was a large variation in weight change responses of the participants. In addition, although significant gender differences were reported in initial weight loss, with boys reducing their adjusted BMI by 62 ± 18% compared to 48 ± 16% in girls, no gender differences were found at follow-up.

Residential camps

A number of residential weight loss summer camp programmes have provided another form of specialist treatment for obese children (Braet and Van Winckel, 2000; Gately et al., 2000a, 2005; Nichols et al., 1989; Rohrbacher, 1973). In addition to the summer camp programmes documented in the scientific literature, there are a range of commercially run programmes, mainly in the US, that do not provide any peer-reviewed evidence to support their approach and have therefore have not been considered. The duration of the programmes ranged from 10 days (Braet and Van Winckel, 2000) to eight weeks (Gately et al., 2000a) and similar to inpatient treatment interventions varied in their diet, physical activity and behaviour modification components. Although using different outcome measures, the short-term results of these interventions are as impressive as the inpatient programmes, including: −13.7 kg (54), −12.1 kg (53), −4.4 kg/m² (57), −18% overweight (Braet and Van Winckel, 2000). In addition, where follow-up data are available, all programmes reported successful outcomes from baseline measurements: −11.1 kg at six months (Rohrbacher, 1973), −2.6 kg/m² at one year (Gately et al., 2000b), −15% overweight at 4.6 years (Braet and Van Winckel, 2000).

Gately (Gately et al., 2005) recently reported findings from the first four years (1999–2002) of an ongoing six-week non-profit residential weight loss camp in the UK. The results of 185 children who attended the weight loss camp were compared to 94 (38 overweight and 56 normal weight) non-camp attendees who undertook unmonitored summer vacation activities. Children who attended the camp on average lost 6 kg, reduced their BMI by 2.4 kg/m² and reduced their SDS (standard deviation score) BMI by 0.28 units. Measurements using Air Displacement Plethysmography (Dempster and Aitkens, 1995) revealed the diet and physical activity programme was able to produce significant decreases in FM (from 42.7 ± 14.4 kg to 37.1 ± 12.6 kg) while maintaining FFM (from 46.2 ± 10.4 kg to 45.7 ± 10.8 kg). Furthermore, significant improvements were also recorded in a range of other physical and mental health variables, including blood pressure (from 119 ± 8 mm Hg to 112 ± 9 mm Hg systolic and from 71 ± 6 mm Hg to 66 ± 8 mm Hg diastolic), submaximal aerobic fitness (from 2.0 ± 0.5 L/min to 2.3 ± 0.6 L/min) and self-esteem (from 2.56 ± 0.63 to 2.77 ± 0.58). Multivariate analysis of covariance revealed significant pre to post differences between campers and the non-camp attending comparison groups across all measures. No gender differences were observed between the intervention group during the eight-week intervention programme.

Inpatient treatment programmes summary

The presented outcomes demonstrate the potential of both residential weight loss camps and inpatient treatment programmes as forms of effective treatment programmes for obese children and adolescents. However, despite impressive short-term outcomes illustrating that it is possible to decrease FM and preserve LBM, while improving both physical fitness and mental health, these intervention programmes posses a number of limitations, namely: variations in intervention content, assessment and outcome measure, small sample sizes, and in several cases limited follow-up data and high costs. Additionally, their reproducibility is limited by the lack of specific programme details. Despite these factors they may be useful to provide an intensive and efficient treatment for the large number of obese children who require greater attention than population-based preventative interventions will provide and/or for those children whom previous outpatient treatment had failed. Further research is required to discover what factors have the greatest impact on a child's ability to maintain or continue weight loss after such interventions.

Conclusion

As outlined in the introduction these data tend to focus on both boys and girls rather than the intended group for this book, boys. There are a couple of probable reasons why gender differences are not described. First, in the context of intervention studies, the main effects associated with the intended outcomes are not achieved. Therefore further analyses by gender are unlikely to be explored and/or reported. In addition, few researchers report the details of the interventions, highlighting that interventions are not sophisticated enough to appropriately differentiate between boys and girls. Clearly this is a problem when one is looking to understand more about the impact of interventions on one particular group. With such an evidence base on which to base our findings it is not surprising it was difficult to communicate the data specifically on boys. It is clear that levels of childhood obesity continue to increase, at a time when the systems in place to tackle obesity are poor and the evidence base on which to guide public health officials is weak. The likely outcome at this time is that at best obesity levels will continue to increase in line with the rates that have been observed during the last 15 years. Significant global action is required in order to initially slow down the rates of increase and ultimately reduce the rates of weight problems in children. It is hoped that guidance from the WHO *Global Strategy on Diet, Physical Activity and Health* (2004), and the National Institute for Health and Clinical

Excellence (NICE, 2006) guidance on obesity will provide greater momentum to undertake the efforts required to tackle the global epidemic of being overweight and obese.

References

Archibald EH, Harrison J, Pencharz P. Body composition changes in obese adolescents on a protein sparing modified fast. *Ped Res.* 1981; **15**: 440–5.

Braet C. Patient characteristics as predictors of weight loss after an obesity treatment for children. *Obesity.* 2006; **14**(1): 148–55.

Braet C, Tanghe A, Decaluwe V, Moens E, Rosseel Y. Inpatient treatment for children with obesity: weight loss, psychological well-being, and eating behavior. *J Pediatr Psychol.* 2004; **29**(7): 519–29.

Braet C, Van Winckel M. Long-term follow-up of a cognitive behavioural treatment program for obese children. *Behav Ther.* 2000; **31**: 55–74.

Brown MR, Klish WJ, Hollander J *et al.* A high protein, low calorie liquid diet in the treatment of very obese adolescents: long-term effect on lean body mass. *Am J Clin Nutr.* 1983; **38**(1): 20–31.

Bundred P, Kitchiner D, Buchan I. Prevalence of overweight and obese children between 1989 and 1998: population based series of cross sectional studies. *BMJ.* 2001; **322**(7282): 1–4.

Campbell K, Waters E, O'Meara S *et al.* Interventions for preventing obesity in childhood: a systematic review. *Obes Rev.* 2001; **2**: 149–57.

Canning H, Mayer J. Obesity: its possible effect on college acceptance. *N Engl J Med.* 1966; **275**: 1172–4.

Canning H, Mayer J. Obesity: an influence on high school performance? *Am J Clin Nutr.* 1967; **20**: 352–4.

Chinn S, Rona RJ. Prevalence and trends in overweight and obesity in three cross sectional studies of British children, 1974–94. *BMJ.* 2001; **322**: 24–6.

Cole TJ, Bellizzi MC, Flegal KM, Dietz WH. Establishing a standard definition for childhood overweight and obesity worldwide: international survey. *BMJ.* 2000; **320**: 1240–3.

Cramer P, Steinwert T. Thin is good, fat is bad: how early does it begin? *J Appl Dev Psychol.* 1998; **19**: 429–51.

Dao HH, Frelut ML, Oberlin F, Peres G, Bourgeois P, Navarro J. Effects of a multidisciplinary weight loss intervention on body composition in obese adolescents. *Int J Obes.* 2004a; **28**: 290–9.

Dao HH, Felut M-L, Peres G *et al.* Effects of a multidisciplinary weight loss intervention on anaerobic and aerobic aptitudes in severely obese adolescents. *Int J Obes.* 2004b; **28**: 870–8.

Deforche B, Bourdeaudhuij ID, Debode P *et al.* Changes in fat mass, fat-free mass and aerobic fitness in severely obese children and adolescents following a residential treatment programme. *Eur J Pediatr.* 2003; **162**: 616–22.

Deforche B, Bourdeaudhuij ID, Tanghe A *et al.* Role of physical activity and eating in weight control after treatment in severely obese children and adolescents. *Acta Paediatrica.* 2005; **94**: 464–70.

Dempster P, Aitkens S. A new air displacement method for the determination of human body composition. *Med Sci Sports Exerc.* 1995; **27**(12): 1692–7.

Department of Health. *Health Survey of England.* London: The Stationery Office; 2003.

Department of Health. *Health Survey of England.* London: The Stationery Office; 2004.

Dietz WH, Schoeller DA. Optimal dietary therapy for obese adolescents: comparison of protein plus glucose and protein plus fat. *J Ped.* 1982; **100**: 638–44.

Doak CM, Visscher TLS, Renders CM, Seidell JC. The prevention of overweight and obesity in children and adolescents: a review of interventions and programmes. *Obes Rev.* 2006; **7**: 111–36.

Endo H, Takagi Y, Nozue T, Kuwahata K, Uemasu F, Kobayashi A. Beneficial effects of dietary intervention on serum lipid and Apolipoprotein levels in obese children. *Am J Dis Child.* 1992; **146**: 303–5.

Floodmark C-E, Marcus C, Britton M. Interventions to prevent obesity in children and adolescents: a systematic review. *Int J Obes.* 2006; **30**: 579–89.

Freedman DS, Dietz WH, Srinivasan SR, Berenson GS. The relation of overweight to cardiovascular risk factors among children and adolescents: the Bogalusa Heart Study. *Pediatrics*. 1999; **103**(6): 1175–82.

Freedman DS, Khan LK, Serdula MK, Dietz WH, Srinivasan SR, Berenson GS. Inter-relationship among childhood BMI, childhood height, and adult obesity: the Bogalusa Heart Study. *Int J Obes*. 2004; **28**: 10–6.

Fulton JE, McGuire MT, Caspersen CJ, Dietz WH. Interventions for weight loss and weight gain prevention among youth: current issues. *Sports Med*. 2001; **31**: 153–65.

Gately PJ, Cooke CB, Butterly RJ, Knight C, Carroll S. The effects of an eight week diet, exercise, behavior and educational program on a sample of children attending a weight loss camp. *Ped Exerc Sci*. 2000a; **12**: 413–23.

Gately PJ, Cooke CB, Butterly RJ, Mackreth P, Carroll S. The effects of an eight-week physical activity, diet and behavior modification program on a sample of children attending a weight loss camp with a 10-month follow up. *Int J Obes*. 2000b; **24**: 1445–52.

Gately PJ, Cooke CB, Barth JH, Bewick BM, Radley D, Hill AJ. Residential weight loss programs can work: a cohort study of acute outcomes for overweight and obese children. *Pediatrics*. 2005; **116**: 73–7.

Health Select Committee. *Health Select Committee Report on Obesity*. House of Commons. London: The Stationery Office; 2004.

James J, Thomas P, Cavan D, Kerr D. Preventing childhood obesity by reducing consumption of carbonated drinks: cluster randomised controlled trial. *BMJ*. 2004; **328**(7540): 1237.

Janssen I, Craige W, Boyce WF, Pickett W. Associations between overweight and obesity with bullying behaviors in school-aged children. *Pediatrics*. 2004; **113**(5): 1187–94.

Karris L. Prejudice against obese renters. *J Soc Psychol*. 1977; **101**: 159–60.

Lobstein T, Baur L, Uauy R. Obesity in children and young people: a crisis in public health. *Obes Rev*. 2004; **5**(S1): 4–85.

Malina RM, Bouchard C. *Growth, Maturation, and Physical Activity*. Champaign, IL: Human Kinetics; 1991.

McCarthy D, Ellis SM, Cole TJ. Central overweight and obesity in British youth aged 11–16 years: cross sectional surveys of waist circumference. *BMJ*. 2003; **326**(7390): 624.

Mullen MC, Shield J. *Childhood and Adolescent Overweight: the health professional's guide to identification, treatment, and prevention*. Chicago, IL: American Dietetic Association; 2004.

National Audit Office. *Tackling Obesity in England. Report by the Comptroller and Auditor General*. London: The Stationery Office; 2001.

National Institute for Health and Clinical Excellence. *Obesity*. London: NICE; 2006. www.nice.org.uk/guidance/CG43

Nichols JF, Bigelow DM, Canine KM. Short-term weight loss and exercise training effects on glucose-induced thermogenesis in obese adolescent males during hypocaloric feeding. *Int J Obes*. 1989; **13**(5): 683–90.

Pena M, Bacallao J, Barta L, Amador M, Johnston FE. Fiber and exercise in the treatment of obese adolescents. *J Adolesc Health Care*. 1989; **10**(1): 30–4.

Reilly JJ, Dorosty AR, Emmett PM. Prevalence of overweight and obesity in British children: cohort study. *BMJ*. 1999; **319**(7216): 1039.

Reilly JJ, Methven E, McDowell ZC *et al*. Health consequences of obesity. *Arch Dis Child*. 2003; **88**: 748–52.

Resnicow K, Robinson TN. School-based cardiovascular disease prevention studies: review and synthesis. *Ann Epidemiol*. 1997; **S7**: S14–17.

Rohrbacher R. Influence of a special camp program for obese boys on weight loss, self-concept, and body image. *Res Q*. 1973; **44**(2): 150–7.

Rolland-Cachera MF, Thibault H, Souberbielle JC *et al*. Massive obesity in adolescents: dietary interventions and behaviours associated with weight regain at 2 y follow-up. *Int J Obes*. 2004; **28**: 514–19.

Rudolf MC, Sahota P, Barth JH, Walker J. Increasing prevalence of obesity in primary school children: cohort study. *BMJ*. 2001; **322**(7294): 1094–5.

Rudolf MCJ, Greenwood DC, Cole TJ *et al*. Rising obesity and expanding waistlines in schoolchildren: a cohort study. *Arch Dis Child*. 2004; **89**: 235–7.

Sahota P, Rudolf MCJ, Dixey R, Hill AJ, Barth JH, Cade J. Randomised controlled trial of primary school based intervention to reduce risk factors for obesity. *BMJ*. 2001a; **323**: 1–5.

Sahota P, Rudolf MCJ, Dixey R, Hill AJ, Barth JH, Cade J. Evaluation of implementation and effect of primary school based intervention to reduce risk factors for obesity. *BMJ*. 2001b; **232**: 1–4.

Scottish Intercollegiate Guidelines Network (SIGN). *Management of Obesity in Children and Young People*. Edinburgh: SIGN; 2003.

Staffieri JR. A study of social stereotype of body image in children. *J Pers Soc Psychol*. 1967; **7**: 101–4.

Stallings VA, Archibald EH, Pencharz PB. Potassium, magnesium, and calcium balance in obese adolescents on a protein-sparing modified fast. *Am J Clin Nutr*. 1988; **47**(2): 220–4.

Stang JS, Story M, Kalina B. School-based weight management services: perceptions and practices of school nurses and administrators. *Am J Health Promot*. 1997; **11**(3): 183–5.

Story M. School-based approaches for preventing and treating obesity. *Int J Obes*. 1999; **23**(S2): S43–51.

Summerbell C, Ashton V, Campbell K, Edmunds L, Kelly S, Waters E. Interventions for treating obesity in children. *Cochrane Database Systematic Review*. 2003; **3**: CD001872.

Summerbell E, Waters E, Edmunds LD, Kelly S, Brown T, Campbell K. Interventions for preventing obesity in children. *Cochrane Database Systematic Review*. 2005; **3**: CD001871.

Swinburn B, Egger G. Preventive strategies against weight gain and obesity. *Obes Rev*. 2002; **3**(4): 289–301.

Wabitsch M, Braun U, Heinze E *et al*. Body composition in 5–18-y-old obese children and adolescents before and after weight reduction as assessed by deuterium dilution and bioelectrical impedance analysis. *Am J Clin Nutr*. 1996; **64**: 1–6.

Walker LLM, Gately PJ, Bewick BM, Hill AJ. Children's weight-loss camps; psychological benefit or jeopardy? *Int J Obes*. 2003; **27**: 748–54.

Wanless D. *Securing Our Future Health. Taking a long term view*. London: HM Treasury, Public Enquiry Unit; 2002.

Warren JM, Henry CJK, Lightowler SM *et al*. Evaluation of a pilot school programme aimed at the prevention of obesity in children. *Health Promot Int*. 2003; **18**(4): 287–96.

World Health Organization (WHO). *Global Strategy on Diet, Physical Activity and Health*. Geneva: WHO; 2004.

CHAPTER 13

Tackling weight problems in older men

Kate Davidson

The problems associated with being overweight (BMI 25–30 kg/m^2) and obese (BMI > 30 kg/m^2) are not confined to younger generations: older people too increasingly present with major health issues as a result of carrying too much weight. For overweight and obese older men in particular, there are not only physical problems, but also social and emotional consequences. However, morbid obesity (BMI > 40 kg/m^2) in very old age for men, that is over 75 years, is not a major epidemiological problem. This is because the vast majority of these obese men do not survive (Department of Health, 2004). Indeed, there is substantial evidence of reduction in body weight, BMI and mid-upper arm circumference in people aged 75 and over, compared with those under 75 (Forster and Gariballa, 2005). Nevertheless, there is a consensus that obesity has reached global epidemic proportions and that prevalences are particularly high in elderly adults (Janssen *et al.*, 2005). Although the increase of prevalence of obesity is being observed in both developed and less developed regions, most of the literature emanates from the USA, where the trends started earlier than in other parts of the world.

This chapter explores recent trends in older men's weight problem rates in the USA and Europe, and examines some of the research carried out on the physical and emotional outcomes of such trends. It then reports findings from a UK project on older men which examined attitudes to their own health and their relationship with health professionals. Finally it offers some suggestions for health promotion strategies relevant to the lives of men as they age.

In the USA, it was estimated that in 1999–2000, 30.5% of the population over the age of 65 were obese as determined by their BMI (Flegal *et al.*, 2002). This figure had increased from 22.9% in the period 1988–94. In England, the proportion of obese people over the age of 65 in 2003 was 27% (Department of Health, 2004) (*see* Table 13.1). In England, the men were more likely to be overweight (BMI 25–30) than the women (50% compared to 41%) but the women were more likely to be obese (BMI 30+) at 28% compared to 25%, which represents a three-fold increase since the 1980s.

Longitudinal data from Norway (Drøyvold *et al.*, 2006), comparing 1984–86 and

TABLE 13.1 Men's body mass index in mid-life and old age, 2003, England.

BMI (kg/m²)	45–54%	55–64%	65–74%	75+ %
18.5	0	1	0	1
18.6–24.9	24	22	22	29
25–29.9	48	50	49	50
30–39.9	27	26	28	21
Over 40	2	1	1	0
All over 30 (obese)	28	27	29	22
Base numbers	1,073	943	664	369

Source: Department of Health (2004).

TABLE 13.2 The proportion (%) of older men and women overweight or obese (based on both measured and self-reported height and weight), Auckland, 1993.

	65–74 years		75–84 years	
	Men (n = 243)	Women (n = 244)	Men (n = 232)	Women (n = 261)
Obese*				
Measured	15.6	24.1	9.7	10.3
Self-reported	10.3	13.5	6.3	8.9
Overweight**				
Measured	48.4	35.2	47.4	39.7
Self-reported	39.7	35.4	36.0	28.1

*Obese (BMI >30 kg/m²). ** Overweight (BMI 25–30 kg/m²).
Source: Ministry of Health NZ (1993).

1995–97, found that participants who were younger than 50 years at the first survey showed a large increase in body weight. In contrast, the participants who were 70 or older had on average a weight loss. Overall, the proportion classified as obese increased from 6.7 to 15.5% among the males and from 11% to 21% among females. Interestingly, some of the increase can be explained by a reduction in height, which was most pronounced in the oldest age groups.

A reduction in height in later life can also explain the disparity in self-reported and measured BMI of older New Zealanders from the Auckland Heart and Health study in 1993 (Minister of Health NZ, 1993) (*see* Table 13.2). Older people frequently calculate the height they were in their early and mid-years, without recognising that they become shorter as they age. Reduced height of course alters the BMI calculation upwards (Drøyvold *et al.*, 2006).

This brings into question the appropriateness of the BMI measurement for older people. BMI is most commonly used and is particularly relevant for young and middle-aged people. However, it has been argued that BMI may not be the best indicator of risk factors for cardiovascular disease (CVD) in older men and women, as several studies, for example Wannamethee *et al.* (2004) from the UK, Vermeulen (2005), from Belgium and Janssen *et al.* (2005) from Canada, have failed to demonstrate a relationship between a high BMI and mortality in people over the age of 65.

Several hypotheses have been offered to explain this lack of association. One argument is that a higher body fat content may act as a protector or 'reserve' during illness in old age. Rather, waist circumference (WC) is considered a more appropriate measurement because overweight men in particular tend to accumulate abdominal visceral adipose tissue (which indicates fat around the abdominal organs rather than just under the skin) and develop the characteristic 'apple' shape as they age. It is the volume of abdominal rather than subcutaneous fat which is a greater predictor of morbidity and mortality. Racette *et al.* (2006) conclude that increased abdominal adiposity is a strong predictor of insulin resistance (found in type 2 diabetes) in old age, and their findings support the measurement of waist circumference to assess health risk among older adults. In other words, it is the distribution of body fat, as indicated by the waist circumference, rather than the degree of excess weight as measured by the BMI, which may be a better determinant of health risk in later life.

What are the health risk factors?

Overweight and obese middle-aged and older men are more likely to suffer from cardiovascular disease (CVD), high blood pressure and blood cholesterol, type 2 diabetes (non-insulin dependent diabetes mellitus, NIDDM), hypogonadism (reduced testosterone levels) and erectile dysfunction (impotence), sleep apnoea and somatovegetative symptoms (disorders of sleep and appetite) than their slimmer counterparts. Obesity in men tends to peak during middle age (40–65 years) and then reduces over the age of 65, largely because excessively overweight men tend not to survive. Premature death of obese middle-aged people therefore results in an overall decrease in BMI in surviving older adults.

Villareal *et al.* (2005) argue that the appropriate clinical approach to obesity in older adults is controversial, since research has shown that older people may not benefit from weight loss resulting in a reduction in muscle mass and bone density. As discussed above, there is some evidence to suggest that being overweight to some degree in later life can have a health protective effect inasmuch as the BMI value associated with lower mortality is slightly higher than in younger adults. However, Wannamethee *et al.* (2004) warn against misinterpretation of these findings. They point out that the mortality risk associated with increased BMI does increase with age because mortality risk increases with advancing years. The lack of evidence of an association between BMI and mortality after the age of 75 years remains a puzzle. Perhaps those overweight people of 75 plus are part of the small population who 'defy' adverse effects of obesity, rather like the tale of the '40-a-day smoker who lives to be 90'.

Social and emotional effects

On average an obese man will have undergone changes in body composition which include an increase of body fat from 19 to 35%, a 20% loss in lean body mass with an attendant reduction in skeletal muscle power (Tan and Pu, 2002). Although it has been widely recognised for some time, by medical and lay people alike, that excess weight is associated with heart and lung disease, diabetes, bone and joint problems, and some cancers, less attention has been paid to the social and emotional effects of hormonal changes in overweight men. There are studies which have shown an association between low testosterone levels and insulin resistance – that is, a reduced ability to process glucose which leads to type 2 diabetes. What is set up, then, is a vicious circle of weight gain (or inability to lose weight), reduced testosterone levels and the physical consequences, including impotence, which in turn can lead to low self-esteem and depression.

Although somewhat controversial, in the last decade there has been a call for the recognition of an 'andropause' – a male climacteric equivalent to the mid-life menopause experienced by women. The argument stems from the identification of changes in reproductive hormones with advancing age, for both men and women. As discussed above, there is a decrease in testosterone concentration, and research has shown that older men, although many remain fertile into very late life, take longer to achieve a pregnancy, even if their partner is young (Hassan and Killick, 2003). Normal ageing in men is accompanied by a decline in testosterone levels, but obesity depresses the production of testosterone even more markedly and can lead to hypogonadism (Tan and Pu, 2002). Hypogonadism in ageing men is accompanied by symptoms such as decreased libido, erectile dysfunction, loss of energy, periodic sweating, sleep disturbance, increase in fat mass, decrease in lean muscle mass, osteoporosis and mood and memory changes. Testosterone replacement therapy in ageing men may have a role in improving lean body mass and strength, but there have been relatively few studies on hormone replacement for obese men (Tan and Pu, 2002). However, there is evidence to suggest that a combination of testosterone treatment and sildenafil (Viagra) could improve erectile function and impact significantly on the quality of life and self-esteem of sufferers (Shabsigh, 2004).

The relation between energy intake and expenditure is the principal determinant of weight at all ages, but given the biochemical and physiological changes associated with ageing, maintaining a balance has greater relevance in later life. Furthermore, data from longitudinal studies suggest that obese men are more likely to suffer from cardiovascular disease than obese older women (Harris *et al.*, 1997). The current focus on pathological aspects of causality has dominated health research on older men, and less attention has been paid to the meanings of health risk to older men and how these intersect with partnership status and notions of appropriate masculine behaviour. We were interested in unpacking the health behaviours of older men to examine how they are driven by men's socially constructed roles (Davidson and Arber, 2004).

What are older men telling us?

This section reports findings from an Economic and Social Research Council (ESRC) research project[1] carried out in South East England and draws substantially on the published literature from the project. Segments from this literature are reproduced here (Davidson, 2004, 2005; Davidson and Arber, 2003, 2004; Davidson *et al.*, 2003). The project involved 85 community-dwelling men over the age of 65, who were asked about their perceived quality of life, social networks and health behaviours – nutrition, physical activity and well-being.

We collected a purposive sample as we were interested in marital status and living circumstances and so men who lived alone are over-represented (see Davidson *et al.*, 2003, for fuller discussion on the methodological issues). The men were interviewed by an older male social scientist, and a great deal of empathy was perceived between the researcher and his interviewees, demonstrated by their willingness to disclose sexual intimacies and detailed physical limitations, for example their experience of impotence.

We interviewed 30 married/cohabiting, 33 widowed, 10 divorced/separated and 12 never-married men. Half of them were aged between 65 and 74 and half were 75+. The divorced men were the youngest group with an average age of 68, and there were none over the age of 80. This contrasts with the oldest group, the widowers, whose average age was 79 with none under the age of 70. The married/cohabiting men and the never-married men had an average age of 73. The average age of the 85 participants was 75.

Not unlike younger generations, the older men had a widespread knowledge of what constituted good health behaviours, and the consequences of transgressing them. They knew the recommended weekly alcohol limits, they were well aware of the dangers of smoking and could give us chapter and verse on what was meant by a good diet. They stressed the importance of physical activity for fitness and weight control. And, not unlike younger generations, some did not adhere to advice:

> *Jon[2] (72, married): I should walk more. I suppose if I walk round to the post box round the corner, that's the furthest I go during the week. We try and walk at weekends. … I'm a bad lad I know. Like for breakfast, I will get up in the morning and probably have two pots of tea, bad for you, eight cups of tea, eight spoonfuls of sugar – wrong. It used to be 16, but I have cut the sugar down. Lunch I might have a cheese sandwich, bad for me again. But then I have an evening meal. It would be a cooked meal. Last night it was bacon, tonight it will be a small roast. I like a drink, I probably drink too much, more than what I should do.*

Jon was certainly not unusual in knowing what was 'bad' for him. Arthur was obese and had serious cardiovascular problems.

> *Arthur (69, never married): Well, it is obviously related to health [his weight] but I am very conscious of, you know, bad food not being good for me. I think I know what food is definitely bad for me even though I may eat some of it … I would eat a hamburger if I was hungry but I wouldn't go out of my way to eat a hamburger.*

There are also issues of 'denial' rather than ignorance. Despite considerably poor health, Fred continued to take health risks:

> *Fred (78, widowed): Seeing as I have had heart attacks, and by-passes and a few other horrible things … You're not supposed to add sugar and you are not supposed to have salt. So I try and keep within them things … As I say, I might cook some egg, bacon and sausage. I have wishful thinking that the*

vegetable oil that I put in the pan is not going to do me any harm. Probably not true.

Like Fred above, Tom identifies the association between diet, good health and weight, but fails to see it through:

Tom (65, married): Healthwise, we tend to hope that we do it through the varied diet although we have both put on weight in the last five years and both would probably be considered to be a stone overweight.

There is an interesting disjunction between the knowledge these older men have and what they practise:

- I should lose some weight.
- I should walk more.
- I probably drink too much.
- I still like my fried breakfast.
- Smoking is so bad for my chest.

Davidson *et al.* (2003) found that marriage can exert a protective effect on men's physical and psychological well-being, with women taking primary responsibility for monitoring the health of family members, especially a husband in later life. Of the respondents, only six men attended well-man clinics and blood pressure and cholesterol screening sessions (as opposed to diagnostic procedures) and they were all married and tended to be under the age of 75.

Richard (69, married): Well, if there's anything going free to do with health, I usually try to get onto it. I did do a men's health course through Age Concern, a 10-week course about 18 months ago. And if I go to an exhibition somewhere or to an air show, something like that, and they do a blood test and blood pressure, I'll go in and do it, because it's there. My wife gets on at me a bit if I don't take advantage, especially if it's free.

Older lone men, in particular, are less likely to have a 'caretaker' to monitor their health behaviours, or a 'gatekeeper' to encourage health consultation. As a result of rising divorce rates and decreasing remarriage rates, larger numbers of older men will experience solo living in the 21st century. Over two-thirds of older men live with a spouse but demographic trends reveal that an increasing number of older men live alone: in 2001, 29% of men over the age of 65 lived alone compared to 16% in 1971. Among men currently aged 65 and over, 17% are widowed, while only 7% are never-married and 5% are divorced or separated. By 2021, however, it is projected that although the proportion of men aged over 65 who are widowed will fall to 13% mainly because of improvements in mortality, 8% will be never-married, and 13% will be divorced (Government Actuary's Department, 2001), making 34% of men over the age of 65 who are likely to be living alone in 2021.

Reg (70, divorced): Actually, I've been offered one [health screening]. I suppose I ought to, really.

Who, we might ask, will be their caretakers, or gatekeepers for health monitoring?

Older men and health professionals

It is well documented that men, throughout their lives, are less likely to consult health professionals than are women. This stems from men and women's fundamentally different relationship with health and illness. Women consult health professionals when they are not sick: for family planning, pregnancy, children's immunisation and to accompany them if they (the children) are sick, cervical and breast screening, and so on. They subsequently have a positive relationship with health professionals which ameliorates negative aspects of consultation if they themselves are ill. Men, on the other hand, are more likely to avoid consultation since their main contact with a doctor is because there is something wrong. Into the equation is the notion that men should be strong, independent and uncomplaining – in other words, the essence of masculinity.

Our findings revealed three main groups of older men: those who reported that they seldom or never consulted health professionals, those who said they sometimes (five or six times a year) visited the GP surgery, and those who had frequent, at least once a month, contact with a health professional. As discussed below, however, men's reportage of contact does not necessarily conflate with actual contact. A picture emerged that the older married men reported better health and fewer health-damaging behaviours than men who lived alone. Within the latter group, however, there were differences between the widowed, divorced/separated and the never-married men.

Common to each partnership status were men who said they seldom consulted a health professional and, even less frequently, their GP. These men can be categorised into 'sceptics' and 'stoics'.

The *sceptics* used phrases like: 'Most of them are a waste of time'. One said: 'I don't like doctors, I keep as far away from the place … it's not an exact science – you can quote me on that'. This respondent went on to say that meteorology and medicine were about as accurate as each other. Another said that he would rather go to a veterinary surgeon than a doctor 'after the way they treated my wife'. Even if he had cancer, he said, he would put up with it, rather than seek medical help.

The *stoics* said things like:

- 'I think it is like, well, ladies will go to the doctors many, many times more than a man. A man says – "Oh, it came by itself, it will go by itself".'
- 'I don't give in. Even if I felt awful, I wouldn't tell anyone.'
- 'I've always tended to think, well, it's going to go away.'
- ' … a lot of illnesses, people can deal with it themselves.'
- 'You've just got to get through it.'

Most of these 'non-attenders' reported general good health. Some attributed it to heredity and luck, and others to 'looking after themselves'.

> *Andrew (75, married): I am healthy, yes. No, I've never been ill in my life. I always say 'I don't hold with illness'. You know, it's a thing for other people. I think my good health is hereditary.*

> *Rory (84, married): I'm one of these lucky people that have suffered good health all my life. … we are sensible about our eating, we try and do a certain amount of walking exercise each day.*

Peter (70, widowed): I have been wonderfully fit, apart from back trouble since my wife died. I don't drink lots of alcohol, I don't smoke, I live a fairly simple lifestyle, a healthy lifestyle.

Nevertheless, despite saying that they rarely visited a doctor, many of the men reported chronic health conditions. For example, there was a surprisingly high reportage of asthma for which the men were prescribed an inhaler after initial diagnosis. In the UK, it is possible to request a repeat prescription from a surgery without having to see the GP and, while indeed these men were not visiting a doctor, they were still 'receiving treatment'.

There were a number of men who had undergone major treatment/surgery for heart disease (usually a by-pass) or cancer (most commonly prostate), who saw their physician for regular check-ups – from quarterly to biennially. 'They tell you to come back, you have to see them once a year, and he sort of puts the old stethoscope on, asks a few questions and tells you to come back next year.' The men who reported these routine visits did not see them as 'sickness' consultations and tended not to count them as 'going to the doctor', until the interviewer probed, often later in the interview. We termed these *compliance* patients. These men said they rarely went to a doctor when originally asked, and then later disclosed a health condition which required follow-up visits, which they did not view as 'attending the doctor'.

There were men who were very ill, and in need of considerable health professional input. In this group the most frequent story was of what we have termed *domino pathology*, whereby the men said they were 'perfectly healthy' until, say, five years before, and then everything started to go wrong. Interestingly, these stories were most often told by widowers who had cared long term for an ailing wife and could date their health decline from the death of their spouse.

Forrest (81, widowed): I'm now 81 and I'm in poor health, very poor health. Up until the age of 75, I was going fine and then I had a serious cancer operation after my wife died and it's been downhill since.

A few married men also reported some very dramatic health problems, and were very likely to talk about their prevailing ailment(s) at some length, giving graphic details of the history, diagnosis and treatment of their condition. In contrast, the never-married men talked very little about their health, even though they reported prostate and heart problems. Despite the difference in age profile, the younger divorced men were just as likely to report similar serious health problems as the older widowed men, but the widowed men were more likely to have seen a doctor recently, i.e. within the previous three months. Often these visits were recommended by adult children and grandchildren.

Clearly, for older men, marital status and history have a strong influence on health risks and healthy behaviours. The most vulnerable groups were those men who lived alone in their latter years. If the population predictions are accurate and divorce rates in older men are almost trebled by 2021 (Government Actuary's Department, 2001) we consider that more research is needed in this burgeoning group of older men who are the most likely to indulge in health risk behaviours (Davidson and Arber, 2003).

Conclusions

Although about half of the men we interviewed were overweight, only three men were obese and there were no men who were morbidly obese. We cannot generalise from such a small sample of men, but our findings are similar to those of Department of Health Survey of 2003, as shown in Table 13.1, from which we could speculate that obesity is not a serious problem for men over the age of 75 – because they will have died in mid-life or early old age. What emerged from the qualitative analysis was a complex picture of health awareness, health protection strategies and risk taking. Interestingly, most men knew what they 'should' do to maintain good health, both subjectively, by reducing life-threatening practices, and objectively, by undertaking regular health screening such as blood pressure and cholesterol levels. Nevertheless, there was a disjuncture between what they knew, and how they ultimately acted on this knowledge.

While women have routinely visited the doctor throughout the life course, for family planning, pregnancy, or to take their children for clinics, immunisation programmes as well as when they are sick, the men in this study seemed to consider going to the doctor as a sign of weakness (Davidson and Arber, 2003). However, doctor avoidance becomes a vicious circle. The older men interviewed admitted to postponing making an appointment until they were very sick. They then had negative associations with the doctor, who they see when they are in pain, or feel very unwell and, importantly, who may give them bad news about their health. We found that partnered men were more likely to seek help and take appropriate advice following medical consultation than men who lived alone. The presence of a partner seemed to influence both their subjective and objective health behaviours.

To date, most health education has been directed at individuals and has been based on a limited understanding of their social circumstances. We argue that in order to generate substantial and effective changes in the health-related behaviours of older men, interventions need to be sensitive to the economic, biological, social and cultural constructs that shape the expectations and behaviour of men as they age and experience health transitions.

Acknowledgements

I would like to acknowledge the input from my co-researchers on these two projects: Professor Sara Arber, and Mr Tom Daly from the Centre for Research on Ageing and Gender, Department of Sociology, University of Surrey, Guildford.

Notes

1 Economic and Social Research Council: Growing Older Programme. *Older Men: their social worlds and healthy lifestyles.* Award number: L480 25 4033. 2003.
2 All names are anonymised.

References

Davidson K. Why can't a man be more like a woman? Marital status and social networking of older men. *The Journal of Men's Studies.* 2004; **13**(1): 25–43.

Davidson K. Lifestyle and health promotion. In: Heath H, Watson R, editors. *Older People: assessment for health and social care.* London: Age Concern; 2005. p. 74–80.

Davidson K, Arber S. Older men's health: a lifecourse issue? *Men's Health Journal.* 2003; **2**(3): 72–5.

Davidson K, Arber S. Older men, their health behaviours and partnership status. In: Walker A, Hennessy C, editors. *Growing Older: quality of life in old age.* Maidenhead: Open University Press/McGraw Hill; 2004. p. 127–48.

Davidson K, Daly T, Arber S. Exploring the worlds of older men. In: Arber S, Davidson K, Ginn J, editors. *Gender and Ageing: changing roles and relationships.* Maidenhead: Open University Press/ McGraw Hill; 2003. p. 168–85.

Department of Health. *Health Survey of England 2003.* London: HMSO; 2004. www.dh.gov.uk/ PublicationsAndStatistics/PublishedSurvey/HealthSurveyForEngland/fs/en (accessed 21 March 2006).

Drøyvold W, Nilsen T, Krüger Ø *et al.* Change in height, weight and body mass index: longitudinal data from the HUNT Study in Norway. *International Journal of Obesity.* 2006; **30**(6): 935–9.

Flegal K, Carroll M, Ogden C, Johnson C. Prevalence and trends in obesity among US adults, 1999– 2000. *Journal of the American Medical Association.* 2002; **288**(14): 1772–3.

Forster S, Gariballa S. Age as a determinant of nutritional status: a cross sectional study. *Nutrition Journal.* 2005; **4**: 28. www.nutritionj.com/content/4/1/28 (accessed 12 March 2007).

Government Actuary's Department. *Marital Projections: England and Wales.* 2001. www.gad.gov.uk/marital_status_projections/2003/divorce_assumptions.htm (accessed 18 April 2007).

Harris T, Launer L, Madans J, Feldman J. Cohort study of effect of being overweight and change in weight on risk of coronary disease in old age. *British Medical Journal.* 1997; **314**: 1791–4.

Hassan M, Killick S. Effect of male age on fertility: evidence for the decline in male fertility with increasing age. *Fertility and Sterility.* 2003; **79**(3): 1520–7.

Janssen I, Katzmarzyk P, Ross R. Body mass index is inversely related to mortality in older people after adjustment for waist circumference. *Journal of the American Geriatric Society.* 2005; **53**: 2112– 18.

Minister of Health NZ. *Primary Prevention of Cardiovascular Disease in Older New Zealanders.* 1993.

Racette S, Evans E, Weiss E, Hagberg J, Holloszy J. Abdominal adiposity is a stronger predictor of insulin resistance than fitness among 50–95 year olds. *Diabetes Care.* 2006; **29**: 673–8.

Shabsigh R. Testosterone therapy in erectile dysfunction. *The Aging Male.* 2004; **7**(4): 312–18.

Tan R, Pu S. Impact of obesity on hypogonadism in the andropause. *International Journal of Andrology.* 2002; **25**(4): 195–200.

Vermeulen A. The epidemic of obesity: obesity and health of the aging male. *The Aging Male.* 2005; **8**(1): 39–41.

Villareal D, Apovian C, Kushner R, Klein S. Obesity in older adults: technical review and position statement of the American Society for Nutrition and NAASO, The Obesity Society. *American Journal of Clinical Nutrition.* 2005; **82**(5): 923–34.

Wannamethee SG, Shaper AG, Whincup PH. Overweight and obesity and the burden of disease and disability in elderly men. *International Journal of Obesity.* 2004; **38**: 1374–82.

CHAPTER 14

Fit for inclusion: working with overweight and obese men with disabilities

Sue Catton

This chapter explores the incidence of weight problems among disabled people, the components and achievements of the Inclusive Fitness Initiative (IFI) to date and its impact on access to healthy lifestyles for disabled people. It outlines the components delivered by the IFI to provide a proactive response to meet the needs of disabled people in a fitness suite environment and looks at fitness programmes for overweight and obese disabled men. Advice for developing similar programmes and the need for additional research in this area are also addressed.

Defining and measuring disability

The multi-dimensional and dynamic nature of disability makes it inherently difficult to measure. There is currently no definitive measure for disability. As a result a wide variation exists in the survey estimates of the numbers of disabled people in Great Britain. Estimates range from 8.6 million (20%) in the 1996–1997 Disability Survey (Grundy *et al.*, 1999) to 11 million (23%) in more recent estimates of the number of adults covered by the Disability Discrimination Act (Grewal *et al.*, 2002).

The Family Resources Survey 2003–2004 is referenced by the Disability Rights Commission (DRC) stating that the number of disabled adults in Great Britain is currently 9.5 million of which 4.4 million are male, 20% of the male population (Disability Rights Commission, 2006). However, when the figures below are considered, it is evident that in reality the number of people with an impairment is much greater than all the above estimates:
- 9 million deaf or hearing impaired people (Royal National Institute for the Deaf)
- 2 million people with a visual impairment (Royal National Institute of the Blind)
- 1.5 million adults with a learning disability (Mencap)
- 9 million people with arthritis (Arthritis Care)
- one in four people will experience a mental health illness in their life (Goldberg and Huxley, 1992)

- one in six people will have a significant mental health problem at any one time (ONS, 2000).

Disability, as defined for the purpose of the Disability Discrimination Act 1995 (DDA), is:

> *A physical or mental impairment which has a substantial and long term adverse effect on a person's ability to carry out normal day to day activities.*

The statements below further expand on the interpretation of the definition and attempt to highlight the scope of the very wide meaning.

To qualify, a physical or mental impairment must be classified within the World Health Organization's International Classification of Diseases (WHO, 2006) and/or must be any clinically well-recognised or documented condition.

Physical impairment
This includes a weakening or adverse change of a part of the body caused through illness, by accident or from birth, e.g. blindness, deafness, and the paralysis of a limb or severe disfigurement.

Mental impairment
This can include learning disabilities and all recognised mental illnesses.

Substantial
The impairment does not have to be severe. However, it must be more than minor or trivial. Persons with progressive conditions including cancer, multiple sclerosis or HIV infection are all now deemed to be disabled persons, for the purposes of the Act.

Long-term adverse effect
The impairment has lasted, or is likely to last, more than 12 months or for the rest of the person's life.

Normal day-to-day activity
The Act states that an impairment is to be taken to affect the ability of a person to carry out normal day-to-day activities *only* if it affects that person in respect of one or more of the following:
- mobility
- manual dexterity
- physical co-ordination
- continence
- ability to lift, carry or otherwise move everyday objects
- speech, hearing or eyesight
- memory or ability to concentrate, learn or understand; or
- perception of the risk of physical danger.

The DDA definition of disability does not include conditions that could reasonably be reversed such as obesity unless it is caused by a genetic condition. However, obesity often causes disabilities such as type 2 diabetes, mobility problems, an increased risk of both chronic heart disease and cancer, and mental distress (EMHF Fact Sheet).

The profile of disability among men

The *Health Survey for England 2001* found that the profile of disability when compared between genders does not vary significantly until beyond the age of 75 (Bajekal *et al.*, 2003). For men aged 75 to 84, the proportions of the sample reporting at least one disability were significantly lower than those for women (43% versus 51%). When reaching ages of 85 and over, 7 in 10 of both men and women were disabled, but the proportions with serious disability were still lower for men (33%) than women (42%). It is likely that the higher prevalence of disability among women than men in older age groups reflects the shorter survival rates of males with disability.

The most commonly reported type of disability in the survey was locomotor disability (including ambulation and dexterity) with 12% of men (14% of women) reporting it, of which one in four reported a serious disability. The second largest prevalence was in personal care disability using activities for daily living as an indicator, with rates almost half those of locomotor disability for both sexes (6% men, 7% women), followed by hearing disability (6% men, 4% women) and visual impairment (2% men, 3% women) (Bajekal *et al.*, 2003).

When investigating the likely causes of disability there is evidence to suggest that there are gender variances affected by both lifestyle and employment profiles. Of the 25% of males reporting locomotor disability, lifestyle factors at the time of screening and manual social class were both strongly and independently associated with the increased likelihood of locomotor disability 12 to 14 years later (Ebrahim *et al.*, 2000). The study concluded:

> *Smoking, obesity, physical inactivity and heavy drinking in middle age are strong predictors of locomotor disability in later life independent of the presence of diagnosed disease. Leading a healthy lifestyle improves survival and reduces the incidence of disease. It also reduces the risk of locomotor disability and increases the odds of becoming disability free even in the event of developing major cardiovascular disease.*

In the *Health Survey for England 2001*, disabled men (19%) were more likely than disabled women (13%) to report that their condition was a result of an accident, and this gender difference was consistent for all ages except those aged 85 and over. Among those aged 35 to 44, a third of men with disability cited an accident as the cause of their disability compared with just under a fifth (19%) of women (Bajekal *et al.*, 2003). There was no specific questioning around obesity as a cause of disability however.

The incidence of weight problems among disabled people

There has been much research and comment about the increasing prevalence of weight problems, in particular among young people. However, while there is anecdotal evidence, very little research has been conducted into the scale of the problem of obesity among disabled people in the United Kingdom. There has been little research that attempts to place obesity within the context of disability, or analyse the inter-relationship of both as either cause or effect. As a result there is a lack of appreciation and application to address the needs for both the prevention of, and treatment for, weight problems among disabled people.

One of the few comprehensive studies into the area was conducted in the United States. 'Obesity among adults with disabling conditions' (Weil *et al.*, 2002) analysed the prevalence of obesity in adults with physical and sensory impairments and serious mental illness. The research used the 1994 to 1995 National Health Interview Survey of 145,000 respondents, 25,626 of whom had one or more disabilities. The research concluded that among disabled adults within the sample, 24.9% were obese compared to 15.1% among those without disabilities. Mild, moderate and severe obesity were all more prevalent in adults with one or more impairments than for those adults without an impairment. Rates of being overweight were slightly lower among disabled adults than non-disabled adults, except for those who were deaf or had a hearing impairment. Adults with lower limb impairments evidenced the highest incidence of obesity at all levels when compared with other impairment groups. The study confirmed that disabled adults are significantly more likely to be in the obese categories than non-disabled adults.

The overall incidence of obesity in the USA increased significantly from 23.3% between 1998 and 1994 to a figure of 31.1% between 1999 and 2002 (National Center for Health Statistics, 2005) and, based on both the above findings, it could be assumed that the incidence of obese disabled people has risen by a similar ratio.

Weil *et al.* (2002) ascertained that the prevalence of weight problems varies for different impairment groups but no similar studies or comparisons have been conducted to the author's knowledge in the UK. Little data exists for overweight and obese people with physical or hearing impairments and is patchy at best for visual impairments. One US study found that the greatest prevalence of weight problems was among people with arthritis and diabetes. Extreme obesity was also found to be approximately four times higher among disabled people than non-disabled people while all disabled people, regardless of sex and age, had higher rates of obesity when compared to non-disabled people (Rimmer and Wang, 2005). Despite fewer 'obvious' barriers to exercise, adults who were deaf or hard of hearing were also found to be more likely to be obese (Bajekal *et al.*, 2003). Low physical activity levels among individuals who are blind have been associated with increased obesity levels (Weitzman, 1986). People with vision impairments have a higher level of body fat, a factor that increases in frequency with the severity of the vision loss (Jankowski and Evans, 1981).

The recent DRC Interim Report on Health Inequalities (DRC, 2005) has identified that a third of people with schizophrenia and just under a third (30%) of people with bipolar disorder were classified as obese, compared to 21% of the remaining population. (Obesity can be a side effect of medication.) Most data on weight problems among disabled people relate to people with learning disabilities and even these are largely anecdotal. The same survey has revealed that 40% of women, and 35% of men, with learning disabilities in Wales are obese. Other studies from the USA identified that a disproportionate number of adults with a learning disability are classified as obese (Rimmer *et al.*, 1993) and that prevalence to being overweight among persons with Down's syndrome should be considered a major public health concern (Rubin *et al.*, 1997).

The prevalence of being overweight and obese increases with age. In England, about 28% of men aged between 16 and 24 are overweight or obese whereas 76% of men aged 65 to 74 fall into this category (National Audit Office, 2001). Similarly the prevalence of disability increases with age from 12% for young people aged between 16 and 24, to 41% aged 65 to 74, and 55% aged 80 to 84 years (ONS, 2001).

Rationale for the increased incidence of weight problems among disabled people

People with an impairment are more likely to become overweight and obese as a direct effect of their impairment. The role of inactivity as a cause of obesity is well documented (Hardman and Stensel, 2003). It is widely accepted that disabled people are likely to be less physically active due to barriers to participation in addition to factors linked to their impairment, e.g. during relapses of multiple sclerosis. Although some people are genetically more susceptible to obesity than others, the underlying cause of obesity is an imbalance between energy intake and energy expenditure through activity and exercise. Data on the participation of disabled people in physical activity and sport is difficult to find, though Sport England's (2002) National Survey concludes: 'Sports participation rates for disabled adults are significantly lower than for non-disabled adults. This is true for people with a wide range of disabilities.'

The Gary Jelen Sports Foundation (GJSF) commissioned a research project in 1998 that identified the specific barriers that prevented disabled people accessing fitness services in local authority leisure centres.

The main findings (GJSF, 1999) showed that:
- there was a lack of physically accessible facilities
- the fitness equipment in the facilities did not meet the needs of disabled users
- there was a lack of staff training and knowledge in providing fitness services to disabled people
- there was little communication, targeting and marketing of fitness facilities to disabled people
- there was a lack of awareness among disabled people about the benefits of a healthy lifestyle and physical activity.

Low participation numbers may well be as a direct result of the 'medical model' approach to service provision in the fitness industry. Many disabled people, conditioned by attitudes based on the medical model, consider that fitness activities may not be for them. They have been disabled by society in this area and lack confidence in their own ability to take part and access fitness services.

Disabled people are also less likely to eat healthily, e.g. visually impaired people cooking convenience food due to the difficulties associated with preparing food, carers preparing convenience food for people with a learning disability, etc. Disabled people are also less likely to be given proactive health and dietary advice, are less likely to have access to this in the required format and are therefore also less likely to be informed than non-disabled people. Addressing these barriers is however outside the scope of this chapter.

The Inclusive Fitness Initiative – an intervention to improve physical activity levels and health among disabled people

There is currently no co-ordinated framework or action plan aimed at reducing the levels of overweight and obese disabled people in the UK. While many of the interventions and programmes detailed in this book will have a relevance to disabled people, the programmes must be developed to take on board the specific needs of people with different impairments. An example of a programme that has placed disabled people at the centre of the development and delivery mechanism is the Inclusive Fitness Initiative (IFI).

The results of the GJSF (1999) research triggered the development of the IFI, the pilot of which targeted 29 fitness facilities across England between 2001 and 2003. Under the direction of the English Federation of Disability Sport (EFDS), and with the support of £1 million of grant aid from the Sport England Lottery Fund, the IFI worked with not-for-profit fitness facilities, supporting them to become inclusive, providing fitness services for both disabled and non-disabled people in the same environment.

Such was the success of the intervention that a further £5 million was grant-aided by Sport England in 2004 to impact a further 150 facilities. An additional £1.5 million has been contributed by applicant organisations in the form of partnership funding. The IFI is managed and implemented by Sheffield-based sports consultancy, Montgomery Leisure Services, who also conducted the initial GJSF research.

The IFI has supported partners to establish an inclusive culture and communication system within their fitness facilities, delivering appropriate inclusive fitness services to as wide a range of disabled people as possible. The IFI seeks to empower disabled people and give them the confidence that they are able to take part, have the same right to access these services and make healthy lifestyle choices.

By breaking down these barriers, the IFI seeks to endorse the 'social model' to both service providers and service users. The 'social model' underpins the development and delivery of the IFI. The IFI identifies barriers to participation experienced by disabled people when accessing fitness services in a facility. In partnership with facility staff and managers, the IFI stimulates the implementation of an action plan to ensure the modification of the building and the services. By seeking the views of all customers on an ongoing basis, continuous improvement and enhancements can be made.

The IFI has awarded grants in order to support work in the following key areas.

Access

The IFI provides facilities with an access audit for all elements of the building and policies contributing to the delivery of fitness services. It identifies the 'reasonable adjustments' (Disability Discrimination Act, 1995) that must be made to ensure that fitness services can be delivered to all disabled people, regardless of impairment. The audit is delivered by professionals who understand the needs of disabled people in the fitness environment and therefore ensures that the environment is relevant and fit for purpose. It also builds on the feedback received directly from disabled users in this environment on an ongoing basis.

Equipment

The IFI advises fitness equipment manufacturers in the design and production of equipment that is accessible for both disabled and non-disabled people. The equipment is tested by disabled people, and 'accredited' by a panel of experts on the basis of both their feedback and against a set of objective inclusive equipment standards. Grant aid is provided to IFI facilities to purchase equipment that will support a full body workout for the vast majority of disabled people.

Training

Two levels of training are provided for staff in IFI facilities. Level one targets all staff who have direct contact with customers. It is intended to raise staff awareness and understanding of the needs of disabled customers. Level two targets fitness instructors, providing them with the knowledge to implement a safe and effective workout for disabled people. This training is accredited to National Vocational Qualification Level 3. Additionally this is designed to give disabled people the confidence that they can rely upon the advice of fitness instructors. While not specifically targeting obesity, IFI training teaches staff to be more aware of people's barriers to participation, including psychological barriers, and therefore to address this in the way they provide services having a more sensitive approach. As disabled and non-disabled people are 'working out' alongside each other, IFI facilities also appear less threatening to all new users.

Marketing

Facilities are supported by the IFI to ensure that they communicate effectively with both existing and prospective disabled customers. As some people find it difficult to access traditional methods of communication, support is given to facilities to assist them with the identification and implementation of alternative methods and solutions. For many overweight and obese people, fitness suites can seem very intimidating, perhaps more so than to the general population. Fitness suites are often seen as venues for the 'fit, trendy and confident'. The IFI challenges this perception in terms of the marketing material that is produced: inclusive imagery, language in leaflets, etc. The appointment of a member of staff in the role of an Inclusive Activator at all IFI facilities for a minimum 15-month period dispels this notion, provides information in an accessible format and is a 'friendly face' that reaches out to disabled people in their community.

Sport development

The EFDS support IFI facilities to provide additional sporting opportunities for disabled people within the surrounding area of the fitness facility, maximising the choices and opportunities for disabled people taking up physical activity for the first time.

The IFI is a dynamic project, at the cutting edge of inclusive fitness development and also at the forefront of this field internationally. Incredible progress has been made through the commitment of all partners involved. The IFI works at a range of levels to ensure that a non-user of a fitness facility is supported through their change into an independent gym user. It is the inter-relationship of all the above elements that has made the IFI so successful in changing perspectives in the English fitness community.

Physical activity programming for obese disabled people

Fitness instructors at IFI facilities receive their 'Level Two' training from YMCAfit, currently the industry leader in delivering programming advice relating to disabled people. YMCAfit have tutored over 145 'Inclusive Health, Fitness and Physical Activity Disability Training' courses for the IFI programme, providing a huge impetus for the fitness sector to appreciate the exercise programming needs of disabled people and training over 1,440 fitness instructors across England. This training also raises the awareness of the likely needs of obese disabled people in order that they can be specifically provided for in the fitness suite environment.

The American College of Sports Medicine (ACSM) exercise guidelines for reduction in obesity are the same for obese disabled people as for obese non-disabled people (ACSM, 2003). The only difference is that there are additional factors to consider when creating a safe, effective and motivating exercise programme.

As with any client, it is important to ensure that exercise is enjoyable. This can provide the greatest challenge when someone has a heightened level of fear or negativity due to his or her impairment. Fear and misconceptions about personal needs being addressed can build further barriers to exercise for this population group. It is extremely important that the fitness instructor works in partnership with any obese disabled client, to help understand their personal fears and apprehensions, but also to find their personal motivations.

Often addressing improvements in function for everyday life activity can provide a wonderful motivation if impairments in addition to obesity limit independence in activities of daily living, e.g. carrying more bags of shopping, climbing more stairs or walking further.

Educating a disabled person to understand that 'less may be more' is very important. Too often, early motivation is killed off by burnout from over-enthusiasm or a worsening of the impairment. Careful use is made of early motivation to educate the individual about matching their function and fitness levels to a suitable programme. Particular attention is paid to frequency, intensity and duration and how these will progress over the course of the programme. The challenge is to encourage activity without increasing pain levels or setting in early fatigue.

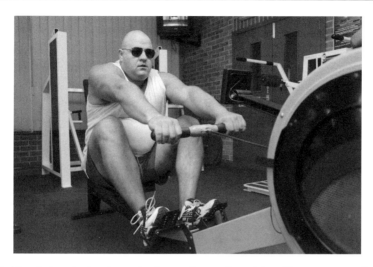

Figure 14.1 Visually impaired male conducting cardiovascular training. Photo courtesy of the Inclusive Fitness Initiative

For those who are paralysed, particularly in the large leg muscles, the challenge is to find the largest muscles of the upper body and get those working. Muscles such as latissimus dorsi, trapezius and pectoralis major are all targeted. Care is taken to avoid overuse injuries in the smaller muscle groups that often get utilised at the same time as these, especially deltoids and the muscles that make up the rotator cuff.

Cardiovascular (CV) training is most effective when employing the large muscle groups, as can be so easily recognised when looking at CV equipment within any fitness suite (for example, *see* Figure 14.1). For disabled people with limited use of leg muscles, upper body ergometers (hand bikes) provide a similarly rhythmic and continuous alternative to conventional lower-body-biased CV equipment. They are also similar in set-up to other CV machines. These factors, as well as the level of independence they offer, make them a popular choice. However, they do not work the largest upper body muscle groups and therefore their use can be limited for some. Other alternatives that are more commonly available in all gyms include the use of conventional resistance equipment, such as seated row and chest press, set to a low resistance with 50+ repetitions employed. In addition, high repetitions of any large muscle group exercise using dumb-bells, resistance bands or body weight only can be very effective.

Repetitive, full-range movements can worsen some impairments, e.g. arthritis. An individual assessment should provide this information and feedback from the client must be gained before, during and after each session. Any increase in pain during the session, later on the same day or on waking the following morning may be an indication that a particular exercise is not suitable. Attention should be paid to encouraging small ranges of movement during warm-ups (if not the whole programme) and introducing only one new exercise per session. In this way the programme can be gradually added to over the sessions without causing unnecessary pain or upset.

Many impairments make it difficult for people to effectively thermo-regulate

TABLE 14.1 Sample programme for obese people without leg function.

Exercise	Time/Reps
Warm-up	
Arm ergometer	8 mins @ 55–65% MHR
Mobility – trunk twists, side bends	6 reps each
Pre stretch as per individual	
Main workout (repeat × 2, either CV then resistance or interspersed)	
CV	
Low row – cable pulley/resistance machine	40 reps @ 60–70% MHR
Chest press – cable pulley/resistance machine	40 reps @ 60–70% MHR
Shadow boxing	2 mins @ 60–70% MHR
Resistance	
Lat pulldown – resistance machine	20 reps @ 90%20 RM
Pec dec – resistance machine	20 reps @ 90%20 RM
Mid row – resistance machine	20 reps @ 90%20 RM
Shoulder press – dumb-bells	20 reps @ 90%20 RM
Seated back extension – band	10 reps @ 70%10 RM
Cool-down	
Arm ergometer	5 mins @ 65–55% MHR
Stretches as per individual	

MHR – maximum heart rate; RM – repetition maximum.

(control their body temperature). As obese people tend to become warm more quickly than non-obese people, especially during exercises involving the large muscle groups, careful monitoring of the disabled person is important. This can be achieved through observation of individual warming-up responses (sweating, flushing) and reminders to maintain hydration levels.

The benefits of resistance training for increasing resting metabolic rate are the same for disabled as for non-disabled obese people. Here again small equipment, such as dumb-bells and resistance tubing, can provide accessible alternatives to more conventional non-accessible resistance equipment. They also provide wonderful opportunities for encouraging additional home based exercise.

Table 14.1 shows a sample exercise programme for obese people without leg function.

The evidence that the IFI approach has worked

The IFI has collated significant qualitative and quantitative data collected from a large sample size (150 facilities). This 'user feedback' personalises the Initiative and enables those working with disabled people to appreciate the positive experiences their clients have from visiting the facility.

Very little data has previously been available in this field and the IFI offers an excellent opportunity to address this issue. Each IFI facility provides usage data for the fitness suite on a monthly basis for 12 months after their 'launch' as part of their

TABLE 14.2 Summary of the reach and impact of the IFI on different impairment groups as a percentage of the total usage of the fitness suite to date (November 2006).

Impairment	Visits	Per cent of total visits by disabled people	Inductions	Per cent of total inductions by disabled people
Learning disability	23,337	14	1,623	15
Physical impairment	42,997	26	2,162	20
Hearing impairment	8,122	5	462	4
Visual impairment	13,762	7	706	7
Not stated	18,398	12	1,803	16
Multi impairment	10,295	6	725	7
Other impairment	51,398	30	3,361	31
Total	168,309	100	10,842	100

grant condition. Data is collected for the number of individual *visits* by disabled people and, based on inductions, the number of *new* disabled users. Facilities are also asked to submit total usage figures (disabled and non-disabled) in order to relate the two figures and track the percentage of usage by disabled people.

IFI facilities are also asked to identify the impairment(s) of their disabled users. This is dependent on the user first identifying that they consider that they have a disability and second agreeing to disclose their impairment at the time of the Physical Activity Readiness Questionnaire. Although this is a very sensitive area, reception and fitness suite staff are given guidance and confidence through the IFI to seek this information in the most sensitive way. On balance disabled people are pleased to support the data collection with the knowledge that this will be used to enhance the future provision of inclusive fitness services.

The overriding feedback from IFI facilities, however, is that as a result of the challenges of collecting quantitative data in this field, the figures presented are considered conservative and that the actual impact of the IFI is likely to be significantly higher than the actual data received.

In summary the IFI has enabled and stimulated to date (November 2006):

- 168,309 visits by disabled people
- an average of 131 visits by disabled people per site per month
- 10,842 new disabled users to the fitness suite environment
- an average of 8.5 new inductions for disabled people per site per month.

Table 14.2 summarises the reach and impact of the IFI on different impairment groups as a percentage of the total usage of the fitness suite to date (November 2006). This data has been used to linearly extrapolate figures forwards to give indicative figures for the whole scheme by March 2007, the end of the monitoring period for all 150 IFI facilities (*see* Table 14.3).

In due course qualitative feedback from users at IFI facilities will be analysed and assessed for differing trends between male and female users. There is however no capacity within the current data collection methods to assess this by the level of obesity or body mass index.

TABLE 14.3 Indicative figures for the whole scheme by March 2007.

	Current based on 1,282 months	Projections for whole scheme Based on 1,800 months
No. of visits by disabled people	168,309	235,800
No. of new inductions for disabled people	10,842	15,300

Where research can influence future interventions

As indicated, there is little research on the actual levels of obesity within the disability population and within different and specific impairment groups. While there is research saying that there is a higher prevalence of overweight people in specific impairment groups, few attempt to quantify this. Until the real extent of the problem is known, how can we know if we are tackling it effectively?

Most projects aimed at disabled people do not focus on health outcomes, since there are inherent difficulties with doing this. For example, health questionnaires are not inclusive. Most tend to start with a question such as 'Can you walk up a flight of stairs?'. There are also problems relating to actually weighing some disabled people. There are not many health clubs or GP surgeries etc. that have scales that wheelchair users can use, for example. Accurately measuring body fat is also difficult as evidenced in other chapters of this publication.

Research programmes that would underpin the development of appropriate future interventions for overweight and obese disabled people could include:

- an assessment of the incidence of weight problems across impairment groups in the UK population
- research to support the design and development of an appropriate health questionnaire, in the required alternative formats, that will effectively measure weight problems within the disabled population
- an assessment of the barriers faced by disabled people (by impairment) in accessing current specific intervention programmes for overweight and obese people
- an assessment of the number of overweight and obese disabled people accessing IFI facilities in England and the physical and social benefits they experience
- a comparative study of the benefits of an appropriate exercise programme across overweight and obese people with different impairment and the resulting health benefits
- to research the appropriateness and reach of existing interventions and strategies for the reduction of weight problems in relation to the needs of disabled people.

The significant network of IFI facilities throughout England now offers an opportunity to easily access the client group required for much of the above research.

IFI implementation principles and advice for delivery agents

The IFI is a turnkey programme that is at the cutting edge of inclusive fitness service delivery. As a result the models, training and delivery all had to be developed essentially from scratch. While the scope of this chapter does not permit an assessment of the individual challenges of each area of delivery, some of the cross-cutting guiding principles that have contributed to the acknowledged success of the IFI programme are listed below. It is hoped that they may stimulate successful interventions in the future in other fields.

- Thoroughly research the issues and current trends.
- Listen to your client group (disabled people) and place their needs at the centre of the development process and delivery mechanisms.
- Deliver a pilot element and be prepared to challenge and question your practices.
- Work in partnership throughout with the identified key influencers and stakeholders.
- Ensure that all partners know their responsibilities.
- Promote the benefits of the programme by using role models and people with first-hand experience of the outcomes.
- Build a delivery team who are personally passionate about the 'product'.
- Be prepared to modify the 'model' action plan and solution to cater for local differences.
- Identify and measure the interventions and impacts, supported by effective data-handling technology.
- Be confident to 'sell the business case' for the intervention.
- Plan in empowerment and sustainability from day one.
- Be prepared to break a cycle of inaction.
- Aspire to change a culture and be prepared to not only take on a challenge but to see it through.

Conclusion

As this book evidences, obesity and being overweight is now one of the most prevalent health conditions among men in the UK. The increased incidence of obesity in the disabled population makes this an even greater priority for health and physical activity professionals. Feedback from both fitness service providers and fitness equipment suppliers and manufacturers involved in the IFI suggest that there is an ongoing need to provide practical support to help them understand and meet the needs of disabled people. The IFI has challenged the way in which they think of service delivery and product development by placing disabled people at the core of the development process. User opinion in this market sector is changing and evolving, therefore demanding more long-term, integral consideration of inclusive services and design issues. Additionally expectations of disabled users are developing, with back-up from strengthening UK legislation.

The IFI has demonstrated that many of the problems faced by disabled people when accessing fitness services are not insurmountable. However, there is very little co-ordinated data that explores the needs of overweight and obese disabled people. The hope is that the IFI will both stimulate and provide an opportunity to more specifically identify and address the needs of overweight and obese disabled men in partnership with delivery agencies in the future.

Acknowledgements

Sara Wicebloom, YMCA Fitness Industry Training, IFI Training Co-ordinator.

References

American College of Sports Medicine. Obesity. Chapter 23 in: *Exercise Management for Persons with Chronic Diseases and Disabilities* (2 e). Indianapolis, IN: American College of Sports Medicine; 2003.

Arthritis Care. www.arthritiscare.org.uk/Home (accessed 12 March 2007).

Bajekal M, Primatesta P, Prior G. Disability among adults. In: *Health Survey for England 2001 – Disability*. London: The Stationery Office; 2003.

Disability Discrimination Act (1995). London: The Stationery Office; 1995. Limited Crown Copyright (2).

Disability Rights Commission (DRC). *Equal Treatment: closing the gap. Interim report of a formal investigation into health inequalities*. Stratford upon Avon: DRC; 2005. p. 9.

Disability Rights Commission (DRC). *Disability Briefing*. Stratford upon Avon: DRC; March 2006. p. 37.

Ebrahim S, Goya Wannamethee S, Whincup P *et al*. Locomotor disability in a cohort of British men, the impact of lifestyle and disease. *International Journal of Epidemiology*. 2000; **29**: 478–86.

European Men's Health Forum (EMHF). *Obesity in Men: a major problem for Europe*. EMHF Fact Sheet. www.emhf.org/resource_images/EMHF_Factsheet_Obesity.pdf (accessed 12 March 2007).

Gary Jelen Sports Foundation (GJSF). *Report on the Findings of the National Survey into Access to Fitness Facilities for Disabled People*. Stoke on Trent: English Federation of Disability Sport and Montgomery Leisure Services Ltd; 1999.

Goldberg D, Huxley P. *Common Mental Disorders: a bio-social model*. Abingdon: Routledge; 1992.

Grewal I, Joy S, Lewis J *et al*. *Disabled for Life? Attitudes towards and experiences of disability in Britain*. Research Report No. 173. Summary (1). London: Department for Work and Pensions; 2002.

Grundy E, Ahlburg D, Ali M *et al*. *Disability in Great Britain: results of the 1996/7 Disability Follow-Up to the Family Resources Survey*. Research Report No. 94. London: Social Research Division, Department for Work and Pensions; 1999.

Hardman AE, Stensel DJ. Obesity and energy balance. In: *Physical Activity and Health. The evidence explained*. Abingdon: Routledge; 2003. p. 114–130.

Jankowski LW, Evans JK. The exercise capacity of blind children. *Journal of Visual Impairment and Blindness*. June 1981; **75**(6): 248–51.

Mencap. www.mencap.org.uk/html/about_learning_disability/learning_disability_facts.asp (accessed 12 March 2007).

National Center for Health Statistics. *Health, United States, 2005 with Chartbook on Trends in the Health of Americans*. Hyattsville, MD: National Center for Health Statistics; 2005.

National Audit Office. *Tackling Obesity in England*. Report by the Comptroller and Auditor General. HC 220 Session 2000–2001. London: National Audit Office; 2001.

Office for National Statistics (ONS). *Psychiatric Morbidity Among Adults Living in Private Households in Great Britain*. London: Office for National Statistics; 2000.

Office for National Statistics (ONS). *Labour Force Survey 2001*. London: ONS, Social and Vital Statistics Division; 2001.

Rimmer JH, Braddock D, Fujiura G. Prevalence of obesity in adults with mental retardation: implications for health promotion and disease prevention. *American Journal of Mental Retardation*. April 1993; **31**(2): 105–10.

Rimmer JH, Wang W. Obesity prevalence among a group of Chicago residents with disabilities. *Arch Phys Med Rehabil.* July 2005; **86**: 1461–4.

Royal National Institute for the Deaf. www.rnid.org.uk/about/ (accessed 12 March 2007).

Royal National Institute of the Blind. www.rnib.org.uk/xpedio/groups/public/documents/PublicWebsite/public_researchstats.hcsp (accessed 12 March 2007).

Rubin SS, Rimmer JH, Chicoine B *et al.* Overweight prevalence in persons with Down Syndrome. *Mental Retardation.* 1997; **36**(3): 175–81.

Sport England. *Adults with a Disability and Sport, National Survey 2000–2001.* Main Report Ref: 2160. London: Sport England; 2002.

Weil E, Wachterman M, McCarthy EP *et al.* Obesity among adults with disabling conditions. *Journal of the American Medical Association.* 2002; **288**(10): 1265–8.

Weitzman DM, Motivation. *Journal of Visual Impairment and Blindness.* 1986; **80**(5): 745–7.

World Health Organization (WHO). *International Statistical Classification of Diseases and Related Health Problems.* 10th Revision. Geneva: WHO; 2006.

CHAPTER 15

Promoting exercise to men

Jim McKenna

Sport and exercise play an important, but diverse, role in promoting the well-being of men, especially in relation to weight control. However, this diversity is no more than is found in men's motivation to initiate and then sustain their involvement. It is precisely this level of diversity that makes effective delivery of physical activity-based health programmes so challenging.

From the outset some clarity about terms is important. 'Physical activity' (PA) reflects any form of bodily movement and so can be considered the parent of sport and exercise. In this chapter 'sport' is used to denote all forms of organised physical activity with a competitive element. 'Exercise' describes organised activity, such as attending circuit training or exercise to music classes. This chapter aims to provide a structure for understanding how to promote physical activity, exercise and sport to men. In this process, specific operational details will not be discussed.

The case for exercising

Exercising reduces risks for as many as 20 of the major diseases that burden public health systems across the world (Booth *et al.*, 2000). Lack of exercise is central to the development of diseases such as heart disease and diabetes. Regular activity can be usefully undertaken to treat conditions with causes beyond inactivity, such as anxiety and depression (Department of Health, 2004). Many of these conditions are over-emphasised in male groups (White and Cash, 2003), yet they demonstrate a dose–response relationship (e.g. Peterson *et al.*, 2005) with PA. Current epidemiological evidence confirms that every instance of activity is associated with some level of risk reduction. Growing evidence also suggests that PA – and therefore exercise and sport – has a similar relationship with important elements of positive health such as improved mental health, emotional well-being and quality of life.

This understanding places renewed value on (a) immediate instances of activity behaviour such as using the stairs instead of the escalators during a shopping trip (Kerr *et al.*, 2001), (b) episodic behaviour such as depicted by the 'weekend warriors' whose interest in sport is limited to a game on a Saturday afternoon or Sunday morning (Min-Lee *et al.*, 2004), and (c) more sustained regular involvement that supports, say, an adult lifetime in body building, hill walking or team sport. This offers promoters at least three different possible messages. Further, if we consider the various combinations of frequency (how many times per week), intensity (how hard), duration (how long) and mode (what type), the range of possible approaches begins to become clear.

Providing up-to-date information may provide an important lever for motivating behaviour change among health-concerned men. For example, one in four men in the 2004 Health Survey for England was classified as obese. However, increasing waist size is an important and emerging marker for reduced levels of activity. Plus, waist size is linked to many of the diseases that threaten men's livelihoods. Further, such increases are now widely regarded as marking increased risk of disease, especially diabetes. In men with type 2 diabetes, risk rose progressively as waists increased beyond 34 inches. Waists of 40 to 62 inches were associated with 12 times the risk (Wang *et al.*, 2005) and with large extra healthcare costs (Cornier *et al.*, 2002). These effects are also evident among boys. Recent work from Leeds showed that boys' waist sizes had increased by 1.5 inches over the past 20 years (Rudolf *et al.*, 2004). For many men reproductive health may be an important issue and those with larger waists are more likely to have higher rates of erectile dysfunction due to a higher risk for cardiovascular disease (Roth *et al.*, 2003).

Understanding behaviour change

Jackson (1997) lists a range of important generic principles for delivering effective behaviour change programmes. These principles derive from a range of theoretical perspectives and provide a clear framework for developing interventions that will recruit and sustain men in more active lifestyles. A range of these will now be addressed.

Acquiring new behaviour is a process not an event

Across the life-course humans continually develop, often through intentional behaviour change. This change can represent a roller-coaster ride and challenges exercise promoters to deliver exercise-based programmes that optimise the process as it is experienced by individual men. Therefore, it is important to understand that what influences initiation, adoption and sustained involvement is likely to shift across groups. We should also anticipate that the same factors act differently as individuals change.

De-marketing the behaviours that support sedentary living may be an important starting point for effective PA promotion. For example, British males currently spend 49% of their free time watching TV (Eurostat, 2004). Freeing this time for more active pursuits may be an important first option for PA promoters. Others may seek to alter harmful work-related attitudes and behaviours. For example, simply agreeing with three or more of these statements provides a further risk factor for weight gain:
(i)   'I feel totally worn out after a day at work'
(ii)   'I feel tired in the morning when I have to get up and go to work'
(iii) 'I have to work too hard'
(iv)   'I feel like I'm totally exhausted'
(v)   'My work is definitely too stressful' and

(vi) 'I worry about my work even when I'm off duty' (Lallukka *et al.*, 2005).

Restricting working hours may be another approach, since working more than 40 hours per week may also contribute to increasing weight. Overtime working increased the risk for injury by 61% more than those putting in a normal eight-hour day (Loomis, 2005).

Theoretical approaches models, such as the transtheoretical model (TTM, Prochaska and DiClemente, 1982), provide a useful framework for understanding the process of change. In all such models, the key constructs offer practitioners important levers for change (McKenna and Davis, 2004). In the TTM approach, individuals pass through different stages of change, from Precontemplation (not thinking about changing and no intention of changing in the near future), Contemplation (thinking seriously about changing in the next 30 days), Preparation (active but only irregularly), Action (regularly and frequently active for less than six months) and Maintenance (regularly and frequently active for longer than six months). This model is helpful in understanding why some behaviourally inactive men – especially those driven by doing-focused elements of masculinity (Robertson, 2003; Robertson and Williamson, 2005) – may be at heightened risk for premature involvement in exercising and, therefore, for dropping out. Table 15.1 shows how the 10 most commonly used processes of change associated with positive behaviour change can be operationalised within PA promotion. The table shows the clear opportunities for men to learn how they can support appropriate and developmental physical activity based on both experiential (cognitive) and behavioural skills.

Clearly, if the process is important, then there is a need for programmes to include periods where men can reflect on that process and also to in-build staff follow-up sessions. Individuals who relapse into inactivity will require substantial investments to help them to become active again. Men may also profit from learning how to manage their exercise experience. This might address use of important mental skills such as self-talk, goal-setting and imagery, both to prepare for, and to do well during, individual bouts of engagement. Exercise staff need time in their working day to follow-up their male clients, even when they are already active, because the effects of previous exercising cannot be stored and every new bout is an achievement.

Exercise specialists also acknowledge the importance of the process of becoming more active. For them, careful planning of the demands of an exercise class will help to control any negative consequences that might accrue from structured exercising. Typically class leaders encourage self-monitoring of heart rate during an exercise class. This is wise for at least one immediate and one more long-term reason. First, perceptions of exertion influence enjoyment, which can influence subsequent involvement. Second, higher-intensity exercise (characterised by high heart rates, being strongly out of breath and increasing heaviness in the limbs) can lead to the development of negative mood states (Ekkekakis *et al.*, 2005) and also with delayed muscle soreness. While there are variations, for low active and/or low fit individuals, this scenario has obvious negative implications for subsequent involvement.

Lifestyle physical activity, where individuals are encouraged to accumulate daily moderate intensity movement, may offer further challenges. With no obvious guides

TABLE 15.1 Operationalising the 10 common processes of change.

Process of change	Tasks/Goals
Experiential*	
Consciousness raising	Increasing information about self and problem and potential solutions
Dramatic relief	Experiencing and expressing feelings about one's problems and solutions; intense emotional reactions to current behaviours
Self re-evaluation	Changing assessment of feelings and thoughts about self and problem
Social liberation	Creating increased social alternatives for behaviours that are not problematic
Social re-evaluation	Changing appraisal of how problem affects others
Behavioural**	
Self liberation	Choosing and committing to act, or belief in ability to change
Counter-conditioning	Changing reactions to stimuli; substituting alternatives for problem behaviours
Stimulus control	Avoiding stimuli that elicit problem behaviours; changing environments
Helping relationships	Enlisting help for change from someone who cares
Reinforcement management	Changing reinforcers and contingencies for a new behaviour; rewarding self, or being rewarded by others, for making changes

*Experiential processes are emphasised in the inactive stages (Precontemplation, and Contemplation).
**Behavioural processes are emphasised in the active stages (Preparation, Action and Maintenance).

for over-use, recent evidence suggests that adults who walk an average of 4,000 to 5,000 steps per day best sustain increases of 2,500 steps/day *before* focusing on public health targets of 10,000 steps per day (Davis *et al.*, 2005). This acknowledges that the exercise process has an essential physicality that is captured by the old Roman motto: '*Make haste, slowly*'.

Psychological factors (notably beliefs and values) influence how people behave

The psychological elements of exercising also follow a process. Jackson (1997) highlights that change often requires learning through sequences (or approximations to 'real life') and this links to an important notion – self-efficacy. Self-efficacy (Bandura, 1997) describes situation-specific confidence and may be illustrated by the difference in confidence that a 35-year-old male may have for negotiating life in a tennis versus a soccer club or participating in a walking group versus an exercise to music class.

Self-efficacy is especially important because increases predict change in physical activity behaviour (Plotnikoff *et al.*, 2001). Clearly, exercise self-efficacy relates very strongly to exercise mode and to context. For this reason it is important to promote acceptable, enjoyable, challenging forms of exercise/sport to attract and retain men. However, because self-efficacy is situation-specific, it is unwise to assume that the confidence to participate in one sport or activity readily transfers to others. Interestingly, compared to females, across stages of change, males typically report higher levels of self-efficacy for exercising regularly, even when it is raining or snowing, when they are tired or have limited time. These are the important factors within self-efficacy and highlight the importance of promoting PA within the wider context of each man's life.

Masculine values also support the 'appeal' of different ways to be active. For example, Gough and Connor (2006) highlight the importance of key values such as rationality, autonomy and strength for male behaviour change. O'Brien *et al.* (2005) note the special reluctance of some men – especially young men – to seek help. For them, help-seeking was only valued, or a realistic prospect, when it restored or preserved other aspects of masculinity. In men suffering from depression, endorsing alternative, but more feminine, concepts, such as creativity, intelligence and sensitivity, was common and this may influence both the appeal and sustainability of different forms of activity (Emslie *et al.*, 2006).

The more beneficial and rewarding the experience, the more likely that it will be repeated

Work is clearly a highly valued way for many men to spend their time. Figures from a *Times* survey in 2004 showed that many men would prefer more money (acquired through working more hours) than more leisure time (Grove, 2004). This highlights their value system and challenges exercise professionals to develop interventions that optimise their work-related interests. The results of a recent randomised controlled trial with cross-over (McKenna and Coulson, 2005) might help. On days when employees exercised (over days when they did not), self-related work performance consistently increased for managing (a) interpersonal demands, (b) time demands and (c) output demands. Clearly, these issues highlight the potential of promoting work-based exercise and/or sport to meet men's career aspirations. Others have highlighted the value of active recreation in contrasting with the stressful demands of work (Robertson, 2003, p. 710). Other studies (e.g. Mutrie *et al.*, 2002) show that active commuting to and/or from work can be effectively promoted among working adults. However, it is also important to use appropriate incentives. The Allied Dunbar National Fitness Survey (ADNFS) (Activity and Health Research, 1992) showed that the phrase 'Do not enjoy physical activity' applied to only 162 (9.3%) adult males.

Pain relief may be an outcome that is more widely promoted to encourage men to become more active. Here the challenge for promoters is to manage the initial discomfort of involvement with 'selling' the undoubted benefits of sustained involvement. Within four months, exercising reduced chronic osteoarthritic knee pain in older overweight and obese men (Bartlett, 2005). These effects were based on small weekly group classes plus a gradual increase in PA to 30 minutes of moderate intensity walking per day. Further, the intervention also emphasised increasing exercise gradually, aiming eventually to accumulate 10,000 steps per day. Small lifestyle changes, such as taking the long route to the toilet at work, or parking on the far side of the car park and using stairs instead of lifts or escalators, were also emphasised to good effect.

A second part of this precept is that the more punishing and unpleasant the behaviour, the less likely that it will be repeated. In this context, it is salutary to consider what men often reject and to learn about our mistakes in promoting PA, exercise or sports. Systems that require men to go to strange venues, like the doctor's surgery, clearly limit engagement. So, too, does a lack of skills. These limitations may not only – or even – be restricted to physical skills.

Despite the immediate pleasure of involvement, sports like five-a-side soccer may be appealing because of relatively unrestrained intensity demands. While on the one hand this can mean substantial rest periods – by standing in goal, for example – the activity demands of general play may be such that it produces delayed stiffness. Subsequently, because of the negative spill-over into other activities, like earning a living, this stiffness – which classically only develops fully after 24 hours – can become understood as a profound Con for further involvement. Under-refined and unskilled movements in confined spaces can also result in injury, meaning that careful adaptation of these highly popular games is needed to recruit middle-aged men back into active living. Currently, only 10% of the men who regularly play the national sport – soccer – in the UK are over 40 years of age (Mori, 2002, p. 22), suggesting that there is considerable potential in this area. Another suggestion is that there is a need to actively intervene to optimise transition experiences out of competitive soccer into other forms of activity. Identifying the key transition events and experiences will help to deliver such interventions.

Behaviour is dependent on context

People influence, and are influenced by, their social environment. Social cohesion, social capital and social inclusion are all part of an emerging construct that links community participation – through bonding and bridging processes (Putnam, 2000) – with notions of trust, shared emotional commitment and reciprocity. At the risk of stereotyping, men especially emphasise doing over being. Many profit from being offered problem-solving approaches within PA promotion (Peterson and Hughey, 2004). However, it is important to note that profiles for health values and behaviours differ markedly across and within countries (White and Cash, 2003).

General practices also offer another 'context' for promoting PA. Men only average three visits per year to their GP (compared with five for women) (Rickards *et al.*, 2004), which underlines the importance of PA promotion within every consultation. Further, more men are using GP services year-on-year, with economically inactive men using these services more than wage earners. However, devolving PA promotion to practice nurses may be unwise as men averaged only one consultation with nurses per year during 2000–2002.

A further 'context' issue is location. Media increasingly highlight 'unhealthy' cities and this may galvanise action in some men. For example, *Men's Fitness* magazine (2 Feb 2006) reported the UK's least healthy cities were (in this order – previous year's position is in brackets):

1 (4)   Bradford
2 (3)   Liverpool
3 (1)   Manchester
4 (2)   Newcastle
5 (5)   Glasgow.

That these cities were also in the top five for two years highlights the need for action and also suggests that effective delivery could reap rich rewards.

Using sport to develop social relationships is an important area of proactive behaviour. Relationships developed within sports can substantially influence how people behave. Indeed, male–male relationships that may begin within sporting settings (e.g. Light and Kirk, 2001) can also be associated with heightened employment opportunities. Setting aside the obvious physical health benefits of exercise, simply having someone to share problems with provides important health benefits for men. Positive elements of social relationships heightened post-coronary survival at six months (Berkman *et al.*, 1992), five years (Williams *et al.*, 1992) and ten years (Eng *et al.*, 2002). Recent UK research found that having a close relationship with a friend or relative in comparison to those without a close confidant halved the risk of a subsequent heart attack in post-coronary patients 12 months after an initial cardiac event (Dickens *et al.*, 2004). Clearly, these confidants can be generated through sport, exercise or physical activity involvement prior to experiencing ill health.

This places a high value on developing a positive social climate and 'working atmosphere' within activity groups. For this reason, instructor, teacher, coach and mentor behaviour are all important for creating a positive learning environment that supports regular involvement. However, social experiences are not universally positive. Equity becomes an important issue where in-group values actively exclude other groups (Robertson, 2003; Welland, 2004). Even the possibility of facing discrimination, prejudice and bias will reduce the likelihood of involvement.

With older adults Rejeski *et al.* (2003) explored group-based physical activity supported by problem-solving for local barriers. Their results showed that males responded with better long-term adherence than women. Values and behaviours also change with experience and as age increases, although there is often an over-concern for cosseting older men who often do not accept that ageing equates to decline. Among 1,710 male respondents in the Allied Dunbar National Fitness Survey (Activity and Health Research, 1992), conducted in the UK, only 128 (6.5%) said that being 'too old' limited their involvement in regular activity. This contrasts with the figures for 'lack of time' (36.4%) and 'not the sporty type' (21.1%). However, and perhaps frustratingly, it is equally important to acknowledge that many men readily reject the positive assumption in this formula: 'men + sport = health' (Robertson, 2003).

Conclusion

This chapter has emphasised the wide range of individualised factors that can be used to develop programmes that attract the sustained interest of active and inactive men. Recent developments within the understanding of the benefits of regular physical activity, however it is achieved, highlight the wide range of approaches that can be developed to increase the appeal of active living for more men, more often.

References

Activity and Health Research. *Allied Dunbar National Fitness Survey: a report on activity levels and fitness levels*. London: Sports Council and Health Education Authority; 1992.

Bandura A. *Self-Efficacy: the exercise of control*. New York: Freeman; 1997.

Bartlett SJ. Relationship among weight loss, body composition, and symptom improvement in overweight persons with knee OA. *American College of Rheumatology Annual Meeting*. 2005; Abstract 1201.

Berkman LF, Leo-Summers L, Horrowitz RI. Emotional support and survival after myocardial infarction: a prospective, population-based study of the elderly. *Annals of Internal Medicine*. 1992; 17: 1003–9.

Booth F, Gordon S, Carlson C, Hamilton M. Waging war on modern chronic diseases: primary prevention through exercise biology. *Journal of Applied Physiology*. 2000; 88: 774–87.

Cornier M-A, Tate CW, Grunwald GK, Bessesen DH. Relationship between waist circumference, body mass index, and medical care costs. *Obesity Research*. 2002; 10: 1167–72.

Davis MG, Code D, McKenna J. 10,000 steps per day or a 2,500 increase: which goal improves low active adults' compliance? *Medicine and Science in Sports and Exercise*. 2005; 37(5)(suppl): S247.

Department of Health. *At Least Five a Week: evidence on the impact of physical activity and its relationship to health: a report from the Chief Medical Officer*. London: The Stationery Office; 2004.

Dickens CM, McGowan L, Percival C *et al*. Lack of a close confidant, but not depression, predicts further cardiac events after myocardial infarction. *Heart*. 2004; 90: 518–22.

Ekkekakis P, Hall EE, Petruzzello SJ. Variation and homogeneity in affective responses to physical activity of varying intensities: an alternative perspective on dose-response based on evolutionary considerations. *Journal of Sports Sciences*. 2005; 23: 477–500.

Emslie C, Ridge D, Ziebland S, Hunt K. Men's accounts of depression: reconstructing or resisting hegemonic masculinity? *Social Science and Medicine*. 2006; 62: 2246–57.

Eng PM, Rimm EB, Fitzmaurice G, Kawachi I. Social ties and changes in social ties in relation to subsequent total and cause-specific mortality and coronary heart disease in men. *American Journal of Epidemiology*. 2002; 155: 700–9.

Eurostat. *How Europeans Spend Their Time. everyday life of men and women. Data from 1998 to 2002*. Luxemburg: Office for Official Publications of the European Communities; 2004.

Gough B, Connor MT. Barriers to healthy eating amongst men: a qualitative analysis. *Social Sciences and Medicine*. 2006; 62: 387–95.

Grove V. *The sad truth: we need more money than time*. London: The Times T2; 22 November 2004.

Jackson C. Behavioural science theory and principles for practice in health education. *Health Education Research: Theory and Practice*. 1997; 12: 143–50.

Kerr J, Eves F, Carroll D. Six-month observational study of prompted stair climbing. *Preventive Medicine*. 2001; 33: 422–7.

Lallukka T, Laaksonen M, Martikainen P, Sarlio-Lähteenkorva S, Lahelma E. Psychosocial working conditions and weight gain among employees. *International Journal of Obesity*. 2005; 29(8): 909–15.

Light R, Kirk D. Australian cultural capital – rugby's social meaning: physical assets, social advantage and independent schools. *Culture, Capital and Society*. 2001; 4: 81–98.

Loomis D. Long work hours and occupational injuries: new evidence on upstream causes. *Occupational and Environmental Medicine*. 2005; 62: 585.

McKenna J, Coulson J. How does exercising at work influence work performance? A randomised cross-over trial. *Medicine and Science in Sports and Exercise*. 2005; 37(5) (suppl): S323.

McKenna J, Davis M. The problem of behaviour change. In: Weitkunat R, Moretti M, Kerr J, editors. *ABC of Behaviour Change*. Edinburgh: Elsevier; 2004. Ch A3, p. 29–40.

Min-Lee I, Sesso HD, Oguma Y, Paffenbarger RS. The 'weekend warrior' and risk of mortality. *American Journal of Epidemiology*. 2004; 160: 636–41.

Mori. *State of the Nation: a survey of English football*. London: The Football Association; 2002.

Mutrie N, Carney C, Blamey A. 'Walk in to work out': a randomised controlled trial of a self-help intervention to promote active commuting. *Journal of Epidemiology and Community Health*. 2002; 56: 407–12.

O'Brien R, Hunt K, Hart G. 'It's caveman stuff, but that is to certain extent how guys still operate': men's accounts of masculinity and help seeking. *Social Science and Medicine*. 2005; **61**: 503–16.

Peterson MD, Rhea MR, Alvar BA. Applications of the dose-response for muscular strength development: a review of meta-analytic efficacy and reliability for designing training prescription. *Journal of Strength and Conditioning Research*. 2005; **19**: 950–8.

Peterson NA, Hughey J. Social cohesion and intrapersonal empowerment: gender as moderator. *Health Education Research; Theory and practice*. 2004; **19**: 533–42.

Plotnikoff RC, Hotz SB, Birkett NJ, Courneya KS. Exercise and the transtheoretical model: a longitudinal test of a population sample. *Preventive Medicine*. 2001; **33**: 441–52.

Prochaska JO, DiClemente CC. Transtheoretical Therapy: toward a more integrative model of change. *Psychotherapy: Therapy, Research and Practice*. 1982; **19**: 276–88.

Putnam D. *Bowling Alone: the collapse and revival of American community*. New York: Simon & Schuster; 2000.

Rejeski J, Brawley LR, Ambrosius WT *et al*. Older adults with chronic disease: benefits of group-mediated counselling in the promotion of physically active lifestyles. *Health Psychology*. 2003; **22**: 414–23.

Rickards L, Fox K, Roberts C *et al*. *Living in Britain. Results from the 2002 General Household Survey*. London: The Stationery Office; 2004. Also available from www.statistics.gov.uk/lib (accessed 12 March 2007).

Robertson S. 'If I let a goal in, they'll beat me up': contradictions in masculinity, sport and health. *Health Education Research: Theory and Practice*. 2003; **18**: 706–16.

Robertson S, Williamson P. Men and health promotion in the UK: ten years further on. *Health Education Research: Theory and Practice*. 2005; **64**: 293–301.

Roth A, Kalter-Leibovici O, Kerbis Y *et al*. Prevalence and risk factors for erectile dysfunction in men with diabetes, hypertension, or both diseases: a community survey among 1,412 Israeli men. *Clinical Cardiology*. 2003; **26**: 25–30.

Rudolf, M, Greenwood DC, Cole J *et al*. Rising obesity and expanding waistlines in schoolchildren: a cohort study. *Archives of Disease in Childhood*. 2004; **89**: 235–7.

Wang Y, Rimm EB, Stampfer MJ, Willett WC, Hu FB. Comparison of abdominal adiposity and overall obesity in predicting risk of type 2 diabetes among men. *American Journal of Clinical Nutrition*. 2005; **81**: 555–63.

Welland I. Men, sport, body performance and the maintenance of 'exclusive masculinity'. *Leisure Studies*. 2004; **21**: 235–47.

White A, Cash K. *A Report on the State of Men's Health Across 17 European Countries*. Brussels: European Men's Health Forum; 2003.

Williams RB, Barefoot JC, Califf RM. Prognostic importance of social and economic resources among medically treated patients with angiographically determined coronary heart disease. *Journal of the American Medical Association*. 1992; **267**: 520–4.

CHAPTER 16

Counselling the man beyond the weight problem

Richard Bryant-Jefferies

Obesity and being overweight are not topics that feature a great deal in the counselling and psychotherapeutic literature, and even less so where the focus is specifically upon obesity in men. Yet we know that male obesity and men being overweight is a growing problem. Obesity in England has grown by almost 400% over the course of the last 25 years. Today, about three-quarters of the adult population are now overweight or obese (around 22% are now obese) (House of Commons, 2004). The *Health Survey for England* for 2003 (Department of Health, 2004) shows that the proportion of men with a desirable BMI (20 to 25) decreased from 37.8% in 1993 to 28.8% in 2003, while the proportion of men categorised as obese (BMI over 30) increased from 13.2% in 1993 to 22.9% in 2003.

Many psychological problems result from obesity. The National Audit Office (NAO) report in 2001, *Tackling Obesity in England*, noted that 'Obese people … are more likely to suffer from a number of psychological problems, including binge-eating, low self-image and confidence, and a sense of isolation and humiliation arising from practical problems'. All of these issues may be helpfully addressed through counselling and psychotherapy but none of them are likely to change quickly, given that they may have become deeply embedded or ingrained over a number of years.

Of course, psychological problems associated with obesity are not simply linked to the *effect* of size or the pattern of eating. The counsellor or therapist will want to consider obesity from the angle of psychological and emotional causation. They will be interested in what factors have contributed to triggering an over-eating urge in the first place, assuming that the man's weight is the result of this and not simply lack of exercise, a lowered metabolism, the side effect of medication, or some other physiological factor. People put on weight for many different reasons, and sometimes this can be to deal with particular experiences in life. We will consider this further later in this chapter.

What needs emphasising is that therapeutic counselling should address the whole person, rather than be symptom- or problem-centred. I have focused on this elsewhere in relation to the perception of, and attitude towards, working with a person with a drink problem (Bryant-Jefferies, 2001) − hence the title of this present chapter. A counselling approach that stresses the importance of forming a therapeutic relationship with the client is vital, particularly as so many problems – and being overweight is no exception to this – have some connection to problematic relational experiences.

Excess weight connects with body image

For many men, size will have been an important factor in terms of their status, their sense of being a man. For many younger men, a major concern is about putting on weight in the sense of 'bulking up' through intense fitness regimes that include exercise, high-energy foods as well as following particular eating patterns. McCabe and Ricciardelli (2001) have pointed out how many men, and particularly adolescents, desire an increase in weight in order that they might meet their ideals of bodily strength and size. Hill (2004) refers to a 'culture of muscularity leaving men at risk of feeling dissatisfied or unhappy with their own physiques'. This marketing of the ideal physique can bring problems other than eating disorders and obsessive exercising. For many it is a factor in contributing to steroid use with all the risks associated with this. Linked to this is the condition of 'body dysmorphia', which in males '… is often referred to as "reverse anorexia" and occurs when an individual thinks he cannot get big or muscular enough. Like an emaciated anorexic who looks in the mirror and sees fat, many overly brawny bodybuilders see parts of their body as being too scrawny' (Cohn, date not known).

Excess weight and bullying

For some men, putting on excess weight (whether muscle or not) could stem from the experience of being bullied. Men may put on weight in order to intimidate others, or in order to feel safe. From being bullied, they may in time become the bully themselves, finding a sense of power and satisfaction in their use of their size to intimidate others. However, this is not the case for everyone. For many who are bullied, the resulting low self-esteem will cause them to withdraw and, in contrast, binge-eating for them could be about comfort, about trying to fill the emotional void inside that has emerged as a result of the bullying and rejection they have experienced. Isolation can be an effect, and if a person withdraws from social contact because of their size, either through lack of mobility or embarrassment, further complications may then arise, for instance agoraphobia. And where someone is agoraphobic they are less likely to be out walking or taking other forms of exercise, which adds to the risk of further weight increase.

CASE STUDY 1

Reginald is in his fifties. He was always quite shy, particularly as a child. He lived in an area where he was the only black child, and had to cope with a lot of racist taunting. He didn't join in the activities that the white kids got involved in. He preferred to stay at home. He didn't eat excessively then, there wasn't much opportunity. Money was tight. But later, when he left home, things did change, but he never regained his confidence. Kept himself to himself. Tended to comfort eat, as much out of boredom as anything else. And he drank heavily as well. Over the years his weight has continued to increase. He doesn't work any more, he can't get around much.

He doesn't like going out; it's not just the physical effort, it's the anxiety. He doesn't like being outside, open spaces. He feels safe at home. He's 35 stone, and he hates his size, hates himself. He's thought about killing himself. Sometimes suicidal ideas cross his mind, but he doesn't feel it's something he could do, though there have been times when the urge has been stronger.

He knows his weight isn't doing him any good, and he's seen the TV programmes showing how people can have weight removed. He thinks it might be an idea, but it scares him to think about it, and he wonders just how different he'd feel anyway if he wasn't so big.

Reginald feels very lonely sometimes. Neither of his parents are still alive. He'd like someone to talk to, or at least just to be there, some company. He finds himself getting depressed, he can't sleep properly and he often feels tired.

A counsellor could give Reginald the time he needs, the human contact that emotionally and psychologically he is crying out for, offering him empathic understanding will help him to share his anxieties. Receiving unconditional positive regard can help him to begin to develop a little positive self-regard to combat his depressive experiencing. Inside the large physical Reginald is a diminished person that needs relating to therapeutically. The counsellor working with the obese client, while not ignoring size, must be able to empathise with the person, which can be in marked contrast to the physical appearance.

Excess weight and earlier abuse

So, we have men for whom putting on weight will have been a method of creating a more powerful physical appearance to boost their masculine sense of self, and we have men whose weight is the result of, and now a contributing factor in, psychological and emotional withdrawal. Another set of causal experiences, and not often focused on, is men putting on excess weight in order to reduce the risk of sexual attention. Men who experienced sexual abuse may see creating a fat body as a way of minimising risk of further, unwanted attention, and this internal imperative may carry on into, and even throughout, adult life.

CASE STUDY 2

Dave is 32, and has been overweight since his mid-teens. He's 22 stone. He put on weight as a reaction to being sexually abused during his earlier teenage years. For Dave, weight is a defence, a barrier through which he seeks to make himself unattractive to men. The abuse also impacted on his sexual identity. He is heterosexual, and has had a stream of sexual relationships with women, driven to prove to himself that he is, in his mind, 'a heterosexual male'. But he cannot sustain a relationship. He needs to lose weight. He knows it, but the thought of losing that barrier remain a block. Powerful feelings are buried within his structure of self needing release, and he needs to redefine himself and unravel the conditions of worth and distorted self-concept that his traumatic experiencing have left him with.

Dave is unlikely to be able to change his eating pattern or reduce his weight, and certainly not in a sustainable way, until he has addressed the underlying emotions associated with the traumas he experienced. He needs to experience a safe, warmly accepting therapeutic relationship to have a chance of encountering himself and his past, and make sustainable weight loss a possibility. He needs to be able to 'tell his story', release his feelings, try to make sense of what happened, and the thoughts and feelings that he is left with that have shaped his self-concept and his structure of self. It is highly likely that 'conditions of worth' will have been established during the grooming period, and in the intense psychological effect of the abuses on him. How has he internalised his experience and how much has it spread into his nature, his way of being and relating to others?

There will be no 'quick-fix'. Yes, Dave may be able to make changes to his eating pattern to reduce weight, but he will need to address the underlying factors to ensure that change is sustained and sustainable.

Heavy drinking, binge eating and loss

Excess weight and size can also stem from heavy drinking, itself often an effect of a range of psychological, emotional as well as social pressures. Then there is comfort eating, satisfying a need to feel full as a way of counteracting some inner emptiness, perhaps the result of a significant loss in the man's life – a close relative in childhood, contact with his children after a failed marriage, for instance. This could be in the form of binge eating, a reaction to the painful feelings as they emerge more acutely at particular times, or a habitual heavy eating pattern that brings the man a sense of physical satisfaction which may then become addictive in its nature. Such binge eating could be on top of an already established heavy eating pattern, and other emotional factors that are not seen as being connected to eating and weight.

CASE STUDY 3

Gary is 24. He's tall and big – 26 stone. He has been eating fatty, processed foods for as long as he can remember. It was what he was conditioned into. Family meals that invariably included chips and burgers were common, and 'fry-ups' were the norm. He doesn't take much exercise. He feels heavy, his mood is low. He doesn't think he has a problem. His mates have similar eating patterns. His dad recently had a heart attack and died. He was also very overweight. The doctors said his poor diet had contributed to his death. Gary really loved his dad, they were great 'mates', going out to football together. Now he feels lost and he's eating more. He always feels empty inside, regardless of how much he eats. He can't imagine eating different foods, but he's worried, he saw what happened to his father. Yet he can't see himself talking to anyone. Not something you do. He's a man. Men are supposed to be big. It's not a problem. Eating disorders? That's for women, not men. He doesn't want to talk about it, but he's still eating heavily and his weight has started to go up again.

Although he hasn't made the connection himself, other losses in his life are factors contributing to the empty feelings inside himself. He was particularly close to his grand-mother who died when he was 14. He hasn't resolved that loss either. In fact, she was the one person who cooked fresh food, which he enjoyed when he was with her. Gary had a girlfriend around that time as well, but she broke off their relationship a couple of years later, as Gary's size began to increase.

Gary will need to explore the losses in his life and the painful emotions that they have left him with. His eating is a mixture of habit as well as an attempt to resolve an emotional void. He will need to experience a therapeutic relationship with a counsellor who truly accepts him, who can relate to Gary the person, the man, and not simply see him in terms of his weight. He is a man in pain at some deeper level, confused about what he should do. He needs time to make sense of himself, of the factors that have contributed to his eating pattern and his size, so that he can then begin to own his difficulties for himself. He cannot be hurried into changing his eating. This must be in response to what he thinks and feels he needs to do.

Engaging with the whole person

There are, of course, many approaches to counselling and psychotherapy. I have elsewhere presented the rationale of the person-centred approach as an effective psychotherapeutic response to men with problems of obesity and over-eating (Bryant-Jefferies, 2005a, 2005b), focusing on the need for the person to experience the relational qualities of this approach in order to help them come to terms with painful feelings, distorted self-perception and the conditioning of their self-worth that can cause or be the result of being overweight.

Sharman (2004) has described her work using the Cycle of Change model (originally devised for working with smoking and widely used now within substance misuse services) (DiClemente, 2003; DiClemente and Prochaska, 1998; Prochaska and DiClemente, 1982). The Cycle of Change model suggests that people pass through stages. Each stage has certain characteristics and demands particular areas of focus and response in order to help the client move on. This model is closely associated with the development of 'motivational interviewing' (Miller and Rollnick, 2002) which seeks to encourage people to change by helping them recognise their need to change.

From talking to obese men and women, Sharman makes the point that while they often do understand what foods to eat, and what to avoid, and they know exercise will help, the difficulty lies in putting knowledge into action. She realised that 'traditional methods of dieting, as a form of weight control, in the main, do not work'

(2004, p. 20). In establishing the SHINE Project (Self Help Independence Nutrition Exercise) with young people in Sheffield, Sharman has sought to establish not only the three elements outlined in the guidelines for obesity management – nutrition, exercise and behaviour modification – she also includes the application of the 'person-centred approach to enable clients to understand the psychology of their eating problems' (2004, p. 20). She also makes the point that 'radical changes in the treatment and management of obesity are required to promote permanent changes to both lifestyle and attitudes, and the psychology behind obesity needs to be urgently addressed before the epidemic gets out of hand' (2004).

The Health Committee's Obesity Report concluded that:

> *it is vital that advances in medical and surgical treatment of obesity should be supported by equivalent development of services to address the psychological and behavioural aspects of obesity. All those receiving treatment for obesity, whether in a primary or in secondary care setting, should have access to psychological support provided by an appropriate professional, whether this is a psychiatrist, psychologist, psychotherapist, counsellor, or family therapist.*
> (HOUSE OF COMMONS, 2004, PP. 109–10)

A difficulty is that many men who are obese or overweight simply do not see it as a problem. They have not experienced the detrimental effects to their health or, if they have, do not think of it as something to seek help for. It is generally less easy for a man to seek help from a counsellor about a problem of any kind than a woman, and it becomes doubly difficult when the problem is one that, in many men's minds, and in society generally, is associated with being a 'woman's condition'.

However, this is changing. It has to. And while specialist treatment for obesity is sparse, it is developing. Within this developing area of specialist help, counselling must be allowed to play its part for without doubt, obesity and being overweight are seldom simply physical problems, whether the emotional and psychological difficulties are cause or effect, or both. What is particularly important, from a counselling perspective, is that whatever treatment intervention is made, it has to address more than size, eating, lack of exercise, or any other lifestyle choice contributing to excess weight. It has to include the experience of a therapeutic relationship, for instance the presence of empathy, genuineness and authenticity, warm acceptance and unconditional positive regard from the counsellor towards the client, for the client to have the opportunity to feel safe enough to allow himself to engage with and resolve the painful feelings that may be associated with his weight and physical appearance.

As the title of this chapter suggests, the counsellor has to work with the man beyond the weight problem. Behaviour change has to be underpinned by emotional and psychological change – changes to the person's self-concept and structure of self. Inner change makes outer change not just more likely but perhaps, most important, more sustainable. When it comes to reducing hazardous weight, any weight loss achieved has to be sustained to be of significant health benefit.

References

Bryant-Jefferies R. *Counselling the Person Beyond the Alcohol Problem*. London: Jessica Kingsley Publishers; 2001.

Bryant-Jefferies R. *Counselling for Eating Disorders in Men: person-centred dialogues*. Oxford: Radcliffe Publishing; 2005a.

Bryant-Jefferies R. *Counselling for Obesity: person-centred dialogues*. Oxford: Radcliffe Publishing; 2005b.

Cohn L. *Fat is NOT JUST a Feminist Issue Anymore*. Date not known. Gurze Books website: www.gurze.com (accessed 13 March 2007).

Department of Health. *Health Survey for England 2003*. London: DoH; 2004.

DiClemente CC. *Addiction and Change*. New York: The Guilford Press; 2003.

DiClemente C, Prochaska JO. Towards a comprehensive, transtheoretical model of change: stages of change and addictive behaviours. In: Miller W, Heather N, editors. *Treating Addictive Behaviours* (2 e). New York: Plenum; 1998.

Hill M. *Male Eating Disorders on Rise*. 2004. Article published on the Gurze Books website: www.gurze.net (accessed 13 March 2007).

House of Commons. *Health Committee's Report on Obesity*. London: HMSO; 2004.

McCabe MP, Ricciardelli CA. Body image and body change techniques amongst adolescent boys. *European Eating Disorders Review*. 2001; 9: 335–47.

Miller WR, Rollnick S. *Motivational Interviewing* (2 e). New York: Guilford Press; 2002.

National Audit Office. *Tackling Obesity in England*. London: National Audit Office; 2001.

Prochaska JO, DiClemente C. Transtheoretical therapy: towards a more integrative model of change. *Psychotherapy: Theory, Research and Practice*. 1982; 19: 276–88.

Sharman K. From compliance to concordance: a psychological approach to weight management. *Healthcare Counselling and Psychotherapy Journal*. Rugby: BACP; October 2004.

CHAPTER 17

Communicating the risks of obesity to South Asian men

Jenne Dixit

Several factors play a role in the increased obesity in South Asian men. This chapter looks at genetic factors, environmental issues and how cultural influences affect the way men from these communities view themselves and their health.

Before we explore some of these factors, it is important to acknowledge that there are significant health inequalities among people from black and minority ethnic communities (BME) (Acheson, 1998): inequalities relating to disease prevalence, differential access to services and differential delivery of services. Further to the Acheson Report (Acheson, 1998) the Stephen Lawrence Inquiry Report by McPherson (1999) highlighted the continued negative experiences of people from BME groups, notably that these groups were not receiving just and equitable access to services. This report also furnished a definition of institutional racism that goes beyond that offered by previous official inquiries, including those addressing health inequalities (McPherson, 1999).

People from black and minority ethnic groups generally show some positive health behaviours, such as lower alcohol consumption and fewer smokers than those in the white community. However, this does not apply to Bangladeshi men or South Asian women, who have high smoking rates and low exercise levels respectively (Lowdell *et al.*, 2000). Traditionally it was assumed that you were from a wealthy family if you smoked. Smoking among these communities is seen more as a social statement than as a bad habit with detrimental effects on health.

The Health of Ethnic Minority Elders in London Report analysed all available information about older people from ethnic minority groups and identified that mortality rates for diabetes were high in elders from the Caribbean, Africa, Asia and the Middle East. This supported the overwhelming statistical evidence that people from South Asian communities are six times more likely to be diagnosed with diabetes than the white population (Marks, 1996). Furthermore, diabetes has an earlier onset, and earlier diagnosis, in South Asian and African Caribbean people than in the white population. Health outcomes are generally worse with a three- to six-fold higher rate of mortality (Balarajan, 1998). There is also a higher prevalence and incidence of complications secondary to diabetes within these communities. South Asians with diabetes have a two- to three-fold excess of mortality from coronary heart disease (Chaturverdi and Fuller, 1996; Mather *et al.*, 1998).

Men from South Asian communities are further disadvantaged since both mortality and morbidity are increased by socio-economic deprivation. For example, morbidity resulting from diabetes complications is 3.5 times higher in people in lower social classes than those in higher social classes. The government's Social Exclusion Unit states that:

> *Ethnic minority disadvantage cuts across all aspects of deprivation. Taken as a whole, ethnic minority groups are more likely than the rest of the population to live in poor areas, be unemployed, have low incomes, live in poor housing and have poor health and be the victims of crime.* (HOME OFFICE AND NCVO, 2000)

The Royal College of Physicians Report, *Assessing Health Needs of People from Minority Ethnic Groups*, summarised studies which demonstrate the continuing impact of social inequality, deprivation and exclusion on the health status of BME groups (Bahl and Rawaf, 1998).

This inequality in outcome has many causes. Deprivation is strongly associated with higher levels of being overweight or obese, physical inactivity, smoking and poor blood pressure control. Other factors include poorer blood glucose control, lower education, employment and housing status, worse access to services, and referral bias. In addition, those who are socially excluded may experience a sense of hopelessness that will work against them developing confidence to manage their health difficulties.

However, as Nazroo (1997) observes, the focus on the ethnic variation in disease to ascertain the cause of disease tends to examine the cultural and biological attributes. Genetic differences in how the body processes and stores fat can result in high blood fat level and increased storage of fat around the abdomen (or being 'apple-shaped' as opposed to 'pear-shaped'). Genetically people from South Asian communities tend to be apple-shaped and are therefore more likely to be at risk of being obese.

It is important to note that for a South Asian man their waist circumference in indicating increased risk is 35 inches (90 cm) compared with 37 inches (97 cm) for white and black men. This has implications for how men from South Asian communities should be thinking about their weight, however difficult this is in the context of their traditional diet.

Samosas, bhajias, parathas and mittaes can send not only your taste buds soaring but also your cholesterol, blood pressure and waist measurement! Traditional foods consumed in South Asian communities tend to be high in fat and sugar. These sorts of treats, once saved for rare special occasions, are now eaten on a daily basis because they are widely affordable and widely available.

Although these foods are eaten throughout the year, religious or auspicious occasions in South Asian communities are still celebrated by an array of foods usually considered high in fat and sugar. At these times people visit as many friends and family as they can, and at these gatherings food occupies a central place. It is part of South Asian culture to gently 'persuade' people to eat as much as they can, and when plates are emptied more food is always offered. It is generally regarded as bad etiquette to refuse.

Change of environment and change of climate has been known to affect levels of obesity in South Asian communities. For example, there was less obesity in the olden days in India even though the diet has remained the same. It could be argued that with the intensity of the sun, people were able to digest the food better as they are able to 'sweat it out'. In rural areas, there were few or no cars or public transport; people were used to walking for miles or riding bicycles, thus getting a good dose of exercise. Foods consisted of more fresh fruit and vegetables in contrast to today's processed tinned products. Today, things are very different. People are still eating the same foods in a colder climate alongside western fast foods and tend to take little or no exercise.

Another reason why men from South Asian communities are obese is because of the lack of information and education about healthy eating and cooking for South Asian women. Women generally do the cooking in the communities and are more than likely to be taught by their mothers. In the practices of the olden days (which may still be found) measuring tools such as teaspoons and tablespoons were never used. Oil was usually poured from the tin and lumps of ghee were put on food and in cooking at one's discretion. Not only does this mean that there is no control on the amount of fat used in Indian cooking but also men have no control in what they are eating. Furthermore, women (usually of first and second generation) have no desire to use recipes or to change their cooking habits of a lifetime. So although there are murmurs of 'healthy eating' in the community and ideas that Indian food should be 'cooked differently', with less ghee and oil used, women do not necessarily believe that a different method of food preparation will enable the food to still taste the same.

Cultural influences can affect the levels of physical activity people are used to, and women seem worse affected than men. For example, some elderly women from orthodox religions will not be seen out alone (to take long walks) and other women will not attend physical activity classes in leisure centres because of the typical dress code of such classes. There tends to be a lack of awareness generally among South Asian communities about the value of physical activity and the fact that being the right weight for your height helps to manage obesity.

'The size of my stomach represents my good fortune in health and wealth' is something that is still heard among many South Asian men from the first and second generation settled in the UK (Diabetes UK Focus Group, 2004). It is a myth that is passed on from generation to generation, from a time when a family's wealth in India was measured by how much 'ghee' was stored in larders and how many 'mittaes' were distributed to friends and family during religious and auspicious occasions.

It is apparent from this quote that culture can affect the way men from diverse communities view health. Some views overlap, however, and it is interesting that all men will hold similar views no matter what culture or background they come from.

Traditionally men from black and minority ethnic communities were considered as the sole breadwinners. They had no time to be ill and could not afford to take time off to visit the doctor as there might not be a secondary wage coming into the family. For men newly arrived in the country, health was considered less important, as employment, housing, and supporting family took precedent. Men from diverse communities were also under pressure to be seen as the strongest of the family and so health was put on a back burner, with health conditions seen as something that 'will go away in time'.

How men from the communities view healthcare professionals is another factor to consider. Some men from black and minority ethnic communities tend to have a lack of respect and trust for the NHS system. This could stem from not receiving culturally specific care, suffering communication barriers, or simply lack of knowledge about how the NHS works.

Some men from black and minority ethnic communities can be quite religious and may use religious teachings, beliefs and myths to provide answers for their illness. Health conditions may be seen as a 'sin committed in past life'. Most Hindus and Sikhs believe in reincarnation, leading some to believe that they are dealing with past sins committed in their past life in their existing life in the form of an 'illness, wrath or a curse'. Therefore they feel that there is nothing they can do about their health condition and choose not to visit their doctor or take prescribed medication. Some also believe that certain health afflictions 'were written in their destiny', i.e. this was meant to happen to them – they were meant to have a heart attack so there is nothing they can do and no amount of western intervention can benefit them.

How to reach South Asian men

It has been well documented that among the myriad of concerns for planners serving the needs of black and minority ethnic communities is the difficulty of communication 'between them and us' (Rudat, 1994). Furthermore, special considerations need to be made when communicating with men from South Asian communities because they do not comprise one homogenous group. It is most important that we do not assume that all South Asian men are the same or in fact have the same needs. Instead we need to address them according to cultural features such as customs, religion – be they Hindu, Sikh or Muslim – lifestyle, food and language.

It is also important to consider communication routes: mainstream messages communicated through mainstream channels may not reach men in all these communities. For example, there may be communication barriers, alienation from wider society, or the men may feel the message does not reflect their own lifestyle or culture. The messages that need to be got across have to be clear, specific and communicated in a tone, language and emotion that are relevant to individual cultural values and beliefs.

It is also essential to provide and promote culturally and linguistically appropriate information, particularly for people whose first language is not English and who do not have English as a second language. There is a lack of culturally appropriate information, and this leads to widespread communication difficulties coupled with insufficient communication support (King's Fund, 2000; Leedham, 2000).

South Asian men can be divided into two groups:

1 those who are hard to reach, particularly those who are non-English-speaking and older, and

2 those who are part of the wider mainstream society, who do speak English, but obtain information through different communication channels as well as traditional ones.

In order to meet the needs of South Asian men, it is essential to work at a local level to raise awareness of obesity and related healthcare problems.

There is no one single way of communicating. Multiple routes need to be used,

---

BOX 17.1 Case study: Diabetes UK advertising campaign launched September 2006

In the UK, the prevalence of type 2 diabetes is six times as high in the South Asian population as the white population. Type 2 diabetes is seen in people as young as 25 years in BME communities compared with people aged 40 years in the white population.

Research has shown that people diagnosed with type 2 diabetes have often already had the condition for 9 to 12 years without being aware of it. Worse still, they may already be suffering from one of the complications at the time of diagnosis.

To help address this, Diabetes UK ran an awareness campaign in September 2006. It was devised following research undertaken by MORI which indicated the lack of awareness that people have of the risk factors for developing type 2 diabetes. The MORI research showed that, while the black and South Asian people are more likely to develop the condition, they often have a very much lower awareness of the risk factors than the white population, so it was essential that these communities were reached.

Diabetes UK's *Measure Up* campaign aims to encourage people with two or more of the following risk factors to go and get a test for type 2 diabetes: being overweight, being over 25 years old, having diabetes in the family and being of black or South Asian origin.

A very easy way for people to find out if their weight is a risk factor is to measure their waist. *Measure Up* highlights waist measurement as a key indicator of being at risk from diabetes.

Because South Asian Men do not have to be as overweight as the white population to be at risk of developing diabetes (waist measurement of 35 inches for South Asian men compared with 37 inches for white men; the figure for all women is 31.5 inches) Diabetes UK produced a special promotional poster (*see* Figure 17.1) aimed at the South Asian men produced in the five major Asian languages. There was also advertising in some of the key South Asian and black publications.

Diabetes UK hopes that the campaign will also raise awareness of diabetes generally and make the general public more aware of the condition. The campaign will be taken to a local level via four major religious institutions (a mosque, a temple, a gurdwara and a church) to enable healthcare professionals to engage with people from the diverse communities in an environment where they feel secure.

This is the largest and most effective campaign that Diabetes UK has ever run. Activities will include advertising at bus shelters and in the national press, stories in the media, posters at GP surgeries, in pharmacies and information on relevant websites.

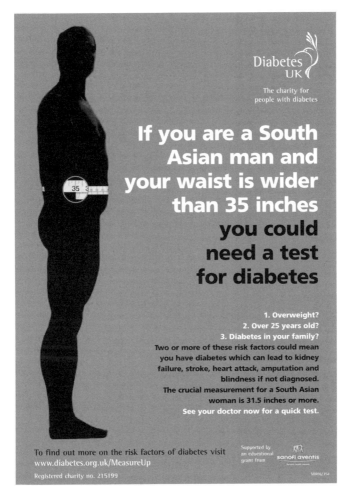

Figure 17.1 Diabetes UK's *Measure Up* campaign.

some PR, some through community development approaches, and so forth. Communication channels include community organisations, leaders (imams and priests), religious institutions (mandhirs and mosques) and the use of the ethnic media. It is also important to inform and educate wives and children to facilitate support to fathers, husbands, and other male members of families. However, it is well known that South Asian men are more likely to take advice from community and religious leaders than listen to their wives so it is beneficial to educate and empower leaders about disease prevention and health promotion. Dissemination of information, e.g. flyers, to religious organisations also works well as people from the communities are likely to pick up information here for themselves, friends or family.

Summary

Multiple factors account for increased obesity in South Asian men. Religious and cultural influences are the strongest contenders and probably the most difficult to dispel. However, with appropriate culturally and linguistic sensitive information communicated via suitable channels, awareness building can help South Asian men have an increased understanding of their health and how they can better manage their health conditions.

References

Acheson SD. Independent inquiry into inequalities in health. HMSO, London; 1998.

Bahl V, Rawaf S, editors. *Assessing Health Needs of People from Minority Ethnic Groups*. London: Royal College of Physicians/Faculty of Public Health Medicine; 1998.

Balarajan R. Trends in mortality from diabetes in England and Wales among those born in the Indian subcontinent and the Caribbean Commonwealth. *Ethnicity & Health*. 1998; 3(1/2): 55–8.

Chaturverdi N, Fuller JH. Ethnic differences in mortality from cardiovascular disease in the UK: do they persist in people with diabetes? *Journal of Epidemiology and Community Health*. 1996; **50**: 139.

Diabetes UK Focus Group. Quote taken from a South Asian man over 40 years old. 2004.

Home Office and NCVO. Bringing Britain together – a national strategy for neighbourhood renewal. 1998. From: *COMPACT Black and Minority Ethnic Voluntary and Community Organisations: a code of good practice*. London: Home Office and NCVO; 2000.

King's Fund. *Testing Times*. London: Audit Commission; 2000.

Leedham I. *Diabetes Health Promotion in Minority Ethnic Communities: report of a research and development programme in Wales*. London: British Diabetic Association; 2000.

Lowdell C, Evandrou M, Bardsley M *et al. Health of Ethnic Minority in Elders in London. Respecting Diversity July 2000*. London: The Health of Londoners Project; 2000.

Marks L. *Counting the Cost*. London: King's Fund; 1996.

Mather HM, Chaturverdi N, Fuller JH. Mortality and morbidity from diabetes in South Asians and Europeans: 11 year follow-up of the Southall Diabetes Survey, London. *Diabetic Medicine*. 1998; **15**: 53–9.

McPherson W. *The Stephen Lawrence Inquiry: report of an inquiry*. London: Home Office; February 1999.

Nazroo J. Health and health services. In: Modood T, Bethoud R, Lakey J *et al.*, editors. *Ethnic Minorities in Britain. Diversity and disadvantage*. London: Policy Studies Institute; 1997.

Rudat K. *Black and Minority Groups in England. Health and lifestyle*. London: Health Education Authority; 1994.

CHAPTER 18

Weight management in men with mental health problems

Alison Sullivan

Mental disorder and weight gain

People with mental disorders appear to be more vulnerable to development of obesity, with studies identifying higher levels of 'relative body weight and excess abdominal adiposity' (Sharpe and Hills, 1998). A recent inpatient survey found that 36% of the male patients were obese compared with a general population prevalence of 17% (Cormac et al., 2005). One community study in 1995 showed that around 26% of people with mental health needs were obese (Seymour, 2003). Weight gain has been described by patients as extremely distressing, and is related to poorer quality of life, and reduced well-being and vitality (Allison et al., 2003).

Mental disorders are responsible for more than 12% of the total global burden of disease, particularly affecting the most productive section of the population, young adults. The most vulnerable are those with adverse circumstances and the least resources (Bradshaw et al., 2005; WHO, 2003). Depression is the commonest mental disorder, affecting at least 5% of the UK population, accounting for about 25% of all general practitioner referrals (Thomas, 2001) and 121 million people affected worldwide (WHO, 2003). In the USA, 2.5% of the population has a diagnosis of schizophrenia (Wirshing, 2004) and 24 million suffer worldwide (WHO, 2003).

Mental illness is associated with an increased risk for development of physical ill health and premature death (Phelan et al., 2001) with life expectancy reduced by 10 years (Allebeck, 1989; Brown, 1997; Brown et al., 2000). Adults with a diagnosis of schizophrenia have about 60% of the excess mortality due to natural causes, the most common being diabetes mellitus (Holt et al., 2004), digestive diseases, circulatory disorders, pharyngeal and lung cancer (Bradshaw et al., 2005). The greater incidence of these conditions is probably linked to unhealthy lifestyle factors (Brown et al., 1999) such as poor diet, smoking and reduced exercise.

Obesity (BMI > 30) is a serious and chronic physical condition where body fat stores are so enlarged that health is impaired caused by taking in more dietary energy than is required (Garrow et al., 2000). Causation and maintenance of obesity have both genetic and environmental components (Devlin et al., 2000).

Medical co-morbidities of obesity include diabetes mellitus, dyslipidaemia, coronary heart disease, congestive heart failure, stroke, cancer of the colon, rectum and prostate, gallstones, osteoarthritis, sleep apnoea (Garrow *et al.*, 2000), hypertension, metabolic syndrome (Devlin *et al.*, 2000; Thakore, 2005) and depression (Wirshing, 2004). 'Obese people are often anxious or depressed, and it is difficult to establish if this is a cause or effect of obesity' (Garrow *et al.*, 2000).

Additionally to adverse medical effects, prevalent societal negative attitudes towards high body weight can result in disadvantages regarding access to education, renting accommodation, relationships and employment. These obstacles can compound social exclusion and other difficulties related to living with a mental disorder, such as compromised neurocognitive and intrapsychic functioning (Rosenheck *et al.*, 2006; Seymour, 2003).

Garrow states that all penalties of obesity decrease with weight loss, with the exception of the risk for gallstones which are facilitated by cholesterol mobilisation from adipose tissue (Garrow *et al.*, 2000). Weight loss reduces blood pressure, improves lipid profile and blood glucose control, with benefits starting at around 5% to 10% loss of body weight (Devlin *et al.*, 2000).

The effect of psychiatric medication on weight

Weight gain and obesity are associated with psychiatric medications that block histamine H_1 (Wirshing *et al.*, 1999), serotonin 5-HT_{2c} and dopamine D_2 receptors (Devlin *et al.*, 2000). Consequently mood stabilisers, antidepressants and antipsychotics (Schwartz *et al.*, 2004), used in the management of psychiatric disorders, are reported to be involved in weight gain.

Mood stabilisers such as lithium are associated with at least 5% of body weight gain in up to two-thirds of patients receiving this medication. Some 25 to 50 per cent of those treated with anticonvulsants, such as carbamazepine and valproic acid, may experience similar rises in body weight (Devlin *et al.*, 2000).

Recent studies show that modest weight gains are associated with the tricyclic antidepressants and monoamine oxidase inhibitors (MAOIs) with larger increases for a small number of patients. The selective serotonin reuptake inhibitors (SSRIs), such as fluoxetine and sertraline, appear not to be associated with weight gain and some patients are reported to have lost weight. However, studies show weight regain after about one year of treatment with a possible overshoot above baseline on long-term treatment (Devlin *et al.*, 2000).

First-generation (typical or conventional) antipsychotics such as chlorpromazine, mesoridazine and thioridazine, and the second generation (atypical or novel) antipsychotics such as olazapine, clozapine, risperidone and quetiapine, are associated with weight gain, carrying differences in weight gain liabilities (Allison *et al.*, 1999; Wirshing *et al.*, 1999). Short-term studies show weight increase occurring rapidly during the acute phase of medication, with a plateau after one to two years of treatment. However, weight gain may continue for a longer period.

Antipsychotics may be regarded as problematic due to the weight gain side effect and resulting increased risk of patient non-adherence (Ackerman and Nolan, 1998;

Devlin *et al.*, 2000; Weiden *et al.*, 2004) which has been 'estimated to increase illness relapse rates five-fold' (Wirshing, 2004).

Weight gain with a central fat distribution is associated with greater morbidity and has been linked to the atypical antipsychotics (Graham *et al.*, 2005; Thakore, 2005), although this may also be the case with other medications. An ethnicity-appropriate girth measurement can be taken to assess degree of central adiposity for some patients.

The range of mental illnesses

Mental illnesses can be crudely grouped into psychoses, such as schizophrenia, and neuroses, such as anxiety neurosis (Thomas, 2001). Diagnostic criteria can be found in the *International Classification of Diseases* (WHO, 2004) and the *Diagnostic and Statistical Manual* of the American Psychiatric Association (2000).

It is generally held that people with a neurotic condition maintain contact with reality whereas those with a psychotic illness may lose insight regarding reality (Thomas, 2001), or aspects of reality, rendering assessment and treatment of weight gain more challenging.

Presence of a mental disorder can render self-care more difficult, due to a range of factors such as symptoms of the disease, poverty due to lack of well-paid employment, poor environment, reduced access to primary healthcare and education around healthy lifestyle, nutrition, food provision and preparation. These factors should be borne in mind when devising treatment plans.

Note: Not all mental disorders have been covered in this chapter. For example male patients with eating disorders or dementias may require help to manage weight changes, meriting specialist nutritional interventions from a registered dietician.

Mood or 'affective' disorders

Depression and mania are mood disorders. Mood can be high (mania), low (depressed) or both, as in bipolar disorder (BPD). These disorders can impact upon food and fluid consumption and preferences (*see* Table 18.1), causing under, over or inappropriate nutritional intake, leading to weight change. Medications to treat mood disorders may also affect nutritional status (*see* Table 18.2), affecting energy intake and body weight.

Psychotic disorders – schizophrenia

Schizophrenia is a psychotic disorder, which can be severe. Causation is not understood, although stressful events in the teens or later in life may be a trigger. It has been reported that 25% of people presenting with schizophrenia can fully recover with no reoccurrence, 50% recover with recurrent episodes and 25% may be seriously disabled requiring ongoing care. The symptoms are classified as 'positive' or 'negative' (Thomas, 2001). *See* Table 18.3.

TABLE 18.1 Nutritional consequences of mood disorders. Italic type denotes factors which may contribute to weight gain.

Mood disorder	Possible influences on food intake	Possible nutritional consequences
Depression	Apathy, disinterest in food Anorexia Sense of guilt or worthlessness causing feelings of not deserving food Loss of thirst sensation Fluid refusal *Distorted food intake* *Carbohydrate craving*	Under-nutrition Weight loss Dehydration, constipation, impacted faeces *Unbalanced diet, weight gain* *Weight gain, obesity*
Anxiety	Frequent loose stools Abdominal pain/discomfort	Selective food avoidance Food refusal
Mania	Drug-side effects causing dry mouth/altered taste Hyperactivity *Increased appetite* *Erratic eating habits*	Difficulties in chewing/swallowing Altered taste sensation Increased energy demands, Weight loss *Excess calories, weight gain* *Unbalanced diet, weight gain*

Adapted from Thomas B, *Manual of Dietetic Practice* 3/e, 2001, with permission of Blackwell Publishing.

TABLE 18.2 Effects of medication and mood disorders. Italic type denotes factors which may contribute to weight gain.

Antidepressants	Typical drugs	Potential nutritional side effects
Tricyclic	Amitryptyline Imipramine Lofepramine Dothiepin Doxepin	Dry mouth (increased fluid intake) Sour metallic taste Constipation, possible diarrhoea Nausea and vomiting, epigastric distress Anorexia (rarely) *Increased appetite and weight gain due to carbohydrate craving*
Selective serotonin reuptake inhibitors (SSRIs)	Citalopram Fluoxetine Fluvoxamine Paroxetine Sertraline	Anorexia Nausea and vomiting Weight loss *Dry mouth (increased fluid intake)* Dyspepsia, diarrhoea
Monoamine oxidase inhibitors (MAOIs)	Isocarboxazid Phenelzine Tranylcypromine	Nausea and vomiting *Dry mouth (increased fluid intake)* Constipation Increased appetite and weight gain Potentiation of action of insulin or oral hypoglycaemic with lowered blood glucose Hypertensive crisis if foods containing tyramine ingested
Mood stabilisers	Lithium	*Weight gain, thirst*

Adapted from Thomas B, *Manual of Dietetic Practice* 3/e, 2001, with permission of Blackwell Publishing.

TABLE 18.3 Nutritional consequences of schizophrenia.

Symptoms of schizophrenia	Potential nutritional consequences
Positive symptoms	
Delusions	Beliefs that foods and/or drinks may be harmful/poisoned leading to request for special diets/foods or food/drink avoidance or refusal. May avoid meals and rely on snack or fast foods.
Hallucinations	May be advised by 'voices' about what to eat and drink. May find some previously liked foods unacceptable. May result in unusual choices or combinations.
Paranoia	Fear that food/drink harmful. May become malnourished due to existing on a small range of 'safe foods'. Suspicious of advice or motives of health professionals.
Agitation	May miss meals and rely on snacking. May eat or drink more frequently.
Hostility	May not accept food/drinks or advice from others. May not follow agreed plan.
Negative symptoms	
Emotional withdrawal	May not want to discuss nutrition and to eat alone, possibly avoiding full meals in favour of quickly eaten snacks.
Social withdrawal	Hard to engage in appropriate shopping or eating behaviours, especially if necessary to shop or dine with others.
Lack of motivation	May eat what is most convenient such as snack or fast foods. May forget to carry or use sweeteners or agreed snack foods. May not adhere to an agreed eating plan.
Inability to cope with daily living tasks	Ability to select appropriate foods/drinks, shop and prepare meals may be impaired. May have low income and poor living conditions.
Difficulty in rational thinking	Make poor food and drink choices. Lack of meals and routine. Poor planning and budgeting. Poor understanding of causes of weight gain and management options.
Poor rapport	Difficult to obtain an accurate assessment, agree a nutritional plan and meaningfully review progress.

Adapted from Thomas B, *Manual of Dietetic Practice* 3/e, 2001, with permission of Blackwell Publishing.

Factors affecting energy balance

Weight gain occurs when more energy is consumed than is required. Energy intake and expenditure affect body weight, with the greater effect generally exerted by intake.

Energy intake

People with mental health needs may have poor quality diets, eat more saturated fat, and less fibre and vegetables than the general population. Intakes of vitamin C and E are also thought to be compromised (McCreadie *et al.*, 1998). Factors that may lead to over-consumption of dietary energy and weight gain include the following.

Illness effects
- Increased appetite (illness effect, medication, boredom, anxiety, low mood or poor self-esteem).
- Poor cognition, planning and decision-making ability, sedation.
- Increased thirst (untreated or poorly controlled diabetes, medication effects, boredom).
- Use of sugar-containing drinks, attempting to boost mental and physical energy levels.
- Impaired satiety, binge eating and food preference (Sharpe and Hills, 2003).

Environment
- Institutional food – ready availability of high-energy meals and snacks or drinks, no selection guidance.
- Ready availability of additional food and drinks (vending machines, hospital shops, etc.).
- Accelerated speed of eating (non-conducive eating environment, staff rushed, short and inappropriately timed meal breaks, use of fast or convenience foods).
- Reduced access to good quality, lower-calorie choices such as fruit and vegetables, low-fat spreads, sweeteners and sugar-free drinks.
- Poor shopping, preparation and storage facilities.
- Inappropriate meal timing (early breakfast, that may be missed, and early supper leaving long evening).
- Speed of eating (unconducive eating environment, staff rushed).
- Reduced access to healthier choices or variety, due to availability, hence need for storage and possible increased cost of items.
- Lack of advice, support and positive role models.

Knowledge/lifestyle
- Selection of poor quality high fat and sugar foods.
- Frequent eating out, 'take-aways', ready prepared meals, snacking.
- Use of sugar-containing drinks.
- Poor financial position.
- Poor shopping, preparation and storage facilities.
- Poor nutritional and food preparation knowledge and skills.
- Poor cognition, planning and decision-making ability.
- Lack of advice, support and positive role models.
- Poor dentition leading to choice of softer, energy-dense foods.

Energy expenditure

People with mental illness may exert low levels of physical activity due to several factors, including lack of motivation and opportunity. Exercise alone is unlikely to control or reduce body weight. However, studies show improved weight maintenance (Devlin *et al.*, 2000) in those exercising. Increased physical activity, especially everyday activities such as walking and using stairs, will increase energy expenditure, increase lean body mass and can contribute to improved physical and mental health.

Illness and other effects

- Illness effects (apathy, listlessness, low mood, low self-esteem, social withdrawal).
- Medication sedation or other effects.
- Pre-existing high body weight.
- Low levels of fitness and exercise capacity.
- Embarrassment/shyness.
- Lack of knowledge about facilities and suitable activities.
- Previous negative experience of exercise.

Environment

- Reduced opportunities for physical activity (household activities, recreational walking).
- Reduced liberty, lack of escorts.
- Lack of suitable environment, e.g. gym, safe walks, health/recreation centres, parks.

Knowledge/lifestyle

- Lack of suitable clothing or knowledge about suitability of clothing.
- Lack of equipment (e.g. pedometer, bicycle, trainers).
- Poor financial position.
- No-one to exercise with.
- Lack of knowledge about facilities and suitable activities.
- Lack of guidance about suitable activities for fitness level.
- Previous negative experience of exercise.
- Poor staff knowledge and skills/attitudes, inappropriate role models.

Assessment

Making an accurate and comprehensive assessment of the patient and issues around weight gain can be especially challenging when working with people who have mental health needs (Devlin *et al.*, 2000; Graham *et al.*, 2005). It may not be possible to complete it in one attempt. However, it is important to get as full an assessment as possible on which to base future individual management plans. Kushner and Blatner (2005) reinforce that 'Understanding the reasons leading to and sustaining the patient's over-weight and obesity... is paramount to designing individualized and targeted treatment'.

An accurate and regular anthropometric assessment, with sensitive feedback of results and implications, can be an important contribution to encouraging a healthier body weight for all people where weight changes are likely, such as those taking medications associated with weight gain.

Assessment includes establishing the degree of overweight and the overall risk status, which can be performed by taking a height, weight and calculation of the BMI. For those below BMI 35 kg/m^2, a waist circumference may also be useful (National Institutes of Health, 2002). Patients with BMI over 35 kg/m^2, and arguably at lower BMI values, may present a challenge to accurate location of a measuring tape due to adiposity masking bones. Also the cut-off values lose usefulness at and beyond this level of obesity (NICE, 2006).

The American Diabetes Association (ADA) consensus statement (2004) advises that people taking second-generation antipsychotics should have height and weight taken and BMI calculated at baseline and a regular weight plus BMI every four weeks for 12 weeks and quarterly thereafter. A baseline and annual waist circumference is also advised.

For all mental health inpatients and community patients, where weight gain is a risk and resources allow, a weekly opportunity for being weighed allows closer monitoring and support. For all mental health patients, calculation of a BMI on admission to the service followed up with regular weighing and healthy lifestyle education, where appropriate, enables early intervention and may increase success of weight management treatment plans. Patients may require referral to a specialist mental health dietician for an individual weight management treatment plan.

Other health risks should be taken into account including physical diseases, cardiovascular risk factors such as personal and family histories, smoking or hypertension, dyslipidaemias and impaired fasting glucose. Some authors consider blood glucose monitoring essential for those taking some second-generation antipsychotics (SGAs) (Lean and Pajonk, 2003; Mir and Taylor, 2001) regardless of body weight.

Some patients may be reluctant to be weighed and have girth measured; therefore time should be taken to explain the benefits to the patient. Developing a culture of normality around regular weighing for all can be helpful in engagement.

Management

'There exists no consensus on whether or how to address obesity in the patient's overall treatment plan' (Devlin *et al.*, 2000). In 2004 the ADA gave guidance for people taking antipsychotics. General obesity management guidance is available based upon studies in non-psychiatric populations (National Institute of Health, National Heart, Lung and Blood Institute, 2002; National Obesity Forum, 2006; Scottish Intercollegiate Guidelines Network, 1996) and there remains no one approach but elements that can be adapted to suit individuals or groups.

Currently there is little guidance about which intervention to choose regarding weight management in psychiatric populations and little gender-specific advice upon which to base interventions for men, with or without mental health needs. Men form the bulk of patient numbers in secure settings. They may require a different approach to that used with women and more gender-specific research is needed. Evidence used to base interventions has generally been established in the mentally well. These strategies may not be directly transferable (Wernecke *et al.*, 2003).

A review of weight management interventions for people with schizophrenia suggested that 'small reductions in weight can be made through pharmacological, behavioural and dietary interventions' (Faulkner *et al.*, 2003). There is limited evidence for efficacy (Wernecke *et al.*, 2003) and Faulkner *et al.* (2003) conclude that 'both dietary and exercise counselling set within a behavioural modification programme is necessary for sustained weight control'.

Sharpe and Hills (2003) state that:

Weight management ... is a unique challenge in patients with psychiatric disorders ... There is widespread agreement that interventions should be proactive and target potential gainers ... Regular monitoring, realistic goal setting and weight control strategies are vital. ... Lifestyle interventions ... may need to be adapted to be most effective; for example, using strategies to counter increased appetite and to enhance physical activity.

They identify the following features of successful weight management programmes:
1 Multidisciplinary approach in the development and implementation of a programme.
2 Tailor programme to individual goals, lifestyle and needs.
3 Provide realistic expectations of weight loss and set achievable goals.
4 Promote long-term gradual change in diet and exercise, appropriate to each individual.
5 Educate about the importance of behaviour change.
6 Encourage patients to consider benefits other than weight loss, for example improved well-being and control of type 2 diabetes, dyslipidaemia and blood pressure.
7 Use strategies to deal with emotional and environmental factors which trigger overeating.
8 Provide appropriate support materials over time as patients needs change.
9 Maintain supportive and empathic attitude towards patients.

Arguably, at any one time, weight loss may not necessarily be advisable or desirable for everyone and should not be insisted upon. For example, some patients report feeling 'less vulnerable' to other patients when having a larger body, regardless of composition. Other patients may be too acutely unwell to deal with the necessary changes.

Weight stabilisation, rather than loss, may be the goal for some patients, especially those experiencing rapid onset weight gain following commencement of medication. Positive dietary change and improvement in other lifestyle factors, such as activity and smoking reduction, can bring health benefits, without weight change.

Patients with special needs such as coeliac disease, food allergies/intolerances, diabetes or eating disorders, should be identified and offered specialist dietetic management.

Dietary therapy
The goals of dietary therapy generally include improvement to the nutritional quality of the diet and eating pattern as well as weight stabilisation or change. For treatment plans that aim for weight loss, Garrow states that an appropriate rate of weight loss is 0.5–1.0 kg/week (1–2 lb/week.). This can be achieved by a calorie deficit of 500–1,000 kcal/day. The first few weeks may give a faster rate due to water and glycogen changes. Greater restrictions lead to difficulties ensuring consumption of adequate essential nutrients (Garrow *et al.*, 2000).

The healthcare team, as a part of lifestyle education, can give first-line healthy eating advice. Patients requiring more focused intervention may be referred to the specialist mental health dietician for an individual plan and follow-up.

Simple changes can lead to effective calorie reductions; for example, patients are often thirsty and may drink large quantities of fluids. A litre of orange juice, full-fat milk or Coke all contain around 500 kcal. If a patient drank a litre of one of these a day, by swapping to water, sugar-free squash or 'diet' carbonated drinks, this would save 500 kcal daily and promote weight reduction in a weight-stable patient.

For inpatients, access to a clear and coded menu, showing low energy or healthy eating choices, should be available at each mealtime. The environment should support dietary change. For example, lower fat milks, non-sucrose sweeteners and reduced fat spreads should be easily accessible when required.

Staff associated with the patient should be aware of any dietary plans and facilitate the agreed behaviour changes. For example, encouraging the use of acceptable products such as sweeteners; ensuring that escorts are available to attend physical activities with patients who need to be accompanied; and ensuring that patients are able to follow their plans.

Physical activity

Physical activity (PA) can contribute to weight reduction as it increases energy expenditure, fitness, lean body mass and insulin sensitivity. However, it is not an effective weight loss strategy, if used alone. For example, the average non-athlete uses only about an extra 5 kcal/minute, or 300 kcal, during one hour of jogging (Garrow *et al.*, 2000).

Studies advise that overweight and obese patients should 'increase their physical activity to 200–300 minutes of moderate activity per week or two 30-minute sessions of moderate activity per week for sedentary individuals' and 'lifestyle activity as opposed to structured exercise may be more attractive to some individuals' (Faulkner *et al.*, 2003).

PA is associated with successful weight maintenance and, if combined with a low-fat, low energy density diet, may allow sufficient decrease in dietary restraint for successful weight maintenance. However, people with a 'BMI > 30 need to persist with long term changes in diet and PA to overcome tendency to regain' (Devlin *et al.*, 2000).

Medication and surgical approaches

Wirshing (2004) warns against knee-jerk switching to an antipsychotic with fewer propensities to increase weight, as this may not be a viable option for the clinically stable patient.

Drugs are available for weight loss; however, pharmacological interventions for patients treated with antipsychotics are generally not supported (Wernecke *et al.*, 2002).

Surgical procedures, such as gastric bypass and gastric stapling, are methods of enforcing dieting rather than alternatives, with the exception of apronectomy, which removes some subcutaneous abdominal fat (Garrow *et al.*, 2000). 'Weight loss medications and bariatric surgery are relatively contraindicated in this [schizophrenic] patient population' (Wirshing, 2004).

A reduction in body weight may impact upon the dose of medication required, including medication for physical and psychiatric conditions. Pharmacists and prescribers should be fully informed about weight changes.

Patient education and health professional training
Weight management may be life-long. Patients might value the opportunity of attending a group with a rolling programme of education and support. Mixed or single-sex groups may require different approaches.

Nutrition, buying and preparing food, bowel health, smoking, physical activity, medication information, dental health, and psychological issues can all be incorporated into the group, dependent on the needs and wants of the participants. Some groups may wish to use the session to go out, for example, on walking, bowling and guided shopping tours. Guest speakers can be invited to add variety and new perspectives. Wirshing suggests that carers and families should also receive education around healthy lifestyles (Wirshing, 2004).

Health professionals delivering training should be appropriately qualified and experienced in group work techniques, teaching and have sound knowledge of the topic that they are to deliver. Groups of overweight patients are likely to include diabetics and an awareness of diabetes management may be useful.

Reviews have identified that further research is required to develop effective healthy lifestyle interventions for mental health populations (Bradshaw *et al.*, 2005). However, if sessions are to run, based upon limited research, it would seem reasonable that they should be planned and critically evaluated after delivery with the aim of continuous improvement.

Patient education can be reinforced by use of activities from the multidisciplinary team, such as quizzes and poster competitions. Incentives such as T-shirts, designed by the group members, may encourage patients to attend a minimum number of sessions, reinforce group identity and give support.

Staff should be trained to measure height and weight, calculate BMI and discuss the health-related implications of results. A sound knowledge of the basics of healthy eating based upon the Balance of Good Health model, from the Food Standards Agency (www.food.gov.uk), gives a clear and consistent message to patients.

Culture and environment
The overweight generally and people with mental health needs can have low self-esteem. A culture of non-judgemental support, positivity towards health and encouragement can be helpful.

The hospital environment can unwittingly encourage obesity due to high availability of energy-dense foods and reduced opportunities to be physically active. While patients are in hospital, there is often opportunity to engage, educate and support people towards selecting and incorporating health-promoting behaviours.

Education of staff who come into contact with patients, in basic healthy lifestyle and encouragement towards health-promoting behaviours, can foster role models from both the staff and patient populations, with potential health benefits all around. In-house publications can be a vehicle for staff and patient lifestyle education.

Occupational health services may wish to offer initiatives such as weight management groups for staff or walking/activity clubs.

The environment can be optimised to facilitate health, for example healthier options in hospital vending machines, shops and at ward level. The eating environment can be modified so that it is as relaxing and enjoyable as possible, with mealtimes adjusted to avoid overlong gaps between meals. Patients may be encouraged to be involved in choosing their meals and to eat slowly, encouraging appropriate detection of satiation. Initiatives such as Better Hospital Food and protected mealtimes are aimed at helping staff to achieve a more enjoyable eating experience for patients.

Patient literature such as posters and leaflets should be of good quality, conveying reliable information, suitable for the readers in terms of content and presentation, in good condition and changed regularly.

For community patients, it may be helpful to explore how shopping, food preparation and storage facilities can be maximised, together with financial considerations and lifestyle change.

References

Ackerman S, Nolan LJ. Bodyweight gain induced by antipsychotropic drugs. *CNS Drugs.* 1998; **9**(2): 135–51.

Allebeck P. Schizophrenia: a life shortening disease. *Schizophrenia Bulletin.* 1989; **15**(1): 81–9.

Allison DB, Mackell JA, McDonnell DD. The impact of weight gain on quality of life among persons with schizophrenia. In: *Psychiatric Services.* 2003; 565–7. http://psychservices.psychiatryonline.org (accessed 13 March 2007).

Allison DB, Mentore JL, Heo M *et al.* Antipsychotic-induced weight gain: a comprehensive research synthesis. *American Journal of Psychiatry.* 1999; **156**(11): 1686–96.

American Diabetes Association. Consensus Development Conference on Antipsychotic Drug and Obesity and Diabetes. *Journal of Clinical Psychiatry.* 2004; **65**: 267–72.

American Psychiatric Association (APA). *Quick Reference to the Diagnostic Criteria from the DSM IV-TR.* Washington, DC: APA; 2000.

Bradshaw T, Lovell K, Harris N. Healthy living interventions and schizophrenia: a systematic review. *Journal of Advanced Nursing.* 2005; **49**(6): 634–54.

Brown S. Excess mortality of schizophrenia: a meta analysis. *British Journal of Psychiatry.* 1997; **171**(12): 502–8.

Brown S, Birtwistle J, Roe I, Thompson C. The unhealthy lifestyle of people with schizophrenia. *Psychological Medicine.* 1999; **29**(3): 697–701.

Brown S, Inskip H, Barrowclough B. Causes of the excess mortality of schizophrenia. *British Journal of Psychiatry.* 2000; **177**: 212–17.

Cormac I, Ferriter M, Benning R, Saul C. Physical health and health risk factors in a population of long-stay psychiatric patients. *Psychiatric Bulletin.* 2005; **29**: 18–20.

Devlin MJ, Yanovski SZ, Wilson GT. Obesity: what mental health professionals need to know. *American Journal of Psychiatry.* 2000; **157**(6): 854–63.

Faulkner G, Soundy AA, Lloyd K. Schizophrenia and weight management: a systematic review of interventions to control weight. *Acta Psychiatrica Scandinavica.* 2003; **108**: 324–32.

Food Standards Agency. *Balance of Good Health.* Information booklet. 2001. www.food.gov.uk/multimedia/pdfs/bghbooklet.pdf#page=6 (accessed 13 March 2007).

Garrow JS, James WPT, Ralph A. *Human Nutrition and Dietetics.* (10 e). Edinburgh: Churchill Livingstone; 2000.

Graham KA, Perkins DO, Edwards LJ *et al.* Effect of Olanzapine on body composition and energy expenditure in adults with first-episode psychosis. *American Journal of Psychiatry*. 2005; **162**(1): 118–23.

Holt RIG, Peveler RC, Byrne CD. Schizophrenia, the metabolic syndrome and diabetes. *Diabetic Medicine*. 2004; **21**(6): 515–23.

Kushner RF, Blatner D. Risk assessment of the overweight and obese patient. *Journal of the American Dietetic Association*. 2005; **105**(5 Suppl 1): S53–62.

Lean MEJ, Pajonk F-G. Patients on atypical antipsychotic drugs: another high risk group for type 2 diabetes. *Diabetes Care*. 2003; **26**(5): 1597–605.

McCreadie R, MacDonald E, Blacklock C *et al.* Dietary intake of schizophrenic patients in Nithsdale, Scotland: case controlled study. *British Medical Journal*. 1998; **317**: 784–5.

Mir S, Taylor D. Atypical antipsychotics and hyperglycaemia. *International Clinical Psychopharmacology*. 2001; **16**(2): 63–74.

National Institute for Health and Clinical Excellence (NICE). *Obesity Guidance on the Prevention, Identification, Assessment and Management of Overweight and Obesity in Adults and Children*. London: NICE; 2006.

National Institute of Health, National Heart, Lung and Blood Institute. *Clinical Guidelines on the Identification, Evaluation and Treatment of Overweight and Obesity in adults*. 2002. www.nhlbi.nih.gov/guidelines/obesity/sum_clin.htm (accessed 13 March 2007).

National Obesity Forum. 2006. www.nationalobesityforum.org.uk

Phelan M, Straddins L, Morrison S. Physical health of people with severe mental illness. *British Medical Journal*. 2001; **322**: 443–4.

Rosenheck R, Leslie D, Keefe R *et al.* Barriers to employment for people with schizophrenia. *American Journal of Psychiatry*. 2006; **163**(3): 411–17.

Schwartz TL, Nihalani N, Jindal S, Virk S, Jones N. Psychiatric medication-induced obesity: a review. *Obesity Reviews*. 2004; **5**(2): 115–21.

Scottish Intercollegiate Guidelines Network. *Obesity in Scotland. Integrating prevention with weight management. A national clinical guideline recommended for use in Scotland*. Edinburgh: SIGN; 1996. www.sign.ac.uk/ (accessed 13 March 2007).

Seymour L. Not all in the mind: the physical health of mental health service users. *Mentality*. 2003; Report No. 2.

Sharpe JK, Hills AP. Anthropometry and adiposity in a group of people with chronic mental illness. *Australian and New Zealand Journal of Psychiatry*. 1998; **32**: 77–81.

Sharpe JK, Hills AP. Atypical antipsychotic weight gain: a major clinical challenge. *Australian and New Zealand Journal of Psychiatry*. 2003; **37**: 705–9.

Thakore JH. Metabolic syndrome and schizophrenia. *British Journal of Psychiatry*. 2005; **186**: 455–6.

Thomas B. *Manual of Dietetic Practice* (3 e). Oxford: Blackwell Publishing; 2001.

Weiden PJ, Mackell JA, McDonnell DD. Obesity as a risk factor for antipsychotic non-compliance. *Schizophrenia Research*. 2004; **66**: 51–7.

Wernecke U, Taylor D, Sanders TAB. Options for pharmacological management of obesity in patients treated with atypical antipsychotics. *International Clinical Psychopharmacology*. 2002; **17**: 145–60.

Wernecke U, Taylor D, Sanders TAB, Wessley S. Behavioural management of antipsychotic induced weight gain: a review. *Acta Psychiatrica Scandinavica*. 2003; **108**: 252–9.

Wirshing DA. Schizophrenia and obesity. *Journal of Clinical Psychiatry*. 2004; **65**(Suppl 18): 13–26.

Wirshing DA, Wirshing WC, Kysar L *et al.* Novel antipsychotics: comparison of weight gain liabilities. *Journal of Clinical Psychiatry*. 1999; **60**(6): 358–63.

World Health Organization (WHO). *Mental Health in Context*. Geneva: WHO; 2003.

World Health Organization (WHO). *Pocket Guide to the ICD-10 Classification of Mental and Behavioural Disorders*. Edinburgh: Churchill Livingstone; 2004.

CHAPTER 19

Working with men via the internet

Jim Pollard

On the face of it, the internet is a perfect medium for delivering services to men. However, success is not guaranteed.

The dramatic explosion of the first dot-com bubble five years ago demonstrates the importance of finding the right fit between the product, the way it is delivered online and the intended target. This is not a given. To use the internet effectively, health communicators need to understand how the internet is used in reality (not how the medium's 'cutting edge' technicians might want it to be used).

This chapter will look at why the internet can be an effective means of reaching men, how it can be done and introduces some of the concerns and issues that reaching men in this way raises.

It is worth clarifying the difference between the worldwide web and the internet as the terms are often wrongly used synonymously. The internet is the medium – the information superhighway, a network of computers – while the worldwide web is one of the products that can be delivered by this medium. Email is another example of a product delivered in this way.

Setting the scene

To demonstrate the way the internet may be used to deliver health information to men, consider the following two case studies.

CASE STUDY BT Work Fit

The BT Work Fit campaign, which the Men's Health Forum (MHF) helped design and deliver, was the UK's biggest workplace health programme and the world's largest online company lifestyle programme. Over a period of four months, nearly 4,400 BT employees lost 10 tonnes of weight between them, an average weight loss of 2.3 kg.

Specifically, 76% of the 5,714 Work Fit participants who entered data twice or more lost an average of 2.3 kg in weight. If the data is analysed for the 2,170 participants (75% male) who it is known were participating for two months or more, the mean weight change was a loss of 1.9 kg and mean waist circumference for this group fell by 1.8 cm.

The proportion of the group who fell into the normal weight category increased by almost 6%, the proportion which was overweight fell by 4% and the proportion which was obese fell by almost 1%. Unsurprisingly, the data also shows that the longer people were actively involved with Work Fit, the greater was their weight loss. This was especially marked after four weeks of participation.

The programme turned the fact that most of the BT staff involved sat at desks using computers for most of their working day to an advantage.

Participants were given pedometers and an information booklet but the programme itself was delivered online. Staff took part as individuals or as members of teams. More than 500 teams took part.

A dedicated intranet site included access to nurses signed up by the Men's Health Forum to act as lifestyle advisers, answer email questions and provide dietary and fitness advice and other health information. Individuals were sent weekly activity programmes and tips for help in lifestyle improvements, such as information on exercise, food and reducing cholesterol.

The success of the BT project has prompted interest from other public sector companies who want to mount similar programmes and the MHF has been in discussion with public health minister, Caroline Flint, about how the Department of Health can back the initiative.* This interest is entirely appropriate. BT launched the programme after it emerged that the company was losing one employee every two weeks to a heart-related illness. CBI (Confederation of British Industry) figures show they are not alone. Absence costs UK employers £12 billion a year, with 168 million working days lost in 2004.

Needless to say, the programme would have cost considerably more – thousands more – to deliver entirely with printed material. It would also have been far less easy for staff to participate.

CASE STUDY malehealth.co.uk

The MHF's malehealth.co.uk website aims to provide fast, free independent health information to men of all ages. Attracting some 65,000 unique visitors every month, it has won awards from the British Medical Association and Royal Society of Medicine.

Clearly, its market share remains limited but it has achieved this level of awareness simply through its online presence and word-of-mouth. There is no advertising budget and indeed the whole project is run on a shoestring without a single full-time member of staff. As a means of distributing information, there is no other medium that is so cost-effective.

Whether through its online surveys or reader feedback, the site also gives the MHF an invaluable direct communication channel with the man in the street.

These two case studies illustrate the importance of different online approaches for different health issues. In the case of diet, most people know what they should be doing,

*As of June 2007 Caroline Flint became Minister of State for Employment and Welfare Reform.

so simply providing raw information is not the main priority; rather it is about getting men to act on what they know. BT Work Fit was ideally suited to the task.

By contrast, malehealth recently added a section called The Tool-kit to its site. Including all the frequently asked questions about the penis, it is constantly consulted as an information resource. An online programme designed with the same end involving teams and personalised emails would not, I would contend, have been so popular with men.

Internet access in the UK

About two-thirds of UK adults use the internet. In October 2005, 64% of adults – and 72% of adult males – in Great Britain had used the internet in the previous three months (National Statistics Omnibus Survey, NSOS, 2005). There is, however, considerable variation by age, region and social class.

While 95% of adults aged 16–24 had used the internet in the previous three months, only 19% of over-65s had (NSOS, 2005). In 2003–4, the last year for which regional data was published, usage was at 64% of adults in London and the South East compared to 43% in the North East of England (NSOS, 2005).

In September 2005, 79% of those in social classes AB were internet users compared to 34% of those in social classes DE. However, this 'digital divide' is narrowing – in December 2003, barely 20% of those in classes DE were internet users. It is interesting to note that the 'digital divide' is already considerably narrower for mobile phones (91% to 77%), suggesting considerable potential for this medium for delivering health messages to men in text form (MORI, 2005).

In October 2005, the three main reasons for not using the internet were lack of interest in the medium (47%), lack of internet connection (44%) and lack of knowledge or confidence in the medium (35%). Cost, it is worth noting, was no longer a major concern (NSOS, 2005).

Most users (86%) access the internet from their own home but there are other significant outlets. These include workplace (43%), another person's house (33%), an educational establishment (16%), public library (10%) and internet 'cafe' (8%). (Figures add up to considerably more than 100 per cent as many users, of course, access the internet from more than one place.)

These statistics show that internet access is far from uniform and that the medium – for all its advantages – is considerably less effective at reaching older men, men in non-white-collar jobs and socially isolated men – exactly the groups that many health campaigns are desperate to target. This must be borne in mind in any health communications strategy.

The internet and health information

A considerable number of men are internet users. More men use the internet (72%) than read a newspaper (70%) (ONS, 2006). But are they using the internet to find health information?

A study carried out in writing this chapter, via the Men's Health Forum's health information website malehealth.co.uk, suggests that for many men, the internet is actually their first port of call for health information. Clearly, given that the survey

TABLE 19.1 Men's first port of call for health information.

Imagine you want some health information. What do you do FIRST?			
Look on the INTERNET	155	70.45%	
Go to the DOCTOR or hospital	23	10.45%	
Go to another HEALTH PROFESSIONAL – please state below	7	3.18%	
Go to a PHARMACIST	2	0.91%	
Go to a HEALTH FOOD STORE	0	0.00%	
Ask a FRIEND	2	0.91%	
Ask a FAMILY member	9	4.09%	
Look in a BOOK at home or buy a book	17	7.73%	
Look in a book at the LIBRARY	1	0.45%	
Other	4	1.82%	

If your first choice doesn't have the answer, what would you do next?			
Look on the INTERNET	43	20.00%	
Go to the DOCTOR or hospital	71	33.02%	
Go to another HEALTH PROFESSIONAL – please state below	12	5.58%	
Go to a PHARMACIST	11	5.12%	
Go to a HEALTH FOOD STORE	0	0.00%	
Ask a FRIEND	15	6.98%	
Ask a FAMILY member	13	6.05%	
Look in a BOOK at home or buy a book	28	13.02%	
Look in a book at the LIBRARY	16	7.44%	
Other	6	2.79%	

was carried out by a health website, there is a strong element of self-selection about the 265 participants but even with this caveat the findings are surprising. Some 70% of respondents said that the internet was the first place that they went to when looking for health information. A further 20% said it was the second (*see* Table 19.1). All told, nine out of 10 respondents saw the internet as their first or second port of call for health information.

Older respondents were marginally less likely to use the internet first but it was still by far the most popular choice.

Despite the size of the sample and the nature of its selection, it is hard to argue that these are not significant findings. Certainly they demonstrate that if men can be tempted to the internet, they are likely to use it to search for health information, and it could play a vital role in men's self-management of weight problems.

TABLE 19.2 Main reasons for using the internet for health information.

What would be your main reasons for using the internet for health information – tick the TWO most important reasons only.			
It's the quickest way	146	36.59%	▉
It's private	80	20.05%	▉
It's free	50	12.53%	▊
There's more information than you can get from a book or medical appointment.	60	15.04%	▊
Links on the internet make it easier to follow a question through.	59	14.79%	▊
Other reason	4	1.00%	|
I never use the internet for health information.	0	0.00%	

TABLE 19.3 Main problems when looking for health information on the internet.

What are the main PROBLEMS when looking for health information on the internet? Tick the TWO main problems only			
The information is not easy to understand	0	0.00%	
It's not easy to find the information you want	2	12.50%	▊
The information is not written for people like me	0	0.00%	
The information is not independent because the sites are trying to sell something or promote a viewpoint	3	18.75%	▊
The information is not free	0	0.00%	
You don't know if the information is accurate	6	37.50%	▉
You don't know if the information is up to date	4	25.00%	▉
Other reason	1	6.25%	▊

The main starting point for a health information search was an internet search engine: 48% used Google, 14% used another search engine. The second most likely starting point was a particular website: 18% chose malehealth.co.uk, 17% NHS Direct and 3% another website.

Those men who chose the internet for health information were invited to tick the two most important reasons for their choice: 37% said that it was the quickest way; 20% that it was private; and 15% that there was more information on the internet than you could get anywhere else (*see* Table 19.2).

Respondents were also asked to identify the two main problems with looking up health information on the internet. Some 28% cited uncertainty about the accuracy of the information and 23% cited uncertainty about whether the information was up to date. Younger users were particularly concerned about accuracy.

One in five (20%) said that there was a problem with the independence of some sites which were selling something or promoting a viewpoint while 16% said that it was not easy to find the information that you wanted (*see* Table 19.3).

The survey concluded by asking respondents whether they would use a website that had none of the problems identified above. Only two respondents said that they would not. The potential is clear.

The advantages of the internet

While the dangers of making gross generalisations around gender are clear, it could nevertheless be argued that the internet offers a tight fit with some aspects of the traditional male gender role. For the man who believes he needs to be strong, silent and reluctant to admit weakness, uncertainty or limitations in his knowledge, the internet has clear benefits.

The internet is quick

Given an up-to-date connection, the internet is as fast as the user's fingers. As lives are become increasingly busy, the internet has clear advantages for the delivery of health information and health services that need not be directly mediated by a health professional.

The internet is private

The internet can be consulted in total confidence. This cannot be said for traditional medical services, attending a weight loss group, or even buying a book or taking one out of the library.

The internet is free

While commercial business models are now appearing on the internet with increasing success, there are few in the fields of health and health information. In fact, the requirement to pay can sometimes be viewed as a warning sign about the nature of the site. Certainly, the quality health information sites remain free.

The internet makes an enormous quantity of information available

It is estimated that the worldwide web contains over 3,000 billion pages and is growing by 25,000 pages an hour (Naughton, 2006). The potential of this is mind-boggling. In the raw sense such quantity is clearly an advantage but the challenge of ordering and understanding this information requires information-handling skills that many users do not have. There is also a tension between quantity of information and speed which frustrated some in the MHF survey.

The internet offers hyperlinks

This advantage follows on from the previous one but does require a separate heading since the reading room at a medical library would also offer a lot of information but it would not be nearly so easy to navigate as that on the internet. Hyperlinks mean that a search can be developed and refined while it is in progress. This 'surfing' is one of the pleasures of the internet and is particularly important with medical or health queries where the lay user rarely has the knowledge to formulate an exact query – or even a general one – at the outset.

The internet can be up to date

Unlike a printed publication or even the very best-trained and best-intentioned health professional, the internet has the potential to be up to the minute. Given the right software and information, web pages can be updated instantly. That is, of course, one reason why the internet has revolutionised news coverage. As medical science advances, much patient information material becomes obsolete. This need not happen with internet-based material.

Providing internet-based health information: the challenges

Information is hard to find

The drawback with the wealth of information available is that it can be very difficult to find the nugget that you're hunting. Using even the simplest site requires certain skills. As the number of pages on the web grows so the search engine and navigational skills required of the user will grow too.

In January 2005, I wrote the following:

> *There are 250 million searches on Google everyday. Do a Google search on 'food' and you'll get 213,000,000 results. Refine that to 'diet' and you'll get 43,600,000. Opt for 'Atkins', the most recent in a long, long list of fad diets, and you'll still get over nine million.* (POLLARD, 2005)

By April 2006, these figures had snowballed to 1,730,000,000 (for 'food'), 262,000,000 (for 'diet' – a six-fold increase) and over 41 million for Atkins. The advice the article went on to give about how to use the internet effectively becomes more important by the day.

This point was also made by respondents to the MHF research. 'There's almost *too* much information,' wrote one. 'Sometimes there's more than you need,' wrote another. 'Sometimes it can take too long to get an answer to the question and sometimes the language is difficult to understand,' wrote a third, a comment which raises another concern.

Information is inappropriate

When giving talks about health on the internet I often joke that if you enter any health condition, however trivial, into an internet search engine you will find, within a couple of clicks, someone who has died from it. Exaggeration for comic effect it may be, but it is not far wrong. The dangers here are obvious.

As one respondent to the MHF survey put it:

> *Often when looking for health related issues, you come across very serious sites. You find several sites dedicated to people who died from the condition greater than you can possibly [expect and you] become more worried than if you had direct access to a specialist.*

Whereas a library classifies information to some extent on the basis of who it is written for, this is not the case on the internet where a search will pull up information designed for the most expert of health professionals alongside information for five-year-olds.

Clearly, the information needs of someone who is overweight will be different from those of someone who has just been diagnosed with an eating disorder or weight-related health problem, the needs of someone who wants basic nutritional information different from those of someone with an allergy, the needs of a parent worried about a child different from those of a health professional.

On the internet, the onus to a considerable extent is on the recipient of the information rather than its provider to ensure, by judicious searching and intelligent site-selection, that the information is at the appropriate level for them at that particular time. Again, this requires some skill.

The appropriateness or otherwise of information was a recurring comment in the MHF research. 'Information can prove either (a) too technical or (b) dumbed down too much,' said one respondent. 'You cannot describe in the right detail or find the answer to your query as well as you could if it were face to face with a professional,' said another. A third raised an interesting point about the provision of written information in general: 'The real information is usually not available – one can get high level stuff but detailed technical info is often not made available. Is this due to the risk of being sued?'

Finally, in the MHF research, users were asked what they liked most about malehealth.co.uk. The most popular answer was that it was 'written by men for men'. The anecdotal evidence is that relatively few health websites know how to talk to or write for men.

Information is of variable quality
The accuracy of information was the single major concern in the MHF survey.

Information is out of date
This was the second biggest concern.

Providing internet-based health information: towards solutions
All of the concerns mentioned in the previous section can be addressed to some degree. Knowing that there is one site that you can go to which will give you good quality, appropriate, up-to-date information, and which can, if it hasn't the answer itself, link you to another site which has, would eliminate nearly all of them. Sites such as NHS Direct, malehealth.co.uk and the health strand of the BBC website aspire to this to varying extents. Unfortunately, not everyone looking for health information on the net alights on these sites.

Kite-marking
Surfers need a sign of quality similar to the British Standards kite-mark or the Soil Association's stamp on organic food. The kite-marking of sites or sections of sites by a respected body could have a major impact.

Currently the not-for-profit Health of the Net (HON) Foundation have a code under which accredited sites must be transparent about their funding, sponsorship and editorial policies and offer clearly dated, attributed and justifiable information. The code does not monitor the information itself, which could be seen as a limitation. Moreover, the HON Code is not a particularly well-known brand anyway.

Kite-marking by a better-known, well-respected body such as, in the UK, the NHS, would have far greater impact. At the time of writing, the future of NHS Direct, the NHS's telephone and online arm, was under discussion. It is arguably not core to the NHS's remit or part of its expertise to run a website. It could, however, improve the quality of health information online at a stroke by offering kite-marks to other sites meeting recognised quality standards. A similar point could be made about the BBC.

This sort of quality control would help reduce the current reliance on search engines. This reliance should decline anyway as the internet develops: brands will become better known, individuals will find their own trusted sites, search skills will improve.

Portals

The channelling of users through portals could also make a big difference. The BT Work Fit programme mentioned above was delivered through the firm's intranet. Why shouldn't every firm's intranet have links to recognised quality sites? Similarly, the home pages that users in educational establishments, libraries, internet cafes and other non-domestic environments encounter when logging on could offer similar links.

Improving search techniques

The challenge, given the current reliance on search engines, is to ensure that quality sites appear as high up search results lists as possible. In the long term, this is best done by educating users in effective searching – the strategy that the MHF has adopted in its men's health manuals published in tandem with Haynes. Ideally, all types of home page – those mentioned above and those of internet service providers – should include basic search tips.

The fatal flaw of search engines

In the short-term, webmasters also need to ensure that their sites are registered with search engines (and that each engine's advice on doing this is followed). The exact way that search engines rank is deliberately shrouded in mystery or, if you prefer, is a commercial confidence. Rather than try to solve the insoluble riddle, health communicators need to encourage the scepticism evident in this respondent to the MHF research: 'You don't know if you are missing out on some better info – it all seems a bit random – and I am suspicious of sponsored sites coming up first.'

The key point to note is that when it comes to finding quality sites, internet search engines are fatally flawed. Search engines add to their databases by going to the pages they already know about and following the links from them. Generally speaking, the more links a site has, the higher the ranking in search results. The idea is that the number of links reflects the popularity and so the usefulness of that site.

This sounds fine in theory but may simply mean that the website has included as many links as possible regardless of the quality or relevance. Many commercial sites have long lists of so-called 'links'. Malehealth.co.uk is inundated with proposed link 'exchanges', many from unsuitable sites. The fact is that if it accepted these offers, the site would probably feature higher on web searches.

Moreover, search engines also tend to prioritise sites which are selling something rather than those offering merely information – a big problem with a controversial subject like diet and weight where there's money to be made – and another way in which sites like malehealth.co.uk suffer.

Inequality of access

As the figures cited under 'Internet access in the UK' above demonstrate, there is a clear 'digital divide' with older, working-class men more likely to be excluded.

Figures from the USA suggest that two other excluded groups may be disabled men and black and minority ethnic men. Under disability discrimination legislation, service providers are obliged to make their websites accessible. This is laudable so long as disabled users are online in the first place. US figures from 2000 – admittedly rather old now – suggest that disabled people are half as likely to have a computer as non-disabled people and half as likely to have internet access (Bruyere, 2000 *see* reference notes at end of chapter).

A report from the USA published in September 2005 found that black people – to use the language of the report – are much less likely to have internet access at home than are white people (40.5% compared to 67.3%) (Fairlie, 2005).

As has already been noted, those excluded by the 'digital divide' are often those groups of men that health communicators would most like to target. Internet access, it could be argued, should be regarded as a health need.

There is, however, one group that health communicators are keen to target who can be found in abundance on the internet: younger men. This suggests that the internet could be a very effective health improvement tool for the future. The challenge is that the internet is a flexible medium which can be used in many ways. Health messages on websites will not reach online gamers or chat-room visitors. Health communicators need to understand exactly how young men are using the internet to reach them effectively.

Internet 'addiction'

The internet may be good for delivering health information but it is equally true that excessive use of the medium itself can become unhealthy. It has been estimated that 6–10% of US internet users are 'addicted' to the medium (Kershaw, 2005a *see* note on p 197). Now it is very easy to become absorbed by the niceties of this debate. Are heavy users really 'addicted' in the strict sense of the term? Are they 'addicted' to the internet itself or to that which it makes more readily available such as pornography, gambling or the opportunity to work all day every day. For men's health communicators this misses the main point.

The tight fit between the internet and some aspects of the traditional male gender role has already been mentioned. This advantage can spill over into a disadvantage when taken to extremes. Solo surfing is, at best, a highly mediated form of social interaction and unlikely to develop the social skills that are such an important part of mental well-being.

Of course, this concern may be overstated. The danger of addiction is frequently the meat of a moral panic. A US report from summer 2005 suggested that while 51%

of US teenagers were online everyday (compared to 42% in 2000), this did not appear to have led to a 'withering of social skills' (Kershaw, 2005). However, the potential risk should not be ignored by health communicators.

Social marketing

The internet can be a key tool in social marketing. A social marketing approach replaces a traditional professional-led approach to selling a health message with one that is more customer-focused and exchange-based.

It's an adult-to-adult discourse. Rather than saying, 'Exercise is good for you', social marketing is a little more subtle, saying, to cite one example, that walking is a good idea because it doubles as a form of transport or can be used to exercise pets or is a way to avoid parking tickets, etc. (French, 2005).

Essentially success is measured not by the number of messages –posters displayed, booklets printed, press mentions, etc. – but by changes in behaviour.

Conclusions

The internet has enormous potential, particularly in the developing social marketing context, for delivering health messages to men. It is quick, private and free. It can allow the skilled user to search an enormous amount of information. It can be right up to date and offers the facility for personal communication though email and online chat.

However, at the time of writing, internet-based formation is often difficult to find. This reflects a lack of skills on the part of many users and the unhelpful way in which commercial search engines operate. As a result the information that is found is often inappropriate. Users are also concerned that information is of variable quality and may be out of date.

Kite-marking, dedicated portals and closer working with ISPs (internet service providers) can meet some of these challenges. In the longer term, improved search-engine skills – and perhaps even improved search engines – will enable more effective searching. However, structural problems around inequality of access mean that at present the internet can only ever be part of a health communications strategy.

Health communicators must recognise the diversity of internet skills and access and plan their strategies accordingly. The latest high-tech online wizardry is not a lot of use if only a small minority of relatively well-off – and therefore relatively healthy – men are able to access it.

References

Bruyere S, Ruiz-Quintanillia SA, Bonney, M. *Implications of the information technology revolution for people with disabilities*. Cornell University Employment and Disability Institute Collection; 2000 http://digitalcommons.ilr.cornell.edu/edicollect/185.

Fairlie RW. Are we really a nation online? Ethnic and racial disparities in access to technology and their consequences. Report, Leadership Conference on Civil Rights Education Fund; 20 September 2005.

French J. Social marketing. *Men's Health Forum magazine*. March 2005; 9.

Kershaw S. Hooked on the web. *New York Times*. 1 December 2005.

MORI. MORI Technology Tracker. December 2005. See www.mori.com/technology/trackerdata.shtml.

National Statistics Omnibus Survey (NSOS). *Adults Who Have Ever Used the Internet by Sex/Age (Great Britain)*. London: Office for National Statistics; 2005.

Naughton J. The age of permanent net revolution. *Observer*. 5 March 2006.

Office for National Statistics (ONS). *Social Trends*. 2006; March: 36.

Pollard J. Weight on the web. In: Banks I (ed) *The HGV Manual*. Yeovil: Haynes; 2005.

CHAPTER 20

Innovation in obesity services for men

Jane DeVille-Almond

Learning and innovation go hand in hand. The arrogance of success is to think that what you did yesterday will be sufficient for tomorrow. (WILLIAM POLLARD, CHAIRMAN OF THE SERVICEMASTER COMPANY, USA)

With around 14,000 male deaths each year directly attributed to obesity in England today, and 65% of men considered overweight or obese, it is fair to say that we have a serious public health issue. The 2004 White Paper *Choosing Health: making healthy choices easier* (Department of Health, 2004) actively encouraged primary care teams to play an increasing role in the government's public health agenda. The White Paper states that traditional methods of improving health are becoming outdated and *new approaches and new action* are needed to secure progress. This means developing innovative practice, working within communities and with a range of agencies outside the NHS to have a much greater public health focus.

As far as obesity is concerned it is perplexing that few men seem to access the services provided in primary care. Few healthcare professionals seem to recognise the importance of catering for the differences between men and women in providing services. The result is that men under 50 access primary care services around half as frequently as women in the same age range. There are reasons why men hate going to their GP's surgery. These include: unhelpful opening hours, a female-dominated environment, difficulty in getting appointments, and the macho embarrassment of actually admitting they have a problem.

In a recent poll I carried out with over 100 truckers, only 13% said they would consider going to the GP for help with their weight. This can be partly attributed to the fact that many men do not see obesity as a problem, so there has been very little demand for 'male-friendly' support. This was further borne out in the truckers poll, where only 10 of the men put themselves in the obese bracket despite 78% with a BMI over 30 or waist measurements over 40 inches.

With so much clinical evidence that men suffering from weight problems are more likely to develop a range of health problems which include high blood pressure, type 2 diabetes, cardiovascular disease, some cancers, osteoarthritis, and respiratory problems, it is time to be innovative in finding ways to engage with men.

So where can we start? First, we should acknowledge our lack of services for men and obesity and address this accordingly. Let's face it, if you're a man who is overweight, has a tendency to drink more than Billy the Fish, smoke like Thomas the Tank Engine, and visit the gym only because they have a happy hour on a Friday night, you are hardly likely to turn up at the 'well-man's clinic', are you?

I decided, as a practice nurse, that rather than spending time getting men into the surgery, I should join them in their own environment, tackling health problems on their home turf. I had begun to realise that men are not going to come looking for something they don't even know they want. Rather, I needed to sell them the dream by attempting to make weight management services accessible, fun and something men want to sign up to.

> *When you innovate, you've got to be prepared for everyone telling you you're nuts.* (LARRY ELLISON, THE MULTI-BILLIONAIRE FOUNDER OF ORACLE)

Pub clinics

In July 1997 I held my first pub surgery at the Moxley Arms, situated in the main high street of Moxley, a socially deprived area in the West Midlands. The aim of the surgery was to establish if men would attend a service if it was offered in their own environment. I had chosen this particular venue as I had heard that the landlord of the pub had attempted to run a Weight Watchers clinic for men during lunch time. Having been in to meet the landlord, we decided to run surgeries during the lunch time and early evening over a period of three days.

During this period we saw over 100 men and found that 72% had one or more long-term undetected health risk. These included body mass indexes over 35, alcohol intakes greater than 150 units per week, diastolic blood pressures over 110, smoking more than 30 cigarettes a day, high cholesterol and blood sugar levels, early and more established symptoms of prostate problems and some worrying drug problems and signs of depression.

The response from the men was amazing. We had expected the men to be irritated that we were infringing on their social drinking time but most were delighted that this service was being offered in such a male-friendly environment.

To ensure that everyone was participating I had all the bar staff wear T-shirts with fun health logos such as, 'If you're a bloke who likes ball sports, start by playing with your own', then three key messages on the back describing how a man should look out for testicular cancer. Other T-shirts covered topics such as erectile dysfunction, prostate awareness and safe sex. These T-shirts not only raised health issues but gave the men permission to discuss health issues without losing their macho image.

Following the success of the surgeries at the Moxley Arms, we took the concept to other pubs in the area with similar results. The old myth that men are not interested in their health was soon dispelled when whole groups of men stood around the bar happily showing each other their record cards and discussing their testicles, prostate and body mass index along with the last night's football game.

As a follow-up we invited 50 men with some of the most severe health risks back to the Moxley Arms six months later to chat about the lifestyle changes they might have been able to make, even very small ones. Thirty-eight turned up for this session, many simply because they still drank in the pub, and we found that several had made significant lifestyle changes.

These included weight losses of 4 stone and 2 stone and several smaller losses. One man had begun seeing a drug councillor, and a newly discovered diabetic had commenced treatment. Smaller changes included starting hypertensive treatment and making small changes in drinking habits, such as substituting some pints of beer with shandy, thus lowering their overall alcohol intake.

Many Health Action Zones and primary care trusts began taking the pub clinics concept forward as part of a strategy to improve men's health so I decided to start looking at other areas where male-friendly clinics might work.

Harley-Davidson showroom bikers and health

Several reports in the national press indicated that there had been a substantial increase in middle-aged male bikers driving up the death and injury rate among bikers. The image of a middle-aged man seeking thrills before old age sets in came to mind. This man would have an increase in spare cash, an expanding midriff and high blood pressure and would probably not understand the implications poor health may have on his ability to handle such a powerful machine.

I decided to hold a 'pit stop' for men at the Harley-Davidson showroom in Chapel Ash, offering health MOTs during an open weekend held once every three months. I saw over 50 men during the two days with many more wishing to be seen.

A staggering 65% failed their MOT, with 55% having a body mass index over 28, 17% over 35, and 5.7% over 40. Some 25 per cent presented with a diastolic blood pressure reading over 95. Over 80% were unsure where their prostate was, or understood the signs and symptoms of prostate problems, and over 90% were unsure about signs and symptoms of bowel cancer. Over 20% did not even know the name or address of their GP.

Many of the men I saw made it clear that the reason they did nothing about their weight and health was that they did not want to go to their GP for help. A weight management service was subsequently set up in the back of the bike shop which had an open-access approach. Although this seemed a great way to run a service it soon became apparent there were pitfalls. Many of the men trying to lose weight would come on different days and times so it was obvious that such a service could not be cost-effective. I decided to just leave a set of scales in the back of the bike shop on a regular basis and let the men get on with it themselves. The results were good with many of the bikers losing weight and encouraging each other to go to the gym. Six of the Harley-Davidson successes subsequently appeared on a BBC2 documentary.

Perhaps we should take a leaf from India where there are really funky scales at all the train stations, almost encouraging people to hop on and find their weight. I believe that if we had something similar in the back of bike shops and other venues men would climb on and hear the truth about their expanding midriffs.

Goodwood Festival of Speed

Following the success of the Harley-Davidson clinic, along with some other nurses I held a men's health surgery at the Goodwood Festival of Speed, specifically targeting male obesity. During the festival weekend there were well over 200,000 people in attendance, the majority being men. The initial concern among the nurses was that it would be difficult to get men into our men's health surgery van so I made the decision simply to go up to fat men with an opening line of, 'You're a bit fat. Do you want to come with me to see the nurse?' Rather than the men being offended, most simply laughed and followed me to the van.

Before long we had a queue of men coming in to be seen and discuss health problems. Over 500 were seen during the two days of the festival. It was obvious to us that obesity was a major concern, along with its long-term health implications. But where could men like these go to get help?

Our presence at Goodwood was all about awareness-raising as we had no possibility to follow up these men as patients. What was interesting was to hear how many of the obese men had not realised the impact that obesity had on their health. We picked up 18 men with severe raised blood sugars, indicating type 2 diabetes, along with many other previously undetected health risk problems.

GI's barber-shop health clinic

In my attempt to think about new places where I could meet men on their terms, I stumbled across what I consider to be the perfect venue: the barber's shop. It has a captive male audience and how many men *don't* go and get their hair cut at some time?

> Peter had just had his hair trimmed and decides to come through to the surgery in the back of the barber's shop for his MOT and a chat about his weight. He doesn't know he's going to discuss his weight yet, but the prospect of having his cholesterol checked free of charge entices him without question. Surprisingly, when Peter gets into the back of the shop he has his own set of health questions that he has been storing up for years.

The barber's shop (GI's) offered a drop-in service once a week for any man wishing to have a full health check, which included height, weight, BMI, waist measurements, blood pressure, peak flow, cholesterol and blood sugar reading, smoking and drinking habits, family history and a discussion around prostate, testicular and bowel awareness. There was also an opportunity to discuss health issues such as sexual health, erectile dysfunction and depression.

Almost 50 men were seen in the first two clinics, and 764 men were seen in the first year. All consultation records were sent to the man's GP, unless otherwise requested, and each patient has his own set of records to keep. Any patient found to have a BMI over 28 was offered membership of GI's 'big boy' clinic which he could attend each time he visited the barber's shop to be weighed and discuss eating habits, exercise and lifestyle changes. Those men requiring further medical interventions to help them reduce weight were advised to see their GP but could continue being monitored at the barber-shop surgery.

The surgery was open to anyone, not just shop customers. It was a free service and was initially sponsored by educational grants provided by several drug companies. I advertised it with posters in the window and shop, flyers in the barber's and on the local radio stations.

We don't give out diet sheets; we just provide simple advice to suit the lifestyle of each client. I encourage each man to set himself an achievable target, even if it is as simple as not going up in weight or sticking to the same clothes size.

The cost of such a clinic is minimal. Apart from the cost of the person running it, it only needs the kind of standard equipment any surgery will have, including a set of accurate scales that measure up to 30 stone, a sphygmomanometer, record cards, a peak-flow meter and appropriate leaflets.

CASE STUDY

John is 33 years old. Two years ago he had to stop football due to a knee injury. This is a common problem among men. Since he has given up sport, at 5 foot 11 inches (181 cm) he has gained 15 kg, going from 82 kg (12 stone 9 lb), which gave him a body mass index of 25, to 95 kg (15 stone), a BMI of 29. His waist measurement was 106 cm and he had confessed to going up two trouser sizes in the last few years.

Following his health check in the barber's I discovered he had a blood pressure of 154/ 102. I advised him to see his GP but he said he did not feel comfortable going to the surgery. I stressed the importance of having his BP re-checked by his doctor but in the mean time suggested he came every week for a weigh-in and BP check at the barber's.

Giving him some simple advice, and making a plan together, John decided where his problems lay. He had parted from his wife the previous year, worked in a job that entailed a great deal of entertaining and often spent hours driving where he regularly snacked. In the first month John's weight had come down 3 kg, bringing his BMI down to 28 and more importantly his BP down to 148/98. His waist measurement had also come down 1 cm to 105 cm. John was delighted, and although his BP remained a little high, he could clearly see the effect the weight loss had on his BP. He is going to continue to come and visit me on a regular basis and promises that he will visit his GP the following month if his blood pressure remains high.

As this case study indicates, high-tech solutions are seldom needed to support a man in making health improvements but simply support and time and perhaps an innovative place to deliver the service.

I can already hear the sighs of readers when I mention the word 'time', for this is often the key reason for not running weight management clinics. But consider the amount of time we spend on other services such as diabetes, hypertension, hypercholesterolaemia, post MI (myocardial infarction), and all the other chronic disorders patients develop often due to or exacerbated by being overweight or obese.

My biggest frustration with GI's barber-shop clinic was trying to integrate it within the local primary care setting and getting local practice nurses to take turns in running the clinic. There is still the philosophy among many GPs and nurses that they only get paid to deal with their own patients and therefore have no interest in the bigger public health picture.

Following a radio show in Ireland I was contacted by Bernard Twomey, a community health service worker in Cork, who wanted help setting up a similar service at a local barber's in Cork town centre – a shop called Baldie Barbers. This proved to be a roaring success. The point about innovation is that good ideas spread.

By now I had realised that by focusing on particular venues for men it made it easier to develop the service to suit the clientele. It helped me understand their habits and lifestyles and I could adapt my information to suit their needs. A perfect example of this can be seen with the truck drivers' surgery.

Lymm Truck Stop surgery

In an event I carried out at Lymm Truck Stop, near Manchester, in 2005 it became clear that many men do not have a clear idea what is meant by obesity. At the truck stop I saw 102 men between the ages of 24 and 65. These were the questions the men were asked before undergoing a health check (height, weight, blood pressure, waist measurement, non-fasting blood sugar and total cholesterol test):

- What is your waist measurement?
- Do you define yourself as thin, just right, overweight or obese?
- Do you worry about your weight?
- Have you ever been to your doctor to lose weight?
- Have you ever used a commercial organisation to lose weight?
- Have you ever considered taking medication to lose weight?

Asked how they defined their own weight, only 10% selected the obese category, despite 58% of the men actually falling into this category. More worrying was the fact that all the men who took part failed to guess their waist measurement, under-estimating what it actually was: 78% had waist measurements of 40 inches or above. The problem is that if men do not see themselves as falling into a risk group then how are we going to get them to consider doing something about it in the first place?

It was clear to me that for most drivers their lifestyle contributed to their obesity problem. Many left home in the middle of the night, eating at truck stops where they often ate unhealthy options and had little opportunity to exercise. Knowing this enabled me to give out information that would fit in with their lifestyle. I attempted to use a texting service with some of the truckers to see if I could encourage them to lose weight via a phone message and weighing them a few months later.

This proved successful with one of the drivers losing 10 lb in two weeks. He continued to lose weight and said, 'It was great. I didn't really change much but the regular reminders via text kept me focused'. I think that we should develop new ways of keeping in touch with our male patients, such as mobile phones, to encourage them to manage their weight, and this has special relevance to men on the move.

The future

In this chapter I have described the benefits of taking men's health services into men's own environments. To take men's health forward it is important that we start working outside the box, making men's health services not only more accessible but also a good experience for men. We need PCTs to show real commitment to improving men's health services. Health professionals should no longer be sitting on the fence but thinking up innovative ways of engaging with their male population.

> *If you're not failing every now and again, it's a sign you're not doing anything very innovative.* (WOODY ALLEN, ACTOR AND FILM PRODUCER)

Reference

Department of Health. *Choosing Health: making healthy choices easier*. White Paper. London: HMSO; 2004.

CHAPTER 21

The Australian experience

Garry Egger

Australia's reputation as a sporting nation over the years has led to a self-image of Australian men as being active, lean and healthy. But while this may have been the case in the 1950s, the new millennium version is far from that (*see* Table 21.1). Over two-thirds (67%) of Australian men over 18 years of age were classified as overweight or obese in 2000 and this is increasing by around 1% per year. In over 35-year-olds the prevalence rises to around 75%, and up to one in three men in this age category either have type 2 diabetes (10%) or the pre-diabetes form (25%), which indicates they are likely to become fully diabetic within a decade or so (Dunstan *et al.*, 2001). Australian men also die, on average, seven years earlier than Australian women (AIHW, 2004). Their death rates are higher for the first 14 major causes of disease (except breast cancer), and they suffer more from disability. In the indigenous population all these effects are exacerbated, with the life expectancy of indigenous men being some 20 years less than that of non-indigenous men (AIHW, 2004).

Given this litany of (mainly preventable) problems, one might expect to see men flocking to enhance their health through the most obvious initiatives such as readily available commercial weight loss programmes. Yet, while these are flooded by anxious women, many of whom are not seriously overweight but who regard themselves as

TABLE 21.1 Age-specific prevalence (%) of overweight by BMI and waist circumference, Australia 2000 (Dunstan *et al.*, 2001).

	Age (years)						
	25–34	35–44	45–54	55–64	65–74	75+	Total
BMI*							
Males	60.5	64.2	72.4	74.0	73.1	63.8	67.4
Females	35.1	44.5	58.1	67.6	68.9	52.2	52.0
Waist****							
Males	40.1	51.3	58.3	66.6	71.2	64.8	55.2
Females	36.6	46.9	59.1	72.7	79.7	67.5	56.5

*BMI > 25 kg/m²
** Waist circumference: males > 94 cm, females > 80 cm.

such, they are almost totally devoid of corpulent males, many of whom are genuinely overweight and at-risk, but who do not see themselves as such. The same applies to many other prophylactic health programmes that have been offered over the years.

It was in this environment that the GutBusters 'Waist Loss' program for men was initiated within Australia's largest steel company (BHP) in 1990 (Egger *et al.*, 1996; Egger *et al.*, 2000) Asked by the corporation to find the way to a man's heart (and liver and kidneys and other potentially ailing organs) a team was put together to scratch the male psyche for an explanation of this apparently irrational behaviour. Our findings, although only subjective, suggested a number of unique characteristics of men that needed to be considered in any attempt to 'sell' health. These have been discussed in detail elsewhere (Aoun *et al.*, 2002; Egger, 2000; Egger and Mowbray, 1993). However, of particular relevance here was the classification of men into four distinct groups in relation to weight control.

Male groups

The following groups were proposed from the findings of focus group research with predominantly blue-collar Australian males aged 30–55.

Weight cyclers are those men who have put on (fat) weight – often after getting married – but who claim to be able to shed this reasonably easily, and who seem to do so regularly. Most have gained and lost fat several times over the years (usually around the stomach) and hence are 'weight cyclers'. When they decide to lose, 'cyclers' do so by changing food habits (mostly nutritionally incorrectly), by not eating breakfast and/or cutting back on lunch, by temporarily cutting out alcohol, or, much less commonly, by a planned increase in exercise. 'Cyclers' appear to be the majority of overweight men. They are predominantly 'android' shaped and correspond to Bouchard's (1991) type II obesity.

Perennials make up a second, apparently smaller group for whom weight loss is more difficult. 'Perennials' have generally been overweight for longer and either have family who are overweight, or are of mesomorphic build and thus regard themselves (sometimes incorrectly) as perennially overweight. 'Perennials' are often more ovoid in shape and correspond more to Bouchard's type I form of obesity. They are perpetually trying to lose fat and are able to do so (with much effort and denial) to a point at which weight loss appears to plateau and further effort seems to be of little avail. Understandably, there appears to be anxiety, frustration, and even pent-up anger among 'perennials' about their inability to permanently lose weight.

Ostriches form a third group who openly accept that they are overweight but – at least outwardly – want to forget about it. This group appears small compared to the above two, and seems to consist of both 'cyclers' and 'perennials' who have developed defences for their inability, unwillingness or apparent lack of concern about losing weight. There seems to be two apparent sub-groups: *pseudo-ostriches* use defensive forms of denial, such as humour, abuse, argument or bravado, to hide what seems to be a genuine anxiety; and *real ostriches* seem genuinely not to care. From our experience in Australia, it appears the latter are a somewhat rare species. However, they should

TABLE 21.2 Identified fat typologies and relevant factors associated with fat groupings (from Egger and Mowbray, 1993).

	'Cyclers'	'Perennials'	'Ostriches'	'Jack Spratts'
Apparent group size	Largest	Small	Small	Smallest
Onset of overweight	Late	Early	Late/early	Never
Main body shape	Android	Ovoid	Android/ovoid	Ectomorph
Weight change	Regular	Irregular	Rare	Never
Attitude to weight loss	Positive	Frustrated	Negative	–
Motivation to lose	Feel better	Fit clothes	Health (if any)	Nil
Ease of losing weight	Easiest	Hardest	Hard	–
Coping mechanisms	Humour	Resignation	Denial	Boast

not be confused with men who are just pre-contemplators, on the 'transtheoretical' model of Prochaska *et al.* (1994).

Jack Spratts make up a fourth group who seem unable to get fat. These have been called the 'whippets of the workforce' and are spoken about in almost mythological terms because of the large amounts they are known to eat and drink without putting on weight. Although 'Jack Spratts' make up only a tiny proportion of middle-aged men, most men appear to know or have known one. Their behaviour is used by some to rationalise their own behaviour and to justify the disbelief, particularly by some 'ostriches', of energy balance in weight control.

A summary of the main parameters identified as being associated with each group is shown in Table 21.2.

The development of GutBusters

As a result of these findings in 1990, it was decided that, in line with the corporate brief, the best way to involve men was to provide assistance in reducing a risk that is obvious, i.e. abdominal obesity. While male stoicism (developed possibly from the Neanderthal fear of losing all from a display of weakness) could hide all pathologies of the inner organs to the outside observer, something as obvious as an abdominal protrusion and the discomfort, heavy breathing and sexual amorphousness coming from this could not. An uncoordinated attack on this (using 'boasting' and denial) had been attempted early in the obesity epidemic by men proudly flashing their added baggage (*see* Figure 21.1). However this was short-lived, as the veracity of the epidemic made such a body shape common place, rather than just the privilege of the powerful or wealthy, as it has been throughout evolution.

Men at the BHP Company responded by attending, in numbers, a six-week GutBuster program established to help them rid themselves of their 'patio over the playground'. In the meantime other offerings for men in heart health, nutrition, exercise, quitting smoking and a myriad of other male-based initiatives were being wound up due to lack of patronage. As a result, the State Health Department, who were partner clients in the GutBuster program, proceeded to expand, and ultimately

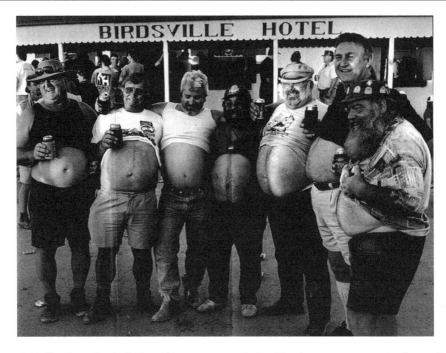

Figure 21.1 The Australian belly 'boast': now an outmoded activity due to excess supply of a previously rare commodity.

smother the programme with bureaucracy. At this stage it was decided that to save the project it would need to be developed commercially. As none of the original developers were business orientated, the programme was purchased (for cost) by Weight Watchers (Australia). During the subsequent eight years during which the programme was run, the net returns were never greater than 2–3% of that received from women. It was decided that this was not profitable enough for a commercial organisation and hence the programme was closed, with no rights returned to the original developers to use the highly popular name, or any materials developed for the programme. The lessons learnt from this, although not evidence-based, were extensive and included many that would not be disclosed by a commercial organisation to protect competitive advantage. Some of these are listed below.

Lessons learnt from the GutBusters program

The biggest problem with men is getting them to admit they have a problem

The fact that there are few (almost no) commercial weight loss programmes specifically targeting men would seem illogical, given the extent of the problem (see Table 21.1) and the size [sic] of the market. The reason, however, is mainly economic. No commercial programme has been able to attract men in large enough numbers to make a stand-alone men's weight loss programme economically viable. Industry and health research suggests that men have difficulty admitting they have a problem with their weight, and therefore do not seek help. Because of the costs resulting from obesity, it should be a priority of public health authorities to understand, and attempt to change this.

Time and repetition is required for men to make a decision

Because many men are typically in the 'pre-contemplative' stage of change (Prochaska *et al.*, 1994) with relation to health issues, they require time and continuous repetition of a message before they are prepared to commit to action. Market research carried out with GutBusters found that adverts for a weight loss programme can be carried around in a man's wallet for 6–9 months before a decision is made to act. Even then, this is only after repeated advertising. Given the ease of attracting females to a weight loss programme (albeit greater difficulty treating the problem), it is understandable that commercial weight loss organisations find the male market economically unviable.

The government health sector finds men's health too hard

The alternative to commercially-based initiatives for men is those undertaken by the government sector health services. The rationale for this is obvious with the huge existing and potential health costs that could be saved by successful prevention of obesity-related disease. Type 2 diabetes alone, for example, has been shown to cost around $US 15,000 per patient in the final year of life with annually escalating costs to this level (Brown *et al.*, 2001). Government sector health services, however, are not structured for the large resources (and patience) required to attract men, and hence most attempts to do this to date have been unsuccessful.

Social proof appears to be important for men

As most marketers are aware, social proof is a key factor of influence in behaviour change. Once people see others performing a behaviour, this provides legitimacy for that behaviour, even to the extent of socially destructive activities such as drug use and suicide (Cialdini, 1994). Perhaps because of the irrational stoicism displayed by men as discussed above, social proof would appear to be of even more relevance to men than to women. To provide visible social proof requires even more resources, exacerbating the problems discussed above.

Appropriate service provision is unclear

All of the above factors make the provision of an appropriate men's weight loss programme problematic. Because they are reluctant to openly declare a problem, men are less likely than women to attend group sessions. A lack of male networking with ageing, compared to that of women, is an added disadvantage in this respect. Because they are often time poor, as a result of occupational ambition, self-study materials also do not seem to be widely accepted as an alternative. Men typically also visit doctors and other health professionals less frequently than women, and hence the opportunity for personal instruction is reduced. It remains to test combinations of these approaches and new initiatives like the internet, video streaming, podcasting and other approaches to see if these difficulties can be overcome.

Men's health issues have little attraction for the media

Obesity in women, children, dogs and cats has been a hot topic for the mass media and public relations (although there are signs that the public is now wearying of this). There is much less interest from the media, however, when it comes to men. The reasons for this are unclear, but personal experience and ongoing feedback from media representatives suggests that it is because men are not seen as 'victims' to the same degree as other target groups. As men have control over many aspects of life, including politics in most western countries, it is suggested that if they really wanted to do something about men's health they would do it. For this reason, there is also little emotional attachment to the welfare of men, as there is with women (who are often mothers), and children. This is a problem that needs to be faced in bringing the plight of male obesity to the public attention.

Once a problem is admitted, the outcome is relatively easy

Weight loss for men, compared to women, is comparatively easy – once they decide to do it! There are physiological, sociological and psychological reasons for this. Physiologically, male fat stores are typically more centrally located and, due to differences in male–female hormones, are more responsive to energy imbalances than female stores. Typical female-pattern gynoid stores are more resistant to fat loss, probably to guarantee survival of the species through pregnancy. Sociologically, men do not come under the same pressure as women to conform to an unrealistic body image (a pressure brought on as much by other women – viz. women's magazines – as men). Psychological issues, such as depression and reduced self-esteem, then occur as a result of these pressures causing vicious cycles in weight loss (Swinburn and Egger, 2004), which seem less potent in men.

Men respond to a 'critical period' in their lives

Marketers profiling overweight men would typically classify them as mostly in the 'pre-contemplative' stage of readiness to change. This may be due to a genuine ignorance or denial of the problem and their own level of severity, to the inability to want to be seen seeking help for such a problem, or to a genuine lack of concern about the issue. A common finding is that middle-aged men do not have particular role models on which behaviour change promotions can be based. They are inhibited by time and family constraints and they are less concerned about ailments where there is a lack of specific obvious symptoms. All this extends the lag time for men in moving between pre-contemplation or contemplation stages to the decision and action stages of readiness to change their behaviour. On the other hand, the lag time is considerably shortened by personal events, such as the sudden death or illness of a family member, friend or acquaintance, scare by a doctor or clinician, or awakening to the risks of reaching a particular age.

Humour is a good mechanism to reach men

Because men appear to have significant defences built up around their body weight, it is necessary to use techniques that can penetrate these in order to get men to become involved in their own health. Humour has been an important part of the

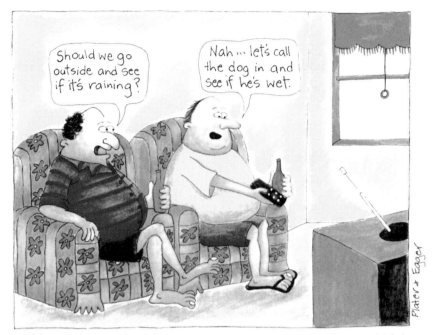

A TYPICAL DISCOURSE BETWEEN MEMBERS OF THE HUMAN ENERGY
CONSERVATION SOCIETY.

Figure 21.2 The light-hearted approach to getting a message to men.

GutBuster and Professor Trim's weight loss programmes for men (Egger, 2002). By being able to laugh at themselves (and others), men are more likely to participate in programmes that may otherwise threaten their self-esteem. Cartoons accompanying meal plans and menus, as well as a light-hearted approach to advertising (*see* Figure 21.2), have helped to increase participation in these programmes in Australia. It is not yet clear whether this approach would hold true across cultures. It is almost certain that it is not true across genders – being overweight is not a laughing matter for females. And pity anyone who tries it!

Is it all futile?

The Australian experience of men's weight control through GutBusters was one of the first of its kind in the world. Its success in creating a cadre of over 100,000 men in the programme showed that men *can* be reached in relation to their weight (and health), and that their success rate in weight loss, once committed, is quite high. However, there is doubt as to whether this can be done commercially, as the costs involved far outweigh the returns, at least over the short-term. It may be that longer-term awareness raising and 'softening up' is required through extensive and ongoing social marketing. Specific targeting of men who have had an 'awakening' to their personal risk might also be preferable to a generic approach to all overweight men.

A related issue is whether the current service provision (i.e. through group weight loss programmes) is appropriate for men. New technology, such as the internet and video streaming, has meant new possibilities, and these are currently being tested in a follow-up program to GutBusters called 'Professor Trim's Weight Loss for Men' (www.professortrim.com). It remains to be seen whether this, or other, approaches can break through the male defence barrier that is currently restricting advances in men's health in general and weight control in particular.

References

Aoun S, Donovan RJ, Johnson L, Egger G. Preventive care in the context of men's health. *Journal of Health Psychology*. 2002; **7**(3): 243–52.

Australian Institute of Health and Welfare (AIHW). *Australia's Health 2004: the ninth biennial report of the Australian Institute of Health and Welfare*. Cat. No. Aus 44. Canberra, Australia: AIHW; 2004.

Bouchard C. Genetic aspects of human obesities. In: Belfiore F, Papalia D, editors. *Proceedings of the Italian Society for the Study of Obesity, Catania Meeting*. Basel: Karger; 1991. p. 303–8.

Brown JB, Nichols GA, Glauber HS *et al*. Health care costs associated with escalation of drug treatment in type 2 diabetes mellitus. *American Journal Health-System Pharmacy*. 2001; **58**(2): 151–7.

Cialdini RB. Interpersonal influence. In: Shavitt S, Brock TC, editors. *Persuasion: psychological insights and perspectives*. Boston: Allyn and Bacon; 1994. p. 195–218.

Dunstan D, Zimmet P, Wellborn T *et al*. *Diabesity and Associated Disorders in Australia: the accelerating epidemic. The Ausdiab Study*. Melbourne: International Diabetes Institute; 2001.

Egger G. What we have learned about men from the GutBuster program. *Australian Journal of Nutrition and Dietetics*. 2000; **57**(1): 46–9.

Egger G. Laughing off fat. *IASSO Obesity Newsletter*. 2002; **4**(1): 19.

Egger G, Bolton A, O'Neill M, Freeman D. Effectiveness of an abdominal obesity reduction program in men: the GutBuster 'waist loss' program. *International Journal of Obesity*. 1996; **20**: 227–35.

Egger G, Dobson A. Clinical measures of obesity and weight loss in men. *International Journal of Obesity*. 2000; **24**(3): 354–7.

Egger G, Mowbray G. A qualitative assessment of obesity and overweight in working men. *Australian Journal of Nutrition and Dietetics*. 1993; **50**(1): 10–14.

Prochaska JO, Norcross JC, DiClemente CC. *Changing for Good*. New York: Avon Books; 1994.

Swinburn B, Egger G. The runaway weight gain train: too many accelerators, not enough brakes. *British Medical Journal*. 2004; **329**(7468): 736–9.

The way forward

David Wilkins

So, what have we learned?

Our starting point has been one that might surprise many people – that, in direct contravention of popular belief, men in the UK are significantly more likely to be overweight than women. Not only that, some underlying causes of being obese and overweight are specific (or largely specific) to men, and the health risks of becoming and remaining overweight are greater in men. Also, perhaps contrary to the popular view, helping a man to lose weight is rather more complicated than placing a hand on his shoulder, looking him squarely in the eye and dispensing the obvious but sadly inadequate 'what you should do my lad, is eat less unhealthy food and take more exercise'. Nothing emerges more clearly from this book than the confirmation that the problem of overweight men has its roots firmly embedded in a rich mix of unhelpful cultural attitudes, adverse circumstances and ingrained behaviours. This makes it difficult for individual men to come to grips with their weight problem and creates a substantial obstacle to those whose job it is to help them.

The desire to eat – we learned at the outset – is controlled by a sophisticated series of physiological mechanisms that are capable of making fine judgements about when we are hungry, when we have eaten enough and what levels of nutrients our bodies need. Potentially, energy input and body shape are in perfect harmony. To use the traditional 'male' metaphor of the body-as-machine, this makes the average bloke sound like he could easily be an E-type Jag with a race-tuned engine. We also learned however, that human beings are equipped with the ability to experience the various sensual pleasures and other powerful psychological associations that come with enjoying food and drink, regardless of whether there is a 'need' to eat or not. In the real world then, our man-as-machine can soon become a clapped-out milk float towing a six-berth caravan.

But so what? What is wrong with men enjoying their food? After all, as several authors point out in this book, food is now tastier, safer, easier to prepare and more abundant (at least in the western world) than at any time in history. Likewise, high levels of strength and stamina are no longer crucial, as they were not so long ago, to a man's ability to earn a living, or to travel, or to otherwise lead a normal daily life. Most men do not expend high levels of physical energy very often because there is simply no need to do so. And, if most of the other blokes are fat too, there is not even the disadvantage of difference. Why then does any of it matter?

The problem is that, although fat men may be traditionally thought of as 'jolly', fat itself is not a jolly substance. It is, as David Haslam points out in Chapter 2, not even an 'inert mass'. Fat is maliciously active, constantly producing toxins, damaging vital organs, straining the body's mechanics and generally reducing the ability to function healthily. These effects are markedly worse in men. Men tend to put on weight around the abdomen, and 'android obesity' (as fat deposited around the waistline is sometimes called), is a predisposing factor for type 2 diabetes and many other thoroughly unpleasant and chronic conditions. The complete list is far too long to repeat here but the more serious are relatively common and are assuredly life-threatening. They include heart disease and a number of cancers. It will suffice to say that being overweight and obese is now causing pain, misery, premature death and economic loss on an unprecedented scale.

This book has explored – directly in some cases, by implication in others – three recurring themes of overarching importance in relation to overweight and obese men.

The first is what we might call – to use jargon for a moment the *'gendered' nature of the problem*. The second is the *political climate*, not only in terms of health policy, but also in terms of the relationship between the kind of society that we make for ourselves and the health of the men who live in it. The third is the pragmatic one – *what can we do about the problem that we know will work?* For those practical types who would jump straight to the third of these, my advice would be not to do so without some understanding of the first two. To be effective, interventions must take account of the evidence base and the broader context. This book has brought together some of the foremost and most experienced thinkers and practitioners in the field and has explored all of these themes wisely and thoroughly.

So, to take the first; what do we mean by a 'gendered' problem and, by extension, how do we arrive at a 'gendered' solution? The Men's Health Forum has propounded the following definition of a 'male health issue':

> *A male health issue is one arising from physiological, psychological, social, cultural or environmental factors that have a specific impact on boys or men and/or where particular interventions are required for boys or men in order to achieve improvements in health and well-being at either the individual or the population level.* (WILKINS & BAKER 2004)

Overweight and obese men conform nicely to this definition. As we have seen, there is a higher incidence of overweight in men in the first place, and the fact of being male then increases the associated health risks.

Several chapters addressed the idea of 'maleness' and its relationship with being overweight. We have read about the increasing complexity of men's sense of their own bodies and how that interacts with their masculinity; about the different ways in which the media influences men and women; and about the subtleties of the relationship between different forms of masculinity and men's generally poor health-seeking behaviour. In the later chapters that deal with approaches and programmes for tackling overweight men, we have seen emerge almost incidentally, numerous male-specific attitudes and behaviours which have a negative impact on men's ability to keep their weight under control. Among many others, these include men's belief that being overweight in later life is 'normal'; men's perception that undue concern with weight is a feminine characteristic; men's lack of knowledge of food, diet and nutrition; men's greater propensity to drink alcohol at health-damaging levels; and men's frequent 'denial' that they have become overweight.

In other words, the occurrence of being overweight in men is inextricably linked with demonstrably male behaviours, attitudes and sensiblities. The only coherent conclusion to draw from this is that if we are to tackle the problem effectively we must acknowledge this masculine dimension.

Such a conclusion brings us neatly to the point where we can address the second of the key themes emerging from this book and ask whether current health policy and provision does indeed manage to do this.

The answer, supported both by the data about the low level of engagement by men in weight loss programmes, and the analysis of the policy-making process in Chapter 3 is regrettably, that we are nowhere near arriving at a 'gender-sensitive' approach. As Alan White points out in that chapter, there is a tension between such an approach and the 'traditional' population-based strategies that are favoured within current UK public health policy. The World Health Organization has been at the forefront of thinking in this area and has developed guidance for the implementation of a 'gender mainstreaming' approach but it has had little influence so far in the UK ('gender mainstreaming' being the term most commonly used internationally for an approach that takes account of men's and women's specific needs in the development of public policy and the provision of public services).

Consequently, there are ingrained inequalities between the sexes in both take-up of services and in health outcomes. These inequalities act largely (but by no means exclusively) to the disadvantage of men. So familiar indeed are these inequalities that their unacceptablility is rarely questioned; they are so much part of the health landscape that we may not even notice them. Furthermore, because it is believed to be 'challenging' to engage with men about health, we may have developed a belief that it is not worth trying. Being overweight in men is a classic example of this situation. The Equality Act 2006 requires health authorities to work towards the achievement of equitable take up of services and equitable outcomes between the sexes. The evidence of this book suggests that as far as overweight and obesity is concerned, compliance with the new legislation will pose very significant problems.

Chapter 3 also draws attention to the focus in much current health policy on delivering 'personal choice'. Such a focus runs the risk of placing undue emphasis on the actions of the individual. Of course, at the most basic level men make choices every day about what to eat for lunch, whether to walk to work or take the car, whether to go for a drink in the evening and so on but, as we noted earlier, they do so within the context of their own world view, heavily influenced as that is by their sense of themselves as men. And if that seems too fanciful, consider the wider political and environmental factors that also impinge upon such apparently banal decisions. Economic considerations often influence the quality of food that people decide to eat, as does the power of the food industry both via advertising and by market-driven considerations that often result in energy-dense nutritional content (and, as has been pointed out by some of our contributors, men and boys often lack useful nutritional knowledge anyway). Economic necessity or the policy of his employer may compel a man to spend long hours in a sedentary job and limit the time and energy he has for physical activity. Fear of crime or a poor local environment may tip the scales in favour of a comfortable car journey rather than a walk or a cycle ride to work. Work-related stress may make it more likely that he heads for the pub on the way home. Alan White quotes the view of the UK Public Health Association that 'choice is a spurious, and largely irrelevant, concept in public health' and that:

> *Public health is principally about organising society for the good of the population's health; at this level of concern, it is no more a matter of individual choice than the weather.*

So far, perhaps, so depressing.

If we pick up the third of our themes however – *what can we do about the problem that we know will work?* – we will see that the majority of the content of this book is in fact, positive, forward-thinking and helpful. It is practical too. Chapters 7 to 21 do two things. First, they offer insights into male attitudes and behaviour that can be taken into account in programme planning and will enhance the likelihood of success. Second, they describe real projects and programmes that have very largely been successful (and where they have been unsuccessful the authors draw lessons that will enable others to avoid encountering the same difficulties). These projects and programmes have in common that they have all sought answers to the fundamental question – 'how can we create something that will appeal specifically to men'.

This has not been easy of course, but it has resulted in workable, transferable day-to-day practice – and not just practice that attracts the 'worried well'. Men have been helped to lose weight in some of the most outwardly unpromising of cultures. In the West of Scotland ('the home of the deep-fried Mars bar' as Jim Leishman so succinctly described it in Chapter 8), the Camelon Centre has found that working class men are more than willing to join weight loss programmes provided they are treated with respect, and that thought is given to such apparently uncontentious issues as the kind of language used (the word 'obese' is particularly unpopular). In Australia, a country widely regarded as having one of the developed world's most unapologetically macho cultures, the 'GutBusters Waist Loss' programme became a highly successful national initiative, eventually reaching 100,000 men from a wide range of socio-economic backgrounds. In Chapter 21 Gary Egger described how that programme used humour to tackle resistance and denial, ultimately demonstrating that many overweight Australian men do indeed want to become fitter and healthier.

Other authors have described how to work with overweight men in particular settings such as the workplace, primary care and community pharmacies. In Chapter 20 Jane DeVille-Almond argued for taking health promotion services out to men wherever they can be found – her own clinics have been delivered in pubs, barber's shops and at biker events. The virtual world has emerged in recent years as having particular potential for reaching men and Jim Pollard in Chapter 19 described how to use the internet to greatest effect. Several chapters addressed the needs of men from particular social groups, including men from minority ethnic communities, older men, men with disabilities and men with mental health problems. Not only are these chapters practical and encouraging, they are studded with real-world observations and learning that we hope will give more people the confidence to take on this pressing issue.

Is this enough?

Well, certainly it is good to know that there is effective practice out there. It is heartening too that there is a developing evidence base and it is the intention that this book should provide a fixed platform for further developments. No real progress can be made, however, without the commitment of politicians, policymakers and health service planners to provide strategic leadership. The need to tackle weight problems in general has been very widely acknowledged; witness the high level investigations, recommendations and guidance published in recent years by the Audit Commission, the Department of Health and the National Institute for Health and Clinical Excellence among others.

The problem has been that none of these has taken account of the need for the gendered perspective, for which this book makes the case. In some ways this is hard to credit, since the evidence of both higher incidence and higher risk in men is pretty much the first thing that anyone looking at population-level data would observe. Add to this the evidence that men are demonstrably less well served by the present range of services and it seems almost absurd not to have taken the matter of gender into account when considering how to tackle the problem. That is the present position however.

(It should perhaps be made clear at this point that none of the contributors to this book has argued for the diminution of policy and services for women in order to shift the focus on to men. Clearly overweight women also have specific needs and no-one would argue that the health of women should be compromised to improve the health of men. A gendered approach to this issue would benefit both sexes and would contribute significantly to improving the health and well-being of the whole population.)

In 2005, the Men's Health Forum published a five point Action Plan (Men's Health Forum, 2005) that sought to identify the underpinning components of a national strategy to tackle the problem of overweight and obese men. The analysis provided by the contributors to this book serves to emphasise the continuing need for such a strategy, and the descriptions of existing initiatives suggest that some of the necessary expertise is already in place. It is well worth reproducing the Action Plan and its introductory paragraph here:

> *The present levels of overweight and obesity in men constitute nothing less than a public health emergency that will continue to get worse unless decisive action is taken in the immediate future. Already two thirds of men are overweight or obese. If current trends continue it is estimated that within five years three men in every four will be so. In short, it could not be plainer that there has been a systematic failure to engage effectively with men about their weight. The consequences of this situation both for individual men and for society as a whole should be regarded as wholly unacceptable by*

health practitioners, and by decision-makers across the whole spectrum of public policy. It is critical that expertise is developed – and developed rapidly in how to enable men to achieve and maintain a healthy weight. Men will otherwise continue to die prematurely, and very large numbers will not experience optimum health and well-being.

The Men's Health Forum calls for the implementation of the following five actions as a matter of urgency:

1 **Politicians, policymakers, practitioners, the media and the public must recognise that weight is a male issue too.** The popular assumption that weight loss is predominantly a women's concern is one of the critical reasons for lack of progress on this issue. This assumption almost certainly results in poorer services for men and underpins an unhelpful degree of resigned acceptance among health professionals. Most of all, it perpetuates a myth which affects men themselves and it may indeed help to explain why excess weight is so much more common in men than women. It is important, however, that any such shift in perception does not rely on the premise that the most important reason for losing weight is to achieve a popular ideal of physical perfection. The idealisation of body-shape has undoubtedly had damaging consequences for women – not least in its association with eating disorders.

2 **Men's attitudes to weight and weight loss need to be more fully understood.** It is clear that the existing, broadly 'unisex', approach is failing men. Unless there is some recognition that helping men to achieve and maintain a healthy weight requires a 'male-sensitive' approach then men will continue to gain weight and will remain resistant to support services. The paucity of existing knowledge in this area means that achieving such an understanding will require investment in a comprehensive and dedicated research programme. As well as exploring men's attitudes and considering how best to work with men, such a research programme could aim also (for example) to answer questions about why so many men tend to gain weight in their twenties and thirties and look at the particular role of alcohol consumption in male weight gain. Such a programme should be instituted as soon as possible.

3 **There must be investment in new 'male sensitive' approaches, particularly in primary care and health promotion.** Although working with men on weight issues is not a well-developed field, there is some practical experience here and there across the country that offers a basis for beginning to tackle the problem. It is important that projects that work effectively with men are properly evaluated and that good practice is widely disseminated. There is an increasing belief among those who have worked to improve the health of men in other fields, that men can be persuaded to take their health seriously provided they are approached in the right way. It is arguable that a step change might be achieved by simply making routine health checks (weight, waist circumference, blood pressure, blood cholesterol etc) more widely and easily available (i.e. not just in clinical settings) and by promoting that availability in a way that will encourage male take up.

4 **It is essential to develop work on weight issues with boys in pre-schools, schools and community settings.** This is vital, not just because of the increasing levels of overweight and obese children, but also because the establishment of a healthy lifestyle before adulthood is likely to reduce the risks of later becoming overweight. Initiatives such as the provision of healthier school meals, reducing opportunities for consuming sweets and sugary drinks in schools and a greater emphasis on physical activity will clearly make a difference. It seems probable that acting to reduce advertising of 'junk' foodstuffs direct to children would also be helpful. As in the case of adults however, attention must also be paid to attitudes and behaviours specific to boys and to developing interventions that are more likely to appeal to them.

5 **A cross-cutting national strategy on overweight and obesity is urgently needed. Such a strategy should focus on men and women separately.** It is short-sighted and demonstrably ineffective to concentrate solely on solutions targeted at individuals, important though these are. Lifestyle programmes, health promotion initiatives and pharmaceutical interventions are essential components of the way forward but the problem of being overweight can be tackled effectively *only* by 'joined-up' solutions. Such an approach should focus directly on the prevention of being overweight and obese, not on co-morbidities. Most importantly, the strategy should take central account of the differences between the sexes in order to benefit both men and women. In the case of men, such a strategy should, for example, encompass action on work/life balance; link strategies on alcohol consumption with action on weight; develop educational provision specifically targeted at boys and encourage employers to develop opportunities for staff to become more physically active and eat a healthier diet.

It isn't going to be cheap or easy. Investment is needed. An overt commitment to improve the health of our men and boys is needed. Political leadership is needed. But no-one would seriously dispute that tackling overweight men *now* is crucial for the future health of the nation. We cannot rely on exhortations to individuals to eat less or exercise more. A considered, concerted and comprehensive approach is the only way forward. Some expertise is out there and we could develop more. Some of the structural frameworks are already in place and there will soon be legislative impetus to ensure that the needs of men and boys are properly addressed. The implementation of the recommendations above would go a long way towards making a difference to public health. It remains true that we cannot hope to improve the health of all unless we learn how to improve the health of men.

References

Men's Health Forum. *Hazardous Waist: Tackling the epidemic of excess weight in men.* Men's Health Forum, London; 2005.

Wilkins D and Baker P. *Getting It Sorted: A Policy Programme for Men's Health.* Men's Health Forum, London; 2004.

The Men's Health Forum

The Men's Health Forum (MHF) is a well-established, respected and influential charity at the cutting-edge of policy development in male health in England and Wales. Our over-arching objective is the achievement of a 'gender-sensitive' approach to every aspect of health policy and practice, nationally and locally.

Our vision is a future in which all men and boys have an equal opportunity to attain the highest possible level of health and wellbeing. We believe that policies and services aimed at improving male health should also take full account of inequalities, including those linked to social class, ethnicity, religion, age, disability and sexuality.

We aim to achieve improvements in male health through:
- policy development
- research
- providing information and consultancy services
- developing health information resources for 'the man in the street'
- stimulating professional and public debate
- working with MPs and Government
- developing innovative and imaginative projects
- professional training
- collaborating with the widest possible range of interested organisations and individuals
- organising the annual National Men's Health Week

The MHF has recently focused on a number of key public health issues, including male overweight/obesity, the high incidence of cancer in men, chlamydia screening, mental health and wellbeing, and long-term health conditions. We are working to make primary care, including pharmacy, more accessible to men and we see workplace health services as central to improvements in male health. We have also pioneered the development of 'male friendly' health information, both paper-based and online.

Further information about the MHF's work can be found at www.mens healthforum.org.uk. The MHF's unique consumer health information site for men is www.malehealth.co.uk.

The MHF can be contacted at:
Tavistock House, Tavistock Square, London WC1H 9HR, UK.
Tel: +44 (0)20 7388 4449; fax: +44 (0)20 7388 4477; email: office@menshealth forum.org.uk

Index

abdominal fat 8–9
  health risks 15
  and metabolic syndrome 8
access issues, work situations
  104–6
Acheson, SD 166
Ackerman, S and Nolan, LJ
  174–5
activity levels *see* physical
  activity levels
advertising campaigns
  aimed at children 7
  industry expenditures 25
  promoting energy dense
  foods 6, 24–5
  see also health education
age and body (dis)satisfaction
  41–2
agoraphobia 160–1
alcohol use 8, 83, 162–3
Allen, Woody 204
Allied Dunbar National
  Fitness Survey (ADNFS)
  154, 156
Allison, DB *et al.* 173, 174
American College of Sports
  Medicine (ACSM)
  guidelines 142
Anderson, AS 30
Andersson, I and Rossner, S
  98
'android' obesity 15
  see also abdominal fat
'andropause' 128
anti-obesity drugs
  evidence studies 70
  mechanisms of action 14
antidepressants 174, 176
antipsychotics 174–5, 176
anxiety disorders 176
Aoun, S *et al.* 206
appetite regulation 13–14
'apple' fat deposition patterns
  see abdominal fat

APPLES (Active Programme
  Promoting Lifestyle in
  Schools) 117
Archibald, EH *et al.* 119
assessment methods 77
  with children 112–13
  with mentally ill patients
  179–80
  with older people 126–7
  see also waist circumference
  measures
Atkins diet 20
attitudes to weight
  health providers 5–6
  male perspectives 3–5, 17–
  18, 43–5, 78–9, 90,
  206–7
attractiveness ratings
  evolutionary perspectives
  40
  socio-cultural influences
  39–40
Australian experiences 205–
  12
  GutBuster programme 4,
  5, 207–12
  male attitudes 206–7
Australian Institute of
  Health and Welfare
  (AIHW) 206

back pain 9
Bagley, C and Tremblay, P 59
Bahl, V and Rawaf, S 167
Bajekal, M *et al.* 137–8
Balarajan, R 166
Bandura, A 153
Banting, William 20
barber shop clinics 201–3
Bartlett, SJ 154
behaviour change 151–3
  context dependency 155–6
  psychological factors 153–
  5

use of counselling
  approaches 163–4
Bem Sex Role Inventory
  (BSRI) 56
Benwell, B 61
Berger, J 37
Berkman, LF *et al.* 156
Billig, M 60
Binge Eating Disorder
  (BED) 26
binge eating patterns 162–3
black and ethnic minorities
  see ethnicity and weight
  problems
blindness 138
blood pressure and obesity
  16, 80
blood tests 81
BMI (body mass index)
  charts 78
  child assessments 112–13,
  114–15
  gender comparisons 3
  older people 126–7
  registers 32, 67
body (dis)satisfaction
  measures 38
body dysmorphia 41, 160
body image and men 160
  background and societal
  context 36–7
  concept definitions 36
  cultural trends and
  changes 39–40
  feminisation issues 37, 38–
  9, 42–3
  self-evaluations and
  dissatisfactions 41–2
  stigma of 'obesity' 78–80
  treatment implications 42–
  5
  see also male attitudes to
  weight
body image and women 37–8

body size
male attitudes 3–5, 41–2
and masculinity 41
Bogalusa Heart Study
(Freedman *et al.* 1999)
115
Booth, F *et al.* 150
Bordo, S 37
Borys, JM and Boute, D 107
Bouchard, C 206
Bradshaw, T *et al.* 173, 183
Braet, C and Van Winckel,
M 120
Braet, C *et al.* 119, 120
brand influences 50
Bray, GA *et al.* 12
British Heart Foundation 6
Brodie, DA *et al.* 40
Brown, JB *et al.* 209
Brown, JD *et al.* 39–40
Brown, MR *et al.* 119
Brown, S 173
Brown, S *et al.* 173
Bruch, H 37
Bruyere, S *et al.* 195
Bryant-Jefferies, R 159–60,
163
BT Work Fit campaign 186–
7
bullying 160
Bundred, P *et al.* 114
Bungum, T *et al.* 107
Buss, DM 40
Buss, DM and Schmitt, DP
40
Bye, C *et al.* 98

Cafri, G and Thompson, JK
38, 41
Cafri, G *et al.* 38–9, 41
Camelon Centre (Scotland)
76, 216
expansion programmes 76–
86
campaigns and promotions
see health education;
public health; weight loss
programmes
Campbell, K *et al.* 70, 116
cancer risk 9, 17
Canning, H and Mayer, J 115
Canoy, D *et al.* 71
canteen food 107
CAP (Common Agricultural
Policy) 25
Cardan, Dick Humelbergius
Secundus 20
cardiovascular disease (CVD)
8–9

in children 115
early interventions 117
mortality rates 16
physiological mechanisms
16
cardiovascular training 143
Carlisle, D 5
Carpenter, KM *et al.* 18
Cash, TF 36
changing behaviour 151–3
dependency on contexts
155–6
psychological factors 153–5
use of counselling
approaches 163–4
Chan, JM *et al.* 17
Chaturverdi, N and Fuller,
JH 167
childhood abuse, and adult
obesity 161–2
children
cholesterol levels 16
government policies 29–32
legacies of sexual abuse
161–2
measurement and
assessment 112–13
physical activity levels 25–
6
prevalence of weight
problems 113–15
treatment evidence studies
70
trends in weight 6
Chinn, S and Rona, RJ 114
cholecystokinin 13–14
cholesterol 16
Choosing a Better Diet report
(DoH 2005) 30
Choosing Health (DoH
2004a) 29–30, 92, 198
CHOPPS (Christchurch
Obesity Prevention
Project in Schools) 118
Cialdini, RB 209
Clegg, A *et al.* 70
clinical guidelines 32, 67–8,
70
clinics *see* weight
management clinics
Cochrane Reviews,
childhood obesity
prevention programmes
116–17
Cohn, L 160
Colditz, GA *et al.* 17
Cole, TJ *et al.* 113
Collinson, DL and Hearn, J
56

colorectal cancer 9
Colquitt, J *et al.* 70
COMA (Committee on
Medical Aspects of Food
Policy) 8
comfort eating 162–3
commercial incentives and
policy drivers 24–6
commercial slimming groups
92–101
*Commissioning a Patient Led
Service* (DoH 2005) 68
Committee on Medical
Aspects of Food Policy
(COMA) 8
Common Agricultural Policy
(CAP) 25
Community Pharmacy
Research Consortium
(CPRC) 87–8
'competitive' weight loss 83–
4
Connell, RW 56–7
Connell, RW and
Messerschmidt, JW 56,
58
convenience foods,
advertising and promotion
6–7, 24–5
Cornaro, L 12–13, 21
Cornier, M-A *et al.* 151
Cosmides, L and Tooby, J 40
Cottam, R 26
counselling men with weight
problems 159–64
Counterweight programme 5,
78
Cramer, P and Steinwert, T
115
Crossley, ML 59
Crow Magazine 18
Crowther, R *et al.* 30
Crozier, Adam 109–10
cultural influences 167–9
curries and Asian foods 167–
8
Cycle of Change model
(DiClemente and
Prochaska) 163
cytokines 14

daily energy requirements 8
Dalziel, Alison 76
Dao, HH *et al.* 119–20
Davidson, K and Arber, S
128, 133
Davidson, K *et al.* 128–33
Davis, MG *et al.* 153
Deforche, B *et al.* 119, 120

dementia 9
demographic trends 3
Dempster, P and Aitkins, S 120
denial reactions 4, 208–9
depression
  and body weight 18, 175–6
  health education campaigns 52, 180–4
Derbyshire, H 23
Developing Patient Partnerships (DPP) 107
DeVille-Almond, Jane 69, 198–204
Devlin, MJ et al. 173–4, 178–9, 182
'diabesity' 17
diabetes (type II)
  causes 16–17
  emotional effects 128
  and ethnicity 15, 166–7
  undiagnosed 17
Diabetes UK, advertising campaigns 170–1
diary keeping 82
Dickins, CM et al. 156
DiClemente, CC 163
diet industry 19–20
dieticians, role in management programmes 72
dieting
  as gendered activity 4–5
  see also healthy eating
Dietz, WH and Schoeller, DA 119
Disability Discrimination Act–1995 105, 136
disability issues 104–6, 135–48
  assessment and definitions 135–7
  characteristics of men with disabilities 137–40
  incidence of obesity 137–9
  Inclusive Fitness Initiative (IFI) 140–8
'disordered eating' paradigm 37–8
divorce rates 130
Doak, CM et al. 116
'domino pathology' 132
Dr Foster organisation 69–70
Drøyvold, W et al. 125–6
drug regimes (psychotropic)
  impact on weight 174–5
  see also anti-obesity drugs
Drummond, MJN 42

Dubois-Arber, F et al. 53
Duchaine, B et al. 40
Duggan, SJ and McCreary, DR 39
Dunstan, D et al. 205

EAR (Estimated Average Requirements) for men 8
Eat Smart campaign 118
eating disordered syndrome 41
Eating Disorders Association (EDA) 37
eating habits 82
  binge/comfort patterns 162–3
  see also healthy eating
Ebrahim, S et al. 137
Economic and Social Research Council (ESRC), research project 128–33
Edley, N and Wetherell, N 56
education deficits see knowledge about healthy lifestyles
educational programmes see health education; healthy eating; weight loss programmes
Edwards, D and Potter, J 44
Egger, G 4–5, 43, 206, 211
Egger, G and Mowbray, G 206–7
Egger, G et al. 206
Ekkekakis, P et al. 152
Ellis, BJ 40
Ellison, Larry 199
email communication 71
employment see work and obesity
employment law 105–6
Emslie, C et al. 154
endocannabinoid system 14
Endo, H et al. 119
energy balance, and mental disorders 177–9
energy intake surveys 8
energy requirements, for men 8
energy utilisation 14
energy-dense foods, advertising and promotion 6–7, 24–5
Eng, PM et al. 156
Equal Opportunities Commission 23
Equality Act–2006 23–4, 215

see also Gender Equity Act–2007
ethnicity and weight problems 6, 166–9
  in South Asian men 166–72
European Commission (EC) responses 28
  see also Common Agricultural Policy (CAP)
evolutionary perspectives, body image and sexual selection 40
exercise regimes
  evidence studies 70
  motivating change 151–3
  for people with disabilities 141–8
  promotion strategies 150–6
  stiffness and negative effects 155
  see also physical activity levels; sport activities

Fairlie, RW 195
Fallon, A 39
Fallon, A and Rozin, P 38
fat
  deposition patterns 8–9, 15
  physiological properties 14, 15–16
fat mass (FM) calculations 113
'fatmanslim' internet campaign (UK) 53
Faulkner, G et al. 180, 182
Featherstone, M 39
feminisation of body image concerns 38–9, 42–3
Finland, North Karelia project 28
Fisher, E et al. 39
'five-a-side' soccer 155
Flegal, K et al. 125
Floodmark, C-E et al. 116
Food Commission 30
food industry 6–7
  commercial incentives and policy drivers 24–6
  responses to public health policy recommendations 28
  see also marketing activities
Food Optimising approaches 94
food replacement programmes, pharmacy-led 88

Food Standards Agency 30
food subsidies 25
food types, high-fat/high-
    sugar products 6–7
football 155
Forster, S and Gariballa, S
    125
Dr Foster organisation 69–70
Foucalt, M 59
Freedman, DS *et al.* 112, 115
French, J 196
Friedman, MA and Brownell,
    KD 37
fruit and vegetable
    consumption, in schools
    25
Fulton, JE *et al.* 116
funding for obesity
    management 70, 75, 88–9,
    219

Gainer, B 49
Gangestad, SW 40
Garrow, JS *et al.* 173–4, 181–
    2
Gary Jelen Sports
    Foundation (GJSF) 139
gastric surgery, evidence
    studies 70
gastrointestinal conditions, in
    obese children 115
Gately, PJ 114, 115, 120
Gately, PJ *et al.* 120
gender equality, defined 23
gender equity, defined 23
Gender Equity Act–2007 68
gender mainstreaming 23–4,
    33–4
gender stereotyping and
    weight 4
    feminisation of body
        image concerns 36–9,
        42–3
General Household Survey
    (2003), on alcohol intake
    8
General Medical Services
    (GMS) Contract 32, 67
genetic influences 14
ghrelin 13
Gill, R *et al.* 39, 57
Gillon, E 44
Gilman, S 18
GI's barber-shop clinics 201–
    3
Glanz, K *et al.* 49
Glenny, AM *et al.* 70
*Global Strategy on Diet,
    Physical Activity and*

Health (WHO 2004) 27,
    121
Goldstein, DJ 80
Goodwood Festival of Speed
    201
Google search engine 190,
    192
Gough, B 55, 58, 60–2
Gough, B and Connor, MT
    55, 154
Gough, B and Edwards, G
    58
government-led campaigns
    see health education;
    policy strategies; public
    health
GP consultations
    engagement strategies 71–
    2
    practitioner gender 69
    reluctance to attend 15, 55,
        62, 131–2, 168–9, 198
GP management of obesity
    and gender stereotyping
        issues 42–5
    policy guidance 32
    promoting exercise 155
    see also primary care
        obesity management;
        weight management
        clinics
Graham, KA *et al.* 179
Grewal, I *et al.* 135
group approaches
    benefits 83–4, 156
    participation issues 78
Grundy, E *et al.* 135
guidelines *see* clinical
    guidelines; policy
    strategies
GutBusters programme 4, 5,
    207–12
    lessons learnt 208–11
Guthrie, JF *et al.* 49
'gynoid' obesity 15

Haddock, CK *et al.* 70
Halberstram, J 56
Halliwell, E and Dittmar, H
    37
Hamill, Iain 99–102
Hardman, AE and Stensel,
    DJ 139
Harley-Davidson bikers 200–
    1
Harris, T *et al.* 128
Haslam, D *et al.* 13, 15
Hassan, M and Killick, S 128
health checks, non-

attendance issues 15
health education
    effectiveness issues 108
    evidence studies 70–1
    gendered perspectives 48–9
    prevention campaigns 70–
        1
    social marketing strategies
        50–1, 52–4
    workplace settings 107–9
    see also exercise regimes;
        healthy eating
Health of Ethnic Minority
    Elders in London report
    (Lowdell *et al.* 2000) 166
Health of the Nation (DoH
    1991) 3, 29
Health of the Net (HON)
    193–4
health promotion *see* health
    education
health risks 8–9, 15–17
    in children and young
        people 115
    in older people 127
health screening 130
Health Select Committee
    (2004) recommendations
    5
Health Survey for England
    (2001) 137
Health Survey for England
    (2002) 6
Health Survey for England
    (2003) 114, 159
healthcare professionals
    roles in weight loss
        programmes 72–3
    training issues 81
    see also GP consultations;
        practice nurses
healthcare providers, attitudes
    towards male obesity 5–6
healthy eating
    knowledge levels 5, 129–
        30, 168
    and 'masculinity' 60–1
    principles for weight loss
        programmes 81–2
    public policy vs. personal
        choice 26–41
    and the slimming industry
        94–7
    see also weight loss
        programmes
Healthy Schools Programme
    29–30
heart disease 8–9
    mortality rates 16

physiological mechanisms 14, 16
hegemonic masculinities 57–9
  and suppression of the feminine 61–2
Helmchen, L 7
Heshka, S *et al.* 98
high-fat/high-sugar products, advertising and promotion 6–7, 24–5
Hill, M 160
historical perspectives 12–13
Hogarth, T *et al.* 7
Hollway, W 57
Hollway, W and Jefferson, T 61
Holt, RIG *et al.* 173
homophobia 58–9
homosexuality
  and body dissatisfaction 42
  and depression 59
  oppressive practices 58
hormonal control of appetite 13–14
Hospers, HJ and Jansen, A 41
hospital foods 183–4
hospital-based weight loss programmes, children 119–20
human rights issues 24–5
humour and obesity 17–18, 210–11
hunger, physiological mechanisms 13–14
hypercoagulability 16
hyperinsulinaemia 16
hypertension, risk factors 16
hypogonadism 128

Inclusive Fitness Initiative (IFI) 140-8
Indian food 167–8
inflammatory responses, role of fat 14
information 'overload' 192
inpatient treatment programmes, for children 119–21
insulin resistance 16–17
interleukin-6 14
International Obesity Task Force (IOTF) 25, 112–13
international perspectives 15
  childhood obesity 113
  childhood treatment programmes 119–20
  obesity rankings 3

see also policy strategies
internet-based programmes and information 53, 96, 186–96
  access in the UK 188
  background 186–8
  benefits 191–2
  challenges 192–3
  problems with addiction 195–6
  quality control 193–4
  solutions to problems 193–6
Ishizaki, M *et al.* 106

Jackson, C 151, 153
Jain, a 70
James, J *et al.* 118
Jameson, T 15, 17
Jankowski, LW and Evans, JK 138
Janssen, I *et al.* 115, 125, 127
Jebb, S 29, 53
Jefferson, T 62
Johnson, M 6
joint replacement surgery 32
Jowell, Tessa 29

Kapur, N *et al.* 62
Karris, L 115
Katz, DL *et al.* 70
Kenrick, DT *et al.* 40
Kerr, J *et al.* 150
Kershaw, S 195–6
Key, T *et al.* 9
kidney cancer 9
Kilminster, S *et al.* 57
Kimmel, M 56
kite-marking 193–4
knowledge about healthy lifestyles 5, 129–30, 200
  internet information 186–96
Kolotkin, RL *et al.* 70
Kushner, RF and Blatner, D 179

Labre, MP 61
Lakka, HM *et al.* 8
Lakkis, J *et al.* 42
Lallukka, T *et al.* 152
Lang, T *et al.* 28
Last Chance Diet 20
Lean, MEJ and Pajonk, F-G 180
learning disabilities 139
Lee, C and Owens, RG 41, 62
Leedham, I 169

legislation, gender equity 23–4, 68
Leishman, Jim 76
Lenz, TL and Hamilton, WR 70
leptin 14
Levine, AS *et al.* 6
Levine, MP and Harrison, K 41
life expectancy
  and obesity 17
  and social class 59
lifestyle issues 19–20
  changing patterns 151–3, 163–4
  impact of government policies 26
  the 'right' to be fat 24–5
  sedentary occupations 55, 151, 203
  social class considerations 59
  see also healthy eating; physical activity levels
Light, R and Kirk, D 156
lithium 176
liver cirrhosis 16
Livingstone, S and Helsper, E 7
Loaded magazine 51
Lobstein, T *et al.* 113
London Marathon 110
long-term weight loss, evidence studies 98–9
Loomis, D 152
low-carbohydrate diets, historical perspectives 20
Lowdell, C *et al.* 166
Lowe, MR *et al.* 97–8
Lymm Truck Stop surgery 203
Lynch, S and Zellner, D 41–2
Lyons, A and Willott, S 61

McCabe, MP and Ricciardelli, CA 160
McCarthy, D *et al.* 114, 115
McCreary, DR 79
McCreary, DR and Sadava, S 4, 49
McCreary, DR and Sasse, DK 38–9
'macho' cultures 60–1
  see also hegemonic masculinities; masculinity
McKenna, J and Coulson, J 154

McKenna, J and Davis, M
152
McPherson, KE and
Turnball, JD 38, 41
McPherson, W 166
McTigue, KM et al. 70
magazines for men 51–2, 61
male attitudes to weight 3–5,
17–18, 43–5
see also body image and men
male body ideals see body
image and men
malehealth.co.uk 187
Malina, RM and Bouchard,
C 113
mania 176
manufacturing influences 6
MAOIs (monoamine oxidase
inhibitors) 174, 176
marketing activities
and gender 49–51
targeting children 7
targeting men 49–51
see also advertising
campaigns
Markey, CN and Markey,
PM 45
Marks, L 166
masculinity
and body image 38–41,
44–5, 160
concepts and dimensions
55–7
infuencing factors 57–9
marginalised identities 58
new definitions 59–61
and physical activity 154
threats and defence
responses 61–2
Mather, HM et al. 167
meal preparation 83
media influences 48–54
food advertising
opportunities 49–51
lack of attention 210
magazines for men 51–2,
61
Men's Fitness magazine 155
Men's Health Forum (MHF)
33–4, 110, 217–19
five action
recommendations 218–
19
website survey 188–93
Men's Health magazine 52, 61
mental health problems and
obesity 138–9, 173–84
general characteristics
173–4

influencing factors 177–84
medication effects 174–5
range of illnesses 175–7
weight management
assessments 179–80
weight management
programmes 180–4
Messner, M 58
metabolic rates 14
metabolic syndrome 8, 17
MHF see Men's Health
Forum (MHF)
micro-activity 19
Miller, WR and Rollnick, S
163
Min-Lee, I et al. 150–1
Mintz, LB and Betz, NE 40
Mir, S and Taylor, D 180
mood disorders 175–6
Moore, H et al. 71
MORI, on diabetes
awareness 170
motivation to lose weight 80
see also changing behaviour
Moxley Arms 199–200
MP5 programme 97
Mullen, MC and Shield, J
115
Murray, M 59
muscle dysmorphia 41
Mutrie, N et al. 154

Nardi, PM 56
National Audit Office 159
'National Charter for Health,
Work and Well-being'
107–8
National Obesity Forum
(NOF) 70
National Opinion Polls
(NOP) survey (2005) 4
Naughton, J 191
Nazroo, J 167
neuropeptide responses 13–14
neurotransmitters 14
New Zealand, obesity trends
126
NHS attitudes towards male
obesity 5–6
NHS Direct 190, 194
NHS 'rationing' practices 32
NICE (National Institute for
Health and Clinical
Excellence) Guidelines on
Obesity 31, 67–8, 70,
121–2
Nichols, JF et al. 120
'non-attenders' 15, 55, 62,
131–2, 168–9, 198

North Karelia project 28
Norway, obesity trends 125–6

'obese', negative connotations
78–9
2000 Obesity: preventing and
managing the global
epidemic (WHO 2000) 27
obesity
health risks 8–9, 15–17
health service attitudes 5–6
historical perspectives 12–
13
international perspectives
3, 15
male attitudes 3–5, 17–18,
43–5, 78–9, 90, 206–7
measurement 3, 15, 71
physiological
characteristics 13–14
policy strategies 24–34,
67–8
prevalence 3, 103–4
treatment rationale 14–15,
104–6
trends 103–4
see also treatments for
obesity; weight loss
programmes
obesity clinics see weight
management clinics
Obesity in Europe report
(IOTF 2002) 25
obesity management
programmes see weight
loss programmes
obesity registers 32, 67
obestatin 13–14
O'Brien, O and White, AK
23
O'Brien, R et al. 154
occupational hazards,
sedentary work patterns 7
occupational health
interventions 20
oesophageal cancer 9
Ogden, J 42
older people and obesity
125–33
current trends 125–7
emotional and social costs
127–8
exercise trends 156
health risks 127–8
healthcare attendance 131–
2
knowledge about healthy
lifestyles 129–30
personal accounts 128–33

2012 Olympics 53
Orbach, S 20, 36–7, 39
Orlistat 70
osteoarthritis 9, 17
Our Healthier Nation (DoH
    1998) 29

Padwal, R *et al.* 70
Parkes, KR 106
participation issues
    engaging men 71–2
    groups and workshops 77–
        8, 83–4
    reluctance to seek help 15,
        55, 62
Pena, M *et al.* 119
Perri, MG *et al.* 97
Peterson, MD *et al.* 150
Peterson, NA and Hughey, J
    155
pharmacies
    role in men's health 87–8
    weight management
        services 88–91
pharmacists
public perceptions 87
role in management
    programmes 72–3
training 89–90
Phelan, M *et al.* 173
physical activity levels 7–8,
    18–19
    barriers 151–2
    and behaviour change
        151–3
    increasing outputs 19, 82–
        3, 150–6
    measurement and
        recording 81, 82
    people with disabilities
        139–40
    policy recommendations
        28–9, 31
    in schools 25–6
    see also sport activities
physical education policies
    25–6
    people with disabilities
        140
    see also exercise regimes
physical effects of obesity *see*
    health risks
physiological characteristics
    of obesity 13–14
Pleck, J 56
Pliner, P *et al.* 38
Plotnikoff, RC *et al.* 153
policy strategies 24–34, 67–8
    European Commission

(EC) responses 28
impact on public health 26
industry drivers and
    commercial pressures
    24–6
vs. individual choice 26–34
within gender
    mainstreaming
    frameworks 23–4, 33–4
World Health
    Organization (WHO)
    27–8
polycystic ovaries 14
Pope, HG *et al.* 38, 40, 41
portion control 82
postmen 106, 109–10
practice nurses
    role in making
        programmes accessible
        199–204
    role in management
        programmes 72, 155
prejudice
    and childhood obesity 115
    and gender concepts 59–61
    workplace situations 104
Prentice, A 22, 32
Prentice, A and Jebb, SA 81
prevalence of obesity 3, 103–
    4
    children and young people
        113–15
prevention campaigns 70–1
    programmes for children
        115–21
    programmes for ethnic
        minorities 170–1
Price, JH *et al.* 1–4
primary care obesity
    management 67–73
    background and policy
        frameworks 67–8
    barriers to participation
        68–9, 131–2
    engagement strategies 71–
        2, 155
    funding 70
    opportunities 68
    setting up clinics 72–3
    specific community-based
        initiatives 69
    studies and reports 69–71
Prochaska, JO and
    DiClemente, CC 152
Prochaska, JO *et al.* 207, 209
Pronk, NP *et al.* 107
prostate cancer 9
prostate disease 14
PSAs (Public Sector

Agreements) on obesity
    30, 31
psychiatric drugs, impact on
    weight 174–5
pub venues and weight loss
    clinics 199–200
public health
    international intervention
        strategies 26–8
    social marketing strategies
        50–1, 52–4
    UK government
        intervention policies
        29–32, 53
Public Sector Agreements
    (PSAs) on obesity 30, 31
Putnam, D 155
Putnam, J *et al.* 107
PYY 3–36 hormone 13–14

quality of life studies, older
    people 128-33
Quality and Outcomes
    Framework (QOF)
    guidelines 32, 67

Racette, S *et al.* 127
Ramsay, Gordon 60
Reeves, R 25
Reilly, JJ *et al.* 112, 114
Rejeski, J *et al.* 156
religious beliefs 169
Renjilian, DR *et al.* 84
Rennie, R *et al.* 8
residential programmes for
    children 119–21
    inpatient treatments 119–
        20
    summer camps 120–1
Resnicow, K and Robinson,
    TN 116, 117
'reverse anorexia' 160
Rickards, L *et al.* 155
Riehman, K 51
Rimmer, JH and Wang, W
    138–9
road traffic accident risks 9,
    17
Robertson, S 152, 154, 156
Robertson, S and Williams,
    P 152
Roehling, MV 104
Rohrbacher, R 120
Rolland-Cachera, MF *et al.*
    119
Rolls, BJ *et al.* 6
Ronti, T *et al.* 13
Rosemary Conley Diet and
    Fitness Clubs 96–7

Rosenheck, R *et al.* 174
Rosmond, R and Bjorntorp, P 4
Roth, A *et al.* 151
Royal College of Physicians (RCP)
  on needs of ethnic minorities 167
  on obesity 32
Royal Mail Group 109–10
Rubin, SS *et al.* 139
Rudat, K 169
Rudolf, MC *et al.* 114
Russell, CJ and Keel, PK 42

'Safe and Sound Challenge' 29
Sahota, P *et al.* 117
salt content, policy recommendations 28
schizophrenia 138, 173, 175, 180
  nutritional consequences 177
schools
  food policies 25
  healthy eating campaigns 29–31
  obesity prevention programmes 117–19
  physical education policies 25–6
Schwartz, MB *et al.* 6
Schwartz, TL *et al.* 174
Scotland
  funding programmes 75
  weight management programmes 75–86
search engines 190, 192–3, 194–5
Segal, L 62
Seidler, V 37
selective serotonin reuptake inhibitors (SSRIs) 174, 176
self-efficacy 153–4
self-esteem and weight 4, 39–42, 79–80
  as outcome measure 98–9
  see also body image and men
self-identity, peer-group comparisons 39–40
serotonin 14
sex discrimination, statutory responses 23–4
sexual abuse 161–2
sexual orientation
  and body dissatisfaction 42

and depression 59
Seymour, L 173, 174
Shabsigh, R 128
Sharman, K 163–4
Sharpe, J-K and Hills, AP 173, 180–1
shift work 106
SHINE (Self Help Independence Nutrition Exercise) Project 164
Sibutramine 70
sick leave 103, 105
SIGN *Guidelines for Obesity in Scotland* (1996) 78, 81
SIGN *Management of Obesity in Children and Young People* (2003) 112
Sims, EAH 17
Singleton, A 59
sleep apnoea 9, 17
Slimming World 93–6
  case studies 99–101
  effectiveness 97–9
SMART goals 83
smoking bans 26
soccer 155
social class
  and life expectancy 59
  and masculinity 57
Social Comparison Theory 39–40
social contexts 6–7
Social Exclusion Unit 167
social marketing 50–1
societal risk factors 25
socio-cultural influences
  body image 39–42
  ethnic minorities 166–9
  work-life balance 7
South Asian men 166–72
Speer, S and Potter, J 60
sport activities 155
  free passes 82
  for people with disabilities 139–40, 140–8
  and social relationships 156
Sport England 139
sports drinks 50
SSRIs 174, 176
Staffieri, JR 115
Stallings, VA *et al.* 119
Stang, JS *et al.* 119
Stibbe, A 61
'Stop Aids' campaign 52–3
Storing Up Problems (RCP 2004) 32
Story, M 116
stroke 8–9
  mortality rates 16

physiological mechanisms 16
Strong, SM *et al.* 42
Stunkard, Dr Albert 18
suicide risk 18
summer camps 120–1
Summerbell, CD *et al.* 70, 116–17
Summerbell, E *et al.* 116
Sunderland, J 60
surgery
  gastric 70
  restrictions due to weight 32
Swinburn, B and Egger, G 108, 116, 210
Swinburn, B *et al.* 3
syndrome X *see* metabolic syndrome

Tackling Obesity in England (National Audit Office 2001) 159
Tan, R and Pu, S 127–8
television watching 151
testosterone levels 128
text messages 203
Thomas, B 173, 175–6
Thomas, PR 81
Thompson, JK 39
Thompson, JK and Stice, E 39
thrombosis formation 16
Tiggemann, M and Wilson-Barrett, E 41
Tolson, A 56
Torgerson, JS *et al.* 98
training for staff 81, 89–90
transtheoretical model (TTM) 152
treatment seeking behaviours15 55, 62, 131–2, 168–9, 198
treatments for obesity
anti-obesity drugs 14, 70
commercial programmes 92–101
exercise promotion programmes 141–8, 150–6
general weight loss programmes 5, 43, 164
group work 75–86, 156
including psychological approaches 163–4
leisure-based clinics 198–204
lifestyle models 20
pharmacy-led approaches 88–91

prevention programmes 70–1, 115–21
primary care programmes 67–73
surgery 70
work-based programmes 20, 103–10, 154–5, 186–7
with children 116–21
tricyclic antidepressants 176
Trivers, RL 40
TROCN-3 training package 89–90
'truckers' 203
Tsai, AG and Wadden, TA 98
TTM *see* transtheoretical model
tumour necrosis factor-α 14
TV watching 151
2012 Olympics 53
Twomey, Bernard 203
Tyson, Mike 62

UK Public Health Association 26, 216
Ulrich, C 25
Ultra Low Calorie Diet (ULCD) 88
unemployment, and 'masculinity' 58
'unhealthy cities' 155
United States, obesity trends 125
US Institute of Medicine 81

Vague, J 15
Vermeulen, A 126–7
very low calorie diets 20
Viagra 128
Vienna Decalaration on Men's Health (EMHF 2005) 33
Villareal, D *et al.* 127

Wabitsch, M *et al.* 119
Wade, TJ 40
Wade, TJ and Cooper, M 40
Waine, C 80
waist:hip ratios (WHR) 72, 73
waist circumference measures 3, 15, 71, 73
and diabetes 17
and metabolic syndrome 17
and older people 127
primary care registers 32, 67
and South Asian men 167

see also abdominal fat; BMI (body mass index)
Walker, LM *et al.* 115
Wang, Y *et al.* 151
Wannamethee, SG *et al.* 126–7
Warren, X *et al.* 118
Watson, J 42
Wee, C *et al.* 6
Weiden, PJ *et al.* 175
weight loss
impact on health 20–1
typical outcomes 84
weight loss drugs *see* anti-obesity drugs
weight loss programmes
general guidance on methods 81–2
male participation rates 5, 42–3
typical outcomes 84
venues and settings 198–204
BT Work Fit campaign 186–7
Camelon Centres (Scotland) 76–86
Counterweight (UK) 5, 78
'*fatmanslim*' internet campaign (UK) 53
GutBusters (Australia) 4, 5, 43, 207–12
pharmacy-led initiatives (UK) 88–91
Rosemary Conley Diet and Fitness Clubs 96–7
Slimming World 93–6
Weight Watchers 96, 97
with disabled men 141–8
with mentally ill patients 180–4
see also prevention campaigns; primary care obesity management; treatments for obesity
weight management clinics
current situation 69–70
setting up programmes 71–3
in 'alternative' venues and settings 198–204
in Scotland 76–86
weight measurements *see* assessment methods; BMI (body mass index); waist circumference measures
weight regain 97–8
Weight Watchers 96, 97

effectiveness studies 97–9
Weil, E *et al.* 138
Weitzman, DM 138
Welch, R *et al.* 106
'well-man' clinics 130
Welland, I 156
Wernecke, U *et al.* 180, 182
Wetherell, M and Edley, N 60
Wetherell, M and Potter, J 60
White, A and Cash, K 62, 150, 155
White, AK and Lockyer, L 23
Whitmer, RA *et al.* 9
WHO (World Health Organisation) 27–8
on food subsidies 25
on gender 23, 215
on mental illness 173
on obesity 15, 27–8
Wiener, Leslie 52
Wilkins, D and Baker, P 214
Wilkins, D *et al.* 4
Williams, N and Malik, N 104, 107
Williams, RB *et al.* 156
Willott, S and Griffin, C 58
Wirshing, DA 173–5, 182–3
Wirshing, DA *et al.* 174
Wolf, N 37
women
attitudes towards obesity 18
BMI data 3
work and obesity 104–7
contributing factors 7, 106–7
particular problems 104–6
sickness absences 103
workplace canteens 107
workplace interventions 20, 103–10, 154–5
background and rationale 103–7
general opportunities 108–9
specific programmes 109–10, 186–7

Yelland, C and Tiggemann, M 39
'Yorkie' advertising campaign 50

Zahman, F and Underwood, C 48
Zhu, S *et al.* 9